New Directions in Cultural Policy Research

Series Editor
Eleonora Belfiore
Department of Social Sciences
Loughborough University
Loughborough, UK

New Directions in Cultural Policy Research encourages theoretical and empirical contributions which enrich and develop the field of cultural policy studies. Since its emergence in the 1990s in Australia and the United Kingdom and its eventual diffusion in Europe, the academic field of cultural policy studies has expanded globally as the arts and popular culture have been re-positioned by city, regional, and national governments, and international bodies, from the margins to the centre of social and economic development in both rhetoric and practice. The series invites contributions in all of the following: arts policies, the politics of culture, cultural industries policies (the 'traditiona' arts such as performing and visual arts, crafts), creative industries policies (digital, social media, broadcasting and film, and advertising), urban regeneration and urban cultural policies, regional cultural policies, the politics of cultural and creative labour, the production and consumption of popular culture, arts education policies, cultural heritage and tourism policies, and the history and politics of media and communications policies. The series will reflect current and emerging concerns of the field such as, for example, cultural value, community cultural development, cultural diversity, cultural sustainability, lifestyle culture and eco-culture, planning for the intercultural city, cultural planning, and cultural citizenship.

More information about this series at
http://www.palgrave.com/gp/series/14748

Susan Oman

Understanding Well-being Data

Improving Social and Cultural Policy, Practice and Research

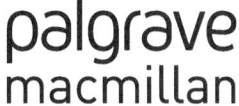

Susan Oman
University of Sheffield
Sheffield, UK

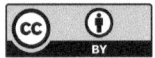

ISSN 2730-924X ISSN 2730-9258 (electronic)
New Directions in Cultural Policy Research
ISBN 978-3-030-72936-3 ISBN 978-3-030-72937-0 (eBook)
https://doi.org/10.1007/978-3-030-72937-0

Cover image: Adam Hester / Getty Images
Cover design: eStudioCalamar

This Palgrave Macmillan imprint is published by the registered company Springer Nature Switzerland AG.
The registered company address is: Gewerbestrasse 11, 6330 Cham, Switzerland

For Robert Johns

Preface: A Personal Note on Why I Wrote the Book

When I left school and wasn't sure that I knew what I was doing with my life, I worked in a call centre. So, when I read Dave Beer introduce his book on the power of data (2016) with his recollections of working in a call centre in the mid- to late 1990s, memories came flooding back. When you logged on to start taking calls, and how many calls you were taking, even when you went to the loo and for a cigarette break and had lunch, were some ways data about you were collected. This data, or *these* data,[1] were used to indicate how well you were doing at your job. They enabled people to make judgements about you.

Crucially, I didn't feel like I knew what I was doing with my life, but as a result of the data collected on me at work, others knew *exactly* what I was doing with moments in my life. Dave Beer's account is an important part of an increasing body of research critiquing the use of data as a form of surveillance. Using data in this way is changing workplace cultures and breaking codes of privacy[2] in broader everyday life that are seen as part of our societal values. It also changes how we feel in day-to-day life in ways we may not immediately recognise.

Using data to monitor people is also referred to as a 'data practice'. These data practices have been shown to make people feel uncomfortable, as they sense they are being watched. In turn, this increases stress and anxiety. These feelings are understandable: these data are about you, but out of your control, and clearly enabling someone else greater control over what you do. The existence of these data changes people's experience of work; it can make them apprehensive of how long they spend going to the toilet or eating a sandwich. Also, despite data's capacity to capture these mundane aspects of your life, these data, and what they look like, remain abstract, somewhat bewildering and hard to grasp.

Moving forward ten years to the mid- to late 2000s, I found myself working with data in a very different way. I was working in a university that trained students in various aspects of theatre and the performing arts. Part of my job was trying to argue the value and impact of the students' work. This task was bigger than that, really; it was to argue the value of training that these students were receiving at the university I worked in, precisely for the impact it had on students and the impact they had on society. A part of making this happen was to 'find data'—often data that could tell a story about well-being. 'We need data to evidence these claims', I was often told.

I believed in the work of the cultural producers I was working for, and with, all those years ago. I was just not so sure about the data and statistics cited in the policy documents that I was being asked to find for funding applications and evaluations. These numbers and the way they are used in arguments about society, culture and value sat uneasily with me. The ones I was borrowing from policy documents didn't make sense to me in a common-sense way, but I also simply didn't *quite* understand them well enough to feel confident that they were evidence. I was also worried about the quality of the data I was collecting myself and their limits. Was I *really* sure that graduates from creative courses were contributing millions to the economy through the soft skills they gain in their training? Was I *really* sure that by simply attending a theatre-in-education workshop that the children involved would experience an improvement in their well-being?

It turned out I wasn't sure enough to feel confident using evidence in ways that were demanded for funding bids and evaluations. It also turned out that it did not necessarily matter, as the fact I cited data as evidence was all that mattered to those who expected numbers in return for funding. The anxiety I felt about the quality of data and evidence I had to use, and the slightly absurd realisation that no one else seemed to care, led me on a journey: leaving this job for another university to become a student myself.

Understanding cultural policy in my masters, I hoped, would help me recognise how I might feel confident in using data and evidence—particularly to argue the social impacts of different types of cultural activity. I hoped it would help me overcome the barriers between me and the numbers and the policy documents that had increasingly become the backbone of my day-to-day job. In actual fact, all that extra critical thinking meant I became even *less* sure and less trustful of data and evidence as they are often used in cultural policy to argue social aims. It also made me less sure that cultural policy means or should mean culture as the arts. Instead it made me *more* sure that society is far more cultural than what is limited by the category 'the arts'. So, I proposed a PhD on well-being data, policy, culture and society (which also didn't help me feel reassured in how evidence and data are used).[3] After which I took two academic fellowships to improve data and data practices in the cultural sector,[4] to now find myself as a Lecturer in Data, AI and Society, as of 2020.

So, this book is written for the me in 2010: the me who was reading the Labour Party's cultural manifesto and cutting and pasting arguments with a sick feeling that I didn't know what I was doing, but I *did know* it felt a bit wrong. It is also written for the me in 2015 as a PhD student editing a conference presentation, when someone looked over my shoulder at an equation I had copy and pasted for a PowerPoint slide to tell me that the equation did not make *sense* to them—it wasn't talking their language. I turned and laughed and said: 'I thought it just didn't make sense to me'.

This book is for so many of the people I have met in the last ten years, who have said, 'I hadn't thought of that' or 'I didn't know that'—when these 'thats' can often be simply explained, but never are. Or maybe they are indeed amazed when they have understood something they thought they could not. It is also for the many people who have to use data in their day-to-day jobs, but feel a bit anxious about it—even if they are unsure why.

This book is also for the me in the 1990s who knew I was being watched at work in some way, and it changed my behaviour. Yet I did not really think of this as anything to do with data at all—which all happened somewhere in sci-fi land. It is for all the people who are maybe interested in how data are such a big part of our lives and our way of being. Whether this is experiencing call centres in the 1990s to Fitbits of the 2010s, the management of resources in World War II or the use of data in the battle against COVID-19.

This book is for my friends who send me links to online articles about data that are misleading or misrepresentative or, worse, shared Facebook posts about ways to happiness and well-being (my pet hate). It is for those I don't know, but who aren't sure about how data about us are used: it isn't all Alexa and deliberating the latest Bill Gates conspiracy theory. In fact, data about us have been used for thousands of years in ways we don't hear about. Even when we know about data collection, as with the UK Census 2021, do we really think about what data they are collecting and why? Who is it for? What do they actually *do*?

This book is for my current Data Science students. Last term one of them told me that 'people don't care about other people's well-being', while another said, 'I really liked the idea of thinking about data with a human element and not just as something a machine would produce'. For those who can do great things with data, how much do we know about whether they think about the people involved? What do people's data help us understand about them? Can it help us be more understanding as a society?

This book is for all my previous students who care so much about their work improving other people's well-being or society in some way. They were often hindered by anxiety surrounding their own research skills and data comprehension. There is often an unacknowledged cultural gap between data and well-being, despite the proliferation of well-being data. This needs addressing.

This book has an agenda for improved data literacy and data competency to address this gap. The book therefore reflects on how understanding well-being data use might help us become a society that is more understanding of each other. The fact that most of the people I list I am writing for are people I have met also means the book retains a mainly UK-specific focus. Perhaps in another ten years, I will be writing about these issues from a different place again. For now, this book is a personal endeavour to reflect on how I have come to understand the issues and to address data literacy in two main ways: first, in research on, in and with cultural and social policy sectors and, second, in the social aspects of data science and data studies. More simply, this might be explained as teaching 'culture and society people' about data and teaching 'data people' about culture and society.

As this review of sociology, as the study of social life and society, points out, everyone has to interpret research in their lives by way of the media, but few of us produce it:

> *to consider more seriously the relationship between research literacy and research competency. All students of sociology at whatever 'levels' and in whatever institutional settings will become long-term consumers of research, but very few of them indeed will ever become producers of it apart from in undergraduate classrooms. In our view, most textbooks (and with honourable exceptions) overemphasise teaching students competency skills, and considerably underemphasize giving them the literacy skills to read, unpack, interpret and evaluate research and the conclusions drawn from it.* (Wise and Stanley 2003)

This book is no textbook, but an overview of how we are equipped to understand data in society and how that helps us understand well-being. The book offers many examples of data collection, and some examples of analysis, that can improve your research skills, should you so need them. However, it was not necessarily written to help people understand how to *do* research, but how to understand data in research. Therefore, it aims to improve understanding of how others use data—and how data can be used. This means we can better appreciate the limits and benefits of assertions regarding what we can understand of people, well-being and data.

This book is for those who feel uncomfortable with data to feel more comfortable with its collection, its expression (basically, those tables and statistics and sometimes squiggly lines) and the language of data. Even for those people who undertake research, or work with data in some way, the language of data can feel so different and alien that this is a barrier to engaging with data. I have found that this is the case with cultural and social policy practitioners, and as we shall see, this affects how people engage with evidence and arguments.

This book is also for people who feel confident with data, but have perhaps been trained to think of data as objective and neutral and to be read as fact. Consequently, the prospect of considering the social contexts of data may feel odd. It is, therefore, also for those who feel comfortable with data to be able to imagine the uncomfortable aspects of data. These include the various questions we should ask about contexts of the data used: where they have come from? Have they already undergone some kind of analysis or cleaning? How they will be used? Context is key to considering the limits to claims made from data about well-being, and, perhaps, even more importantly, how does 'what we do with data' (that we call data practices) affect a person's well-being, or does it have broader negative social impacts?

Caring about well-being doesn't necessarily mean people consider data issues. As I have described, the same is true the other way around: people who care about data don't necessarily consider well-being. It is critical that this book does not reinforce a line of clichés of those who do and do not care about one thing or another, and those who are good at data and those who are not. Rather, there is a culture of misunderstanding that this book aims to help address. This book tackles this gap from the standpoint that just because things are not readily understandable to all does not mean they are hard to understand. Crucial to overcoming this is making it easier to feel more confident that if something about data is incomprehensible, then that may be because the way the data are used is bad, rather than you are not able to grasp what is going on.

As I have discovered a number of times in ten years' researching well-being data, the way data have been used to describe society may not be robust. Also, they may be used to make claims of improving society in some way, when in fact these may not be true. Similarly, the negative social and cultural effects of how data are used to manage and monitor people and society may not be considered. We do not all need to be able to look under the bonnet like a trained mechanic to understand well-being data, but being able to peer in with some confidence may be enough to help us grasp the limits of what we are looking at. Only then can we—as a society—better understand well-being and data: how well-being is captured as data and how data affect well-being.

Sheffield, UK   Susan Oman

Notes

1. A note on data as singular or plural. Most of the time, people talk of data as one thing. Actually, in this book we are going to use data as a plural, as data are rarely one thing, but lots and lots of small things.
2. Legislation is beginning to address these issues. GDPR is an example that offers greater protection, but is currently flawed and cumbersome.
3. My PhD (Oman 2017) was attached to the AHRC-funded project called 'Understanding Everyday Participation: Articulating Cultural Values', 2012–2017 [AH/J005401/1]. This was funded by Arts and Humanities Research Council's Connected Communities Large Project funding. Orthodox models of culture and the creative economy are based on a narrow definition of participation: one that captures engagement with traditional institutions such as museums and galleries but overlooks more informal activities such as community festivals and hobbies. The project aimed to paint a broader picture of how people make their lives through culture and in particular how communities are formed and connected through participation.
4. This research project, initially called 'Social Mobility: The Case of the Arts' was supported by two AHRC-funded projects: Data, Diversity and Inequality in the Creative Industries (or DDI) and What Constitutes 'Good Data' in the Creative Economy? (or Good Data) ran from January to August 2018, January to July in 2019, respectively. Both were funded by the Arts and Humanities Research Council's Creative Economy Engagement Fellowship Scheme (or AHRC CEEF).

References

Beer, D. 2016. *Metric Power*. London: Palgrave Macmillan.
Wise, S., and Stanley, L. 2003. Review Article: "Looking Back and Looking Forward: Some Recent Feminist Sociology Reviewed". *Sociological Research Online* 8 (4): 53–64. https://doi.org/10.5153/sro.822.

Acknowledgements

This book is the result of my experiences of coming to understand well-being, data and the research disciplines and professional practices concerned with them. It is therefore informed by many, many conversations and collaborations—both formal and informal. I am so grateful to everyone who has listened to, read and watched the papers, ideas and reflections that underpin this book. Many discussions over the years have proved essential in developing its positions, arguments and insights. I include those who asked difficult questions when I presented earlier versions of my research (including all the research that does not appear here) and all the students and research participants that pushed me even further on pathways of discovery to further interrogate some of the *whys, whats, wheres, hows* and *whos* of well-being and data that form much of the book. Valuable provocations also came from brilliant people across policy and social and cultural sectors, and different forums from Twitter to meetings to workshops and events. I want to thank everyone who has contributed in this way. You are too many to name individually, but you know who you are.

I also want to thank all my research participants who made the empirical research that informed my understanding and made the case studies in this book so rich. This includes those behind the scenes who helped organise this: the UK's Office for National Statistics (ONS) for agreeing access to their free text data set and my interviewees in the ONS, and those who provided contextual detail for the broader PhD research project. With the Arts Council England (ACE) and the hundreds of people who donated their time across the individual arts organisations, I want to thank their generosity and openness to discovering how things might be improved. I also want to thank those who participated in my PhD focus groups and the third-sector organisations and gatekeepers who allowed this to happen.

This book evolved from almost ten years' research and the formal support that helped make these investigations and explorations possible include:

The PhD research project *All Being Well? Cultures of Participation and the Cult of Measurement* (2017) was supported by the Arts and Humanities Research Council's (AHRC's) Connected Communities Large Project funding for Understanding Everyday Participation: Articulating Cultural Values, 2012–2017 [AH/J005401/1]. The research project, initially titled *Social Mobility: The Case of the Arts*, was supported by two AHRC-funded Creative Economy and Engagement Fellowships on the awards: Data, Diversity and Inequality in the Creative Industries, 2018 [AH/R013322/1]; and What Constitutes 'Good Data' in the Creative Economy? Case studies in media and cultural industries, 2019 [AH/S012109/1]. The project Living With Data: knowledge, experiences and perceptions of data practices is supported by the Nuffield Foundation, 2019–2022 [OSP/43959]. The literature and evidence review for this book were partly facilitated by a Wellcome Trust Seed Award, for Cultural Engagement for Wellbeing, 2015 [201587/Z/16/Z]. In addition to this formal support, I would like to thank my PhD supervisors Andrew Miles, Jackie Stacey and Par Kumaraswami alongside my fellowship mentors Mark Taylor, Kate Oakley, Dave Beer and Helen Kennedy and my MA supervisor, Dave O'Brien. I would also like to thank my brilliant colleagues on the UEP project, these CEEF projects and the Living With Data project for support, camaraderie and inspiration and Nick Ewbank for his encouragement on Cultural Engagement for Wellbeing. This book is open access as a result of Wellcome's further support of this research.

I want to thank Mark Taylor, who collaborated with me on further, unfunded research that features in this book and patiently read my redrafting of this. I am especially indebted to all colleagues, old and new, who I can call friends who read drafts and listened to thoughts and rambles as they became a book: Alex Albert, Caitlin Bentley, Andrew Cox, Sarah Feinstein, Kate Fitzgerald, Nigel Ford, Abi Gilmore, Louise Reardon, Sophie Rutter, Will Shankley, Lauren White and Ros Williams. The biggest thank you is to Charlotte Branchu, my rock in stage one of assembling this book, but also to Leon Tellez Contreras, Itzelle Medina-Perea and Lulu Pinney for helping with figures, referencing and indexing.

Alongside these wonderful people, I want to acknowledge the informal networks that helped me look after my well-being: Lauren White's writing group; my comrades, the cultural policy coven; and more formal networks such as the Cultural Data and Research Network (CDRN).

I would also like to acknowledge all of the relevant research that I was not able to include. The irony of desperately trying to finish a book with a new job in a pandemic is that you have barely any time to read many other books, so new research has emerged that is undoubtedly relevant to the concerns and which are overlooked.

Lastly, special thanks to Dylan James and Frankie Grey for their endless curiosity and advice on project PBW.

Praise for *Understanding Well-being Data*

"Given their power and influence, we might wonder how we feel about data and how data make us feel. In considering the relations between data and well-being, Susan Oman's vital new book considers what data now mean for our lives, opportunities, judgments and, crucially, for our impressions of our selves. Taking a critical approach, this book makes the crucial step of not just thinking of how data shape well-being but also how well-being itself is redefined by data processes."

—Prof. David Beer, Professor of Sociology, *University of York*

"To understand well-being is to understand current cultural policy; it is also to understand the new language of data and metrics at the heart of how culture is governed. *Understanding Well-being Data* offers an essential and accessible guide to the future of the cultural sector, showing both the potential, and the critical limits, of well-being as the new language of cultural and social life."

—Dr Dave O'Brien, Chancellor's Fellow in *Cultural and Creative Industries*

"Susan Oman has written a much-needed book on how social and cultural policy use, for good or ill, data on well-being. She takes nothing for granted, and looks deeply into the centuries-old history of how we have thought about happiness and well-being, and the various ways it might be measured, before turning to its contemporary use as a metric for the impact of arts institutions and policy. It is engagingly written, lively and accessible for all students of culture."

—Michael Rushton, Professor, *O'Neill School of Public and Environmental Affairs, Indiana University*

"*Understanding Well-being Data* is a very timely and valuable book. In a period when we have continually heard politicians claim to be following 'the data' on well-being, this book looks 'under the bonnet' of data collection. It examines the various types of data and information that policy-makers select for use, and how they analyse and interpret them. It shows how understanding the contexts of data and decision-making are critical for policy and practice that aims to do good, or at least prevent harm. It is written in an exemplary accessible and engaging style and provides much food for thought on how data shape society, culture, politics and policy. It deserves to be read by all who are interested in the use and misuse of data and how this impacts everyday lives."

—Professor Ian Bache, *Department of Politics and International Relations, University of Sheffield*

"As a practitioner, now more than ever, we need to critically reflect on our data practices; understanding the contexts of data and decision-making across policy, practice and research is core to this endeavour. This is a timely and accessible book that facilitates important conversations about well-being data and their role in research, policy, culture and society, brought to life through a collection of practical examples."

—Dr Rhianne Jones, *BBC*

CONTENTS

LIST OF FIGURES

LIST OF TABLES

List of Boxes

CHAPTER 1

Introducing Well-being Data

1.1 Introduction to *Understanding Well-being Data*

This book seeks to advance understanding of the role of well-being in social and cultural policy, politics and research. It does this by focussing on ideas, concepts and uses of well-being, as well as differences in types of well-being data. It was written primarily to offer practitioners a view 'under-the-bonnet' of data collection, analyses and uses to see how they actually operate, as well as what happens as a result of their very existence. Its accessible style aims to include students and a more general audience in discussions about data and those about well-being as two crucial issues of our time.

Understanding Well-being Data uses real-life examples, paying particular attention to the ways data are generated, analysed and used, to demonstrate how data practices respond to, and how they shape, society, culture, politics and policy. Its short and longer case studies make this an accessible learning curve, and one that is applicable to experts and novices of all sorts in all our everyday lives. The book focuses on uses of data in culture and society, and how they work as social policy, so that comparisons and contradictions are easy to see.

© The Author(s) 2021   1
S. Oman, *Understanding Well-being Data*,
New Directions in Cultural Policy Research,
https://doi.org/10.1007/978-3-030-72937-0_1

'Following the data' is a now familiar phrase in the UK from its significant role in government communications about COVID-19. The phrase is important, because it demonstrates that the very idea of data is used to justify decisions and policies for the nation's health and well-being. Many across the UK watched various press conferences in 2020 in which its prime minister and other advisors would refer to 'the data' as an objective thing that they were following, rather than various types of data and information that people learn how to use, deliberately collect and generate, and that they interpret and analyse.

The government broadcasts on managing the COVID-19 crisis also included graphs and other data visualisations. Some of these were designed to show a comparison across areas of the country to justify which were under restrictions and which were not. They were badly labelled, making them hard to interpret by those who are data literate, let alone 'the public' being broadcast to. Most people felt more alienated by these uses of data than comforted that they understood what the government was doing—and why. The last one of these press conferences that I personally saw, before finishing this book, was a few days before I was supposed to travel to spend Christmas with loved ones. The whole nation was told that this was no longer to be possible. We were told that the government had followed the data, but that the 'science had changed'.

Of course, 'the science' had not changed at all. Instead, the decisions made, based on human interpretations of data about COVID-19, and other data about the economy and mental health, about schools and universities, about the inequalities of those who can work safely, and those who cannot, were all in a melting pot of pressures involved in decision-making at this level. It was policy that had to change, not the science that had changed, and suddenly one set of data seemed more important than another to those in charge.

So, here we can clearly see that it is not that there is 'the data' as one indisputable thing, but *these data* are not neutral. By which we mean the data are not unbiased, nor impartial. They are collected, read, interpreted and presented and these processes involve many decisions. But, how can data themselves be biased? A good example of bias in data lies in the recent increase in algorithms that are trained using data to automate certain digital processes. Algorithms have actually been with us for centuries (an eighteenth-century happiness algorithm appears in Chap. 2). The word still refers to any form of automated instruction. The majority of algorithms are simpler than most people think and can be a single 'if something is this, then do that' statement that can then be actioned.

Contemporary algorithms tend to be long sequences of these instructions. As you can imagine, with these many instructions and decisions, bias is likely to creep in.

One of the starkest instances of bias can be found in the search engine, which most of us now use all the time. It is a mundane part of our everyday lives that we don't often think about. Search engines have been designed to learn to second guess what we are looking for, as they have a record of, or they 'know' all the searches we have made before this one, alongside all of everyone else's searches.[1] Safia Noble (2018) revealed how these guesses are biased in dangerous ways that are both racist and sexist. As recently as 2011, the first thing that would appear in searches with the term 'black girls' was a link to hardcore porn. You may try and explain this away as an algorithm prioritising some ads over others. Explaining these things away may be—in fact—a part of the problem, of course, when it comes to bias, sexism and racism. It therefore very much deserves attention.

Noble provides much more evidence than this example above, though. Noble shows a variety of ways that the search engine predicted the searcher was looking for derogatory images of black women, even apes, as well as pejorative character traits. Noble 'followed the data' to reveal how data practices are biased, but also revealed our own biases to us. People were shocked when Noble's revelations were published. This shows us that not only are the search engines biased, but that we are. People are biased, in the way some want to believe that we live in a 'post-racial' society, and that we do not need to worry about racism any longer, when actually they are blinded to the fact they are consuming culture, through data, that are both biased and racist.

Data play a large role in society. Critical data studies, like Noble's and throughout this book, where we 'follow the data' to see how it works in context, reveal truths about both data and society. We need to learn from these revelations about data to improve well-being and society.

Subjective and Objective Data

But what if we return to data used by politicians, surely this does not contain evidence of the same biases? A good example is 'the poverty line'. When a politician talks about 'the poverty line', we think that this is an absolute thing. Not necessarily a real thing, like picturing people living under a power line, but that the line represents a measure from data which are objective.

Objective measures of poverty are objective by name, but they are not entirely neutral. So, does that mean they are actually objective? There is no measure of poverty that is conclusive: while it means not having enough resources to cover essential needs, this is a subjective valuation of the words 'essential' and 'enough'. The subjective nature of the word essential has also gained prominence in the UK, as politicians have used it to avoid making clear decisions on what COVID-19 restrictions should entail—despite their data expertise. Instead, people are forced into making their own evaluations on what counts as 'essential' travel, work or food, and therefore what is lawful behaviour under parallel lockdown restrictions in different areas of the UK at different points in time.

Returning to the issue of poverty, in the UK and in most countries, 'enough for essential' tends to mean around 60% of the nation's median income (Francis-Devine 2020). This is classed as 'relative poverty', and it fluctuates. Absolute poverty is adjusted in line with inflation, rather than average living standards. These two different metrics can be used to paint two pictures of the same story, as a topical case demonstrates in Prime Minister's Questions in UK Parliament.

The UK government refused to commit continued support of free school meals in the 2020 summer holidays. This policy decision about children's well-being led to a high-profile campaign and a U-turn (that was repeated again in the Autumn). This controversy and debate included a wider discussion of the current government's impact on child poverty. The leader of the opposition cited that 600,000 more children were living in relative poverty than in 2012 (UK Parliament 2020). Given that the Conservative Coalition took office in 2010, the implication here was that the Conservative governments of the last decade are responsible, and with serious negative effects. The prime minister retorted, 'There are 400,000 fewer families living in poverty now than there were in 2010' (UK Parliament 2020). How can one politician use poverty data to make a claim and the other use poverty data to claim the opposite?

How can data on poverty from the same time period, and cited in such an important setting as parliament, paint such contrary pictures? Each party leader chose slightly different timeframes within this ten-year period and they chose different poverty data. The leader of the opposition chose the poverty data and timeframe that told a story of the greatest negative impact, while the prime minister is thought to have possibly chosen a different timeframe and the other index to argue the exact opposite[2] (BBC 2020). These different indices aren't intended to be fiddled with by politicians, but, actually, some measures will subjectively suit some arguments more than others. This does not mean that they cannot offer a more objective appraisal in other contexts, but as you can see, expert judgements can be subjective when deciding which objective data to use about people's well-being, and in which context.

This use of poverty data is a good example of how well-being data have been used for centuries. Their collection and analysis are motivated by the need to track the health and wealth of society and evaluate the success and progress of social projects and policies. Indeed, these underlying assumptions have been the backbone of social science, statistical and policy work for the last 200 years. Yet, these data are not neutral or entirely objective. They can be used and misused as evidence in forums in which important decisions are made, and yet, we do not often 'follow the data' to appreciate these inconsistencies ourselves.

Understanding well-being data means looking at instances and inconsistencies of their use. It is generated to inform decision-making, which also means it can be used to hold others—particularly those in power—to account. It is also gathered on far smaller scales to appreciate the impact of aspects of society on us: our weight, our work, our children and their schooling. Major events, such as COVID-19, enable the power of well-being data to come to the fore. But these are data about us and are used to evaluate what to do next in a crisis. That is why everyone should feel able to access tools to help them better understand how this all works in society, should they want to; that is why this book tries to offer something for everyone.

1.2   WHO IS THIS BOOK FOR?

For people who work in social and cultural policy and charities, this book offers lots of context to the data they use every day and aims to help *everyday* usage of data in practice. It hopes to speak to people who think they can't do numbers at all. This includes those who think they do not understand the numerical aspects of arguments that use data. It also includes understanding the arguments themselves and potentially their limits.

Capability, capacity and confidence with data are issues for researchers and practitioners working in cultural policy and the sector (DC Research 2017; Oman 2019a, b). Organisations and individuals are affected differently by data-related issues, depending on various matters, including who funds them, how large and 'professionalised' the organisations are, for example (Oman 2019a, b, 2020). Despite increasing emphasis on the importance of data in social policy and cultural policy practice and research, capability, capacity and confidence have not received much attention.[3]

Alongside some evidence of data gaps in social and cultural policy, there is anecdotal evidence that key arguments relating to the value of particular social policy areas remain obscure to some working within them, because of the way data are expressed. For social and cultural policy researchers and students, who are not comfortable with numeric data and the way they are presented, this book aims to open the black box and shed light on what is happening. Looking under the bonnet of data means peering under the cover of the workings, the arguments made, the evidence used and the connection between them and data. Looking at all these components together helps us better understand well-being and data at the same time.

For readers who are happy with analysing data and reading statistics, the book reveals some of the social or political ramifications of data and their uses. How governments 'follow the data' as a way of justifying policy decisions has been foregrounded in COVID-19 times. Revealing the implications of using the idea of data to justify bad, even dangerous decisions, does not mean all is fixed, however. The enduring presence of the pandemic should be the motivation to ask more questions about policy decisions that claim to be fair and equitable based on evidence using specific data, but which are often just the opposite. Understanding well-being data in these broader contexts is therefore critical.

1.3   What Is This Book Trying to Do?

> It's just really hard when you're bogged down in numbers and reports, and you've got a deadline looming, to be sure to know that the statistics you use are correct, or that you're even reading a graph properly.

Someone who uses data all the time said this to me a few years ago. This person's confession in an interview chimed with me and my own imposter syndrome. How can we feel reassured in the data we use and the way others use data? How can we begin to trust ourselves more to know when to trust others?

This whole book reflects on my realisation that—without training and familiarity (and sometimes even with this stuff)—it is really hard to be sure to know that the statistics you cite reflect the 'real world' in some way or that you are interpreting a graph or data visualisation properly. This feels all the more important when these data and arguments are related to people's well-being or social justice. This is the main justification for the value of data in social and cultural policy. Yet data are undervalued at the same time, in that while the importance of data is an absolute, less attention is paid to the data itself: where they are from, who they are about, how they are used. Are well-being data being used appropriately?

Most importantly, the book aims to tell those of you that think you are inherently bad at numbers, that you are not, and this goes for reading graphs or policy documents. Instead, more often than not, it is how these are presented that are flawed or lacking in various ways. People who do research are not always good at communicating it. This is probably, to be honest, mainly because the authors had their own deadline looming, rather than necessarily any immoral practices. But also, sometimes, it can be that people report on their findings without thinking about how to make their findings accessible. This is—of course—why it is important for people who are confident with data to consider those who are not.

There are times, however, when you encounter a bad statistic: one that is misleading or misused. We encounter them all the time in the press and in parliament—and we'll encounter many throughout this book that are linked to well-being. This book might encourage you to realise that you are fully equipped to look for alternative statistics, or to look through the headline findings to understand the data better, and why that statistic sounds inflated or confusing. We have lost confidence in our common sense, which affects confidence in critical thinking and our own resourcefulness to see through the ways that data are used. This book hopes to increase confidence in looking beyond a presented statistic: to look (or at least peer) underneath the bonnet ourselves.

Data of some sort are a vital part of our daily lives, now. Whether we are writing a report with numbers in it, filling in a 'well-being at work' survey or having our BMI measured by our doctor. We have all spent time in COVID-19 working with the data we were given to decide whether our trip to the supermarket was essential *enough*. We are all living and working with data and in contexts that need data. Well-being data are often *our* data, in that they are personal data about us—and their collection requires *our* time and consideration.

When thinking about data, we need to remember the version of us— yes that's you—that encounters data daily. The version of us that ignores those emails asking for our opinions or asking after our well-being because we are too busy, or we feel that whoever is asking for these data don't really care any way. We need to remember that we (well, we here is actually me) will always give an Uber driver 5 stars, irrespective of how safe we felt or kind they were. We need to remember that time we went to a capital city and the highest rated restaurant was McDonald's. We need to think about whether those numbers represent our understanding of the world or not, and if not, then, why not? In a book about well-being data we need to be pragmatic about how different official well-being data are from these more familiar data contexts.

Every day, we interact unthinkingly with metrics, statistics, numbers and data collection all the time. We make common sense, snap judgements that enable us to dismiss them as useful or not to us. What is so different about statistics in a book or in our jobs—or even in research published in reports? Why is it that some people's use of numbers feels incontestable? What is it that means we do not even think to question numbers and their uses? It is a sense of authority and context. So, I hope that with more personal authority and greater appreciation of context gained through reading this book, maybe we can feel more like engaging in and with, not only data as numbers, but ideas of data.

More specifically, this book has six key aims:

- one, to explain the history, politics and contexts of data produced that might be called well-being data;
- two, to explain some of the limitations of these data and the research and policy that have used them;
- three, to describe how changing uses of data have changed how we live in various ways;
- four, to present real-life examples of presentations of data and statistics, to break down how they have been 'made';
- five, to show how numbers can be misrepresentative, why this is a problem and how you should be able to feel confident challenging them; and
- six, to show that data do not capture reality neutrally, but are used to create realities through public decision-making that directly affects personal, community and national well-being.

The examples chosen have been accumulated from my experience of learning to feel more confident with different kinds of data and numbers. They come from my own moments of head scratching and the lost hours on the internet trying to understand why things don't quite seem right; all those times I have asked someone else 'does this make sense?'—to which the other person has sometimes looked puzzled and said, 'actually, no'.

This book also emerges from my feeling uncomfortable with what I was asked to do with data and comfortable to question the status quo. I found myself in a situation where there was an assumption that only numeric data are evidence and that somehow all numeric data were assumed to be evidence. I felt able to challenge the idea that just because data are in a formal-looking report, it is not necessarily 'good data', or factual.

This book also emerges from my realisation that just because things are not readily understandable to all does not mean they are hard to understand. For example, this book also developed from collaborations with academic colleagues who *do* use data well to understand culture and well-being. It also emerges from working in a sector-based data network with colleagues who collect data on what the cultural sector and creative industries are well-known for, as well as what they are less well-known for.

So, let's shake this identity that arts can't do numbers—a phrase I've heard too much. Let's shake this idea that one of my Data Science students shared, that people who do data don't care about well-being. Let's also make sure that the claims made using well-being data in cultural and social research and policy can be substantiated and understood.

1.4   Why Well-being Data?

Well-being data can be about individuals, such as Fitbit data, or population data, such as the census. They include health data and poverty data; information on how we feel, on how we live and how long we live. This book focusses on well-being data for a number of reasons. Firstly, it is easy to assume that well-being data are similar in some way, because they are about the 'same thing': we will look at how diverse well-being data are. It is also through trying to understand 'well-being data' as *a* thing that I came to know data in general.

To come to know well-being data, I had to spend years trawling through books from within and beyond economics, psychology, statistics, policy, politics and philosophy. This was a slow process, and an uncertain process, which fuelled my feelings of imposter syndrome. All these different disciplines used different language that I had to be familiar with. Or worse, the same words to mean different things, which I try to overcome as much as possible in this book. It was years before I slowly gained confidence in my own common sense when reading about either well-being or data. The very idea of data and academic or policy language means we stop trusting our own common sense. We shouldn't. To be honest, some academics do too. They also shouldn't.

Secondly, well-being 'as the aim of all policy-making' (we'll come to this in the next chapter) has unique relevance for areas of social and cultural policy. This is because—in common-sense terms—culture and society are undisputedly about people, and those working in these policy domains often aim to either improve people's quality of life or interrogate what improving lives might actually involve! Unlike other aims of policy, well-being, as a concept, makes sense to those working in it and those affected by it—which is everyone.

Thirdly, well-being is about experience. Some people find it hard enough to explain how they feel with words, let alone using the same words. It is even harder to capture experience with numbers. I mean, for thousands of years, people haven't even agreed on what well-being is *exactly* and statisticians also admit it's impossible to agree on a definition, even, as we shall see! How do you know what you are measuring when you don't know what it is? We'll find out how people have tried and why they have tried.

Fourth, we all have a sense of what well-being is. We also have a sense of doing what is good for us and knowing what has been bad for us or others. We all make decisions daily that are well-being related—that balance of going to the pub versus going to the gym. Maybe it's not getting takeaway coffees and sandwiches for a month to save for a holiday. These decisions we make are based on pleasure and purpose at different moments in time, that's all well-being. We are all well-being experts and we all ignore the evidence (except that app that told me I was happiest in a beer garden with my friends; I listened to that and return to it in Chap. 5).

Fifth, it is also all too easy to forget that not everyone has the same idea of well-being: what makes some people feel better can actually be bad for others.[4] For example, not all religions and cultures will feel as at home in a British pub as I do on a sunny day: not all activities are available or desirable to everyone. Even formal well-being advice from governments and the media in the pandemic has routinely forgotten you can't go for a walk to make you feel better if: you are home alone with three kids, are in the middle of a long shift or are indeed unable to walk. It is important to remember that exposure to well-being solutions is a reminder of what is not available for some, which is inevitably bad for their well-being. We also need to be mindful of when ignoring 'evidence' is better for well-being and that universal solutions do not work.

Lastly, data affect people's well-being. As I've already said, it may seem like data are neutral, but they are used to inform decisions that are political because they affect people—and some people more than others. I ask my students to think about good data and data for good. Good data might be thought of as an issue of quality. In the case of statistics, this means they 'fit their intended use, are based on appropriate data and methods and are not materially misleading' according to the government statistical service (GSS n.d.). The GSS also state that their statistics 'serve the public good', not only because they capture aspects of society, but because they are shared. So, how data and the information they are capable of providing are shared is implicit in an idea of 'good data'. However, more attention should be paid to how this is shared understanding (which is where we shall conclude this book).

1.5   How Are Data Cultural?

Popular culture is constituted by data about popular culture. (Beer and Burrows 2013: 56)

Data issues are bigger than well-being and bigger than social and cultural policy. As we have seen they affect much of how we experience society. In 2015, Helen Kennedy asked 'is data culture?' (2015), ultimately answering yes. We interpret data through journalism and visualisations like graphs, which change the way we understand the world. Data also change the way that we consume the arts and culture.

We might think that data can tell us facts about popular culture, but as Beer and Burrows argued in 2013, data don't just capture culture. In actual fact, data feed back into popular culture, again changing how we feel about things and the decisions we make. Beer and Burrows were diagnosing the digital consumption of music, and the 'digital traces' these processes create. This has been proved empirically in a number of cultural forms,[5] and what they describe is relevant of culture more generally. In other words, they argue that data shape and define culture and have a hand in making culture: they change what we do with our lives in ways we may not notice.

What we listen to, or what we watch, is tracked and stored as data. These data are used to suggest to us what to watch or listen to next (by way of what is called a recommender system). As you might imagine, this *then* changes what shows are thought popular, which are commissioned and recommissioned, the actors in them and who becomes a star. Therefore, data can change what is valuable and this is another obvious way in which we can see some of the biases described by Virginia Noble (2018). What is happening in the virtual world, or how we move around the online world, therefore changes what happens in our offline social world. We saw this relationship play out in the call centre in the opening to this book. What we do, and when, generates data that do more than help us decide what we might want to watch. These data can restrict our behaviour in more sinister ways.

Thus, data are cultural in that they shape our social values and ways of living. They can also shape how we feel, even our access to healthcare or welfare support. Yet, the way we are taught to live with numbers and data in school, and throughout our lives, does not account for these realities. This is why everyday data literacy and comfort with numbers is a social issue, and one that is increasingly acknowledged by government. Not just the parts of government that care about statistics like the GSS (as mentioned in previous section), but data and the data strategy are now the responsibility of the Department for Digital, Culture, Media & Sport. 'Creating a fairer society for all' is one of the key aims of the strategy, which is 'underpinned by public trust', according to the Secretary of State (DCMS 2020).

There has been a lot written about 'trust in numbers' (Porter 1996), but also, trust in how data are used. We trust certain institutions to use data well, while others use them badly; yet trust other institutions, again, to report data honestly and transparently (Steedman et al. 2020; Kennedy et al. 2020). We have already seen how an idea of a poverty rate can be manipulated by politicians to suit their own ends. While politicians themselves exclaim it is only others' numbers we cannot trust. Donald Trump claims that 'negative polls are fake news' (Batchelor 2017) and the UK is told that it has 'had enough of experts' (Gove 2016).

COVID-19 management has resulted in governments telling us how important it is to trust data, but to trust in *their* interpretations of data. People in authority are now dictating how we should *feel* about numbers (and showing us which numbers they want us to feel safe or terrified as a result of). Running in parallel to this rollercoaster of data and trust is the disproportionate faith that we have in the numbers we read on Facebook and other social media. Which presentations of COVID-related deaths do we believe? What makes one more believable than another? Missing from many analyses and discussions of trust and data is how it came to pass that despite the fact that data are everywhere, we do not trust ourselves to use and read data.

Why don't we (the general public) feel able to trust ourselves to understand data and numbers? Are there particular parts of society who feel at greatest disadvantage from this lack of faith in ourselves? Many were taught at school that numbers offer some sort of objective truth: that there is a purity to numbers. We leave school with the feeling that if we don't get them, that's because we *won't* get them. In fact, as you can hopefully see more clearly, all sorts of numbers, statistics and graphs are misused all the time. Sometimes this is to deliberately mislead people, others it is not. Quite frequently, in terms of well-being data though, numbers only suggest what is going on, and they can be interpreted in different ways, if truth be told.

It is hard to navigate which numbers to trust in our everyday lives, but what about the numbers we may use in our working lives—or, as a student writing an essay? For most people, these are not numbers we will have been involved in generating. Even academics, experts and statisticians probably refer to more data generated or analysed by others, than those they may have had a hand in. Instead we all use data to justify our positions, whether that's down the pub to argue about the football, how many man-hours are needed to fix a leaking roof, or for how much, or to a funder for the value of the work we do.

How do we trust which numbers to use in our working lives? Perhaps we trust those that appear in a policy document or from something else we think is a reputable news source. Does citing a published academic paper make us feel like the numbers should be okay, even if we suspect something feels fishy about them? In this book we'll look at how you can better trust yourself with numbers—by feeling more confident in the signs that the numbers are good and not bad. This involves knowing where the data came from, how well explained the approaches to analysing the data are and looking at how it's presented.

1.6   How Should I Use This Book?

The simple answer here is that, like with any book, you should use it how you want. What I wanted to say is that although there is a logical order to this book, which we go into next, not everyone will find all of it useful or interesting. So, as much as this book is about feeling confident in your judgement about data, you should feel confident that if you are not interested in a section of this book, you should feel you can read the next section.

Because this book aims to explain a lot of background detail to give contextual information for different types of data, or ideas about well-being and society, not everything will feel relevant to everyone. For example, you may be interested in the history of well-being data in a general sense (Chap. 2), but feel like you do not have a need to read about the history of decisions behind the OECD well-being indicators in particular (at the end of Chap. 3). If you are that reader, then feel you can skip a section and move onto the shiny new chapter about the recent history of happiness as a new science (Chap. 4) or Big Data (Chap. 5).

Similarly, you may be interested in the first section about well-being data, but less interested in the specific case studies in social and cultural policy. So, why not skim or skip those and jump to the conclusion—where you may find you want to refer back to specific points in previous chapters any way. This book is designed to hopefully allow you to feel confident to read the whole thing in order, like a novel, or refer to sections. It is designed for you to use it how you like.

There are boxes scattered throughout (that you will find after the list of figures). These are used in different ways. Sometimes the material in the box elaborates on the main text and can be skipped if you are not interested. It is often definitional, explaining the difference between two types of economics, or what a variable is, for example. Sometimes a box might present example data, as with the case of some tweets in Chap. 5. Sometimes, reading it will help contextualise what is happening next. Again, the boxes are meant to make it easy to decide whether you want this detail or not.

1.7   Why Is the Book Written in This Order?

This book is a game of two halves, with a post-match pint to digest what we have just watched: the performance of the players and those calls which are on the edge of the rules of the game. The first half is about how different kinds of well-being data (data about well-being) came about. It begins with the historical traditions of philosophy, governance and social science that led to 'well-being data' becoming *a thing* that is useful and looks at the methods, innovations, contexts and limitations of these.

The second half looks at how well-being data are relied on as evidence in social and cultural policy, also how they are used to answer questions beyond the contexts they were collected in. Ideas of a cultural society as a good society have long-shaped social policy and informed future philosophy. We look at how this enabled cultural policy to become an aspect of social policy, before presenting a number of case studies on the relationship between well-being and culture that I have elsewhere (Oman 2015a, 2015b) called the culture–well-being relationship.

The conclusion aims to be a sort of post-match pint down the pub. It reflects on moments of tension, recapping on what has happened and reflecting on how these might be understood from a different position. We end with trying to understand 'understanding' in a number of ways. First, as the ways we understand the world, through data, information, knowledge and wisdom.[6] Second, as a reflection on the work that needs to be done towards a shared understanding of data. Third, how in using well-being data, we may become more understanding of each other.

The First Half

We start by setting up some of the background story to well-being data. Chapter 2, 'Knowing Well-being: A History of Data', puts the concerns of this book into context, these contexts being historical, political and technical. There are different theories of well-being from different times and places, and how these are understood today by researchers, national statisticians and policy-makers affect what data are collected to understand well-being.

We look at the project of measuring well-being as one that wanted to understand how to improve human welfare. We also consider well-being as a tool of policy, as the very idea of it is used to make arguments for one policy decision over another. Or in more real terms, to fund one social project over another. This is deeply connected with developments in national politics and governance, which changed and increased the role of economics in auditing, efficiency and valuation. We consider how these processes led to not only more well-being data, but more well-being data practices. In other words, more uses of more data. This chapter will help the reader think more critically about why and how well-being became such a default 'good idea'—and some of the issues at play here. It will also help think about how striving for a good society became inextricably linked with well-being data.

Chapter 3, 'Looking at Well-being Data in Context', moves more specifically into thinking about the uses of data and measurement in policy, practice and research. The previous chapter's historical focus on measurement as an expression of objectivity and governance is extended here. This chapter is a more focussed appraisal of contexts in which data are collected and used. We think about the role of methods and methodology (explaining what this word means). We look at specific examples of how well-being is measured and how that maps onto philosophical accounts of well-being. This is not a methods textbook, as there are plenty out there that do this job. Instead, this chapter's focus on context, difference and limitations across mundane, critical and authoritative contexts aims to help us think about how we might understand well-being better, or differently.

Therefore, we think about the implications of different kinds of data, starting with how they are collected. Well-being data can be collected in various ways: through administrative processes, such as the recording of births, marriages and deaths, or crime-rates. These data will be used as quantitative data, to understand and develop measures we see in the press, like 'mortality rate'. Quantitative data can also be collected using surveys that allow understanding of more complex aspects of people's lives. Asking people questions means you can know how long it is since they visited their GP (general practitioner), for example, or how far they have to walk to their nearest children's play area. These data are easily turned into numbers to give a picture of how people's lives compare, or how we are doing overall, and can help governments make decisions about how to allocate resources.

Data collected in questionnaires and online surveys can also be qualitative, as can interviews, diaries and observations. Qualitative data are most generally text-based, and so are good to understand how people have described their experiences or opinions; although can also involve image or sound, for that matter. Using qualitative data can allow researchers to understand the complexities of a situation and the specificities of people's personal lives. While quantitative and qualitative approaches tend to be discussed separately, some data collection methods, such as surveys and questionnaires, collect both quantitative data (by ticking a box) and qualitative data (by a free text field), so surveys are able to gather data that offer a bigger picture and more detail at the same time.

Qualitative data often have lots of rich detail about few people in a specific context that have to be interpreted by the person analysing it.

Quantitative data will have been collected so they can be quantified, removing contextual detail for analysis using numbers and comparison across a population. Somewhat confusingly, if you have enough qualitative data, you can quantify them, but this is less common and we look at how and why that can be useful sometimes. While quantitative data also require interpretation, there are standardised mathematical approaches, usually drawing on statistical methods to support these decisions and analyses. This means quantitative approaches are considered to be more neutral and objective. But as we shall see, lots of decisions are needed, and this poses key questions about the idea of objectivity in the data used to make statements about what is good for society and to make arguments that one thing over another will improve well-being.

Chapter 3 is the first chapter where we start to look under the bonnet of well-being data. At some points we get up-close to specific research examples and ideas, including quotes from focus groups and examples of well-being survey questions in an imagined context of evaluating a local community event. We also look at so-called objective well-being indicators (e.g. mortality rate) that feature in well-being metrics, like the OECD's Better Life Index. We 'follow these data' using qualitative data in reports to think about how objective these measures really are. We will reflect on the distinction between objective well-being, as something experts decide is important to well-being, such as an aspect of health, and subjective well-being measures which involved asking people how they feel. All data and ways of using them have pros and cons, which is why context is important. Understanding how different data work in different contexts is key to well-being data and key to data for well-being.

'Discovering "the New Science of Happiness" and Subjective Well-being' is the title of Chap. 4. Here we consider the formation of happiness as something that can be measured. Happiness is part of a broader academic concept called 'subjective well-being'—as an idea of how well-being is felt. Subjective well-being becomes extremely influential in the well-being agenda and we look at the role that these new measures hold. The chapter begins by describing how 'happiness' became a 'new science' including the different academics, politicians and fields of study involved. It describes the evolution of positive psychology and happiness economics and their influence in the realm of policy-making.

Disciplines like psychology and economics often group subjective well-being data into different types. They refer to evaluation, experience and eudaimonic[7] measures. This chapter does the same to explore what these mean in practice, and how they are used or useful to understand specific aspects of the human experience, which is then used in evidence for policy-making. Again, specific examples of the contexts in which these sorts of data are collected and used reveal their limits, as well as contradictions in their use. We then focus on subjective well-being measures in the UK and the Office for National Statistics' (ONS') Measuring National Well-being Programme.

Looking at the invention of subjective well-being measures in the UK offers context behind the ubiquity of well-being measurement practices. Understanding the recent history behind, and breaking down the different ways of measuring a *particular idea* of well-being, is vital to appreciate the limitations of such projects. While the innovations and limitations of well-being data remain unaddressed, their positive contribution for society can never be fully realised. This chapter's comprehensive survey and critical lens aim to offer tools to promote better understanding of subjective well-being and happiness data, their capacity to change culture and society, and the limits of their application in areas of social and cultural policy and practice.

Chapter 5 looks at Big Data, which is an enormous topic to try and cover in one chapter. 'Getting a Sense of Big Data and Well-being' asks many questions, beginning with: what do we even mean by the term?—how are data big? The amount of data on individuals that is now collected is quite simply mind-boggling. The International Data Corporation (IDC) predicts that by 2025, the total amount of digital data created worldwide will rise to 163 zettabytes (Coughlin 2018). That is 10^{21} (1,000,000,000,000,000,000,000 bytes) or one trillion gigabytes. The European Commission forecasted the European 'data market' to be worth as much as €106.8 billion by 2020 (Ram and Murgia 2019). We can therefore see that not only have the amounts of data increased, but their economic value has as well. It is, therefore, even harder to maintain that all uses of well-being data enable neutral decisions about how society is managed, when it is being called 'the new oil' (The Economist 2017).

We begin by asking the question: 'What even *is* Big Data?' We look at what the term means, as well as what Big Data *are* and what they can *do*, including how as soon as someone tries to define *it*, somehow that definition is not quite right. Emergent technologies from all walks of life are producing and collecting and analysing data about us as we move about the online and offline world. This means that more can be known about people—which we discover means that data are a double-edged sword for well-being.

Big Data are often attributed with much power—by those in favour of their use, and those who actively work to limit the negative possibilities of these new data and how they are used. The chapter demystifies Big Data by putting them into historical and a number of practical contexts. For example, smaller organisations, in the arts and social sector, use data mining in small, mundane and often unobtrusive ways (Kennedy 2016; Oman 2013). It is possible to use data in research like this in a way that is ethical and without much software skill or financial resource. We revisit a practical example of a manageable project I undertook to reanalyse Twitter data using a hashtag that was started by a Mass Observation project[8] to understand what makes people happy. As a spoiler, there are many cats.

Mass Observation was a project originally established by an anthropologist, a poet and a filmmaker in 1937[9] who wanted to record everyday life in Britain. The project emerged at a time where there was a desire for more detail in data, and around the same time as social surveys were becoming more complex to understand more detail about people's everyday lives, particularly around World War II. More data were wanted to understand quality of life and manage populations beyond the administrative data collected on mass-scale, like the census.

Most countries now undertake a census of sorts, and in the UK, the ONS have collected its census data every ten years since 1801. The new 'enthusiasm for numbers' in the early to mid-nineteenth century (Hacking 1991, 186; Porter 1986, 1996) coincided with a growing infrastructure to collect and analyse data. This desire for numbers, and the data processes that were required to provide them, led to the 'great explosion of numbers that made the term statistics' (Porter 1986, 11). In this 'avalanche of numbers', 'nation-states classified, counted and tabulated their subjects anew' (Hacking 1990, 2; 1991, 186). Censuses date back far farther, of course, and the ONS' website offers an interesting history of censuses in the UK, back to the Domesday book ordered by the Norman (French) King, William the Conqueror in 1086 (ONS 2016). Again, censuses precede these European data moments by some 4000 years in both Egypt and China, who recorded who lived where how wealthy they were. The Romans held regular censuses to keep track of their expanding—and then contracting—empire. Further back still, the clay tablets of Sumerian script (Harford 2017) might be considered a dataset of Big Data from 6000 years ago. The promise of Big Data is therefore not new.

We look at the promise of Big Data to predict a pandemic, reflecting on the obvious failings of Big Data to forecast COVID-19's impact in a way that could have averted international crisis. We also look at a company that claims to have predicted the pandemic, yet failed to stop it: is it possible that the commercial value of the intelligence they had was a barrier to more effective global prevention? We start some years before that, in 2009 with the failings of Google Flu Trends (GFT), which promised to beat the slow infrastructures of health services and testing in the US. GFT analysed what people searched for on Google, analysing what, where and when people typed symptoms into the search. Yet, this did not work for a number of reasons tied to a lack of capacity to understand context.

Back in the UK, I took part in a home testing programme that the media said would 'clear up [the] "Wild West" of Covid-19 estimates' (Devlin 2020). In what has been called the 'largest testing study for Coronavirus' (Ipsos Mori 2020), tests were posted to you, using the UK's traditional Royal Mail postal system. That all worked fine for me, but there were a series of steps registering different barcodes and I found myself wondering how accessible this was for everyone (when I say everyone, I often think of my once tech-savvy Dad, who'd have been bewildered at this whole process). As a result of these steps, a courier was ordered to collect the test, but failed after three attempts (that I describe in more detail in the chapter). A neighbour told me in passing that this particular courier company was infamous for not bothering to try and collect from my high-rise flats, probably because the buzzer has never worked and it can take too long for a resident to come down. This looks bad for the drivers' performance data, which are meant to encourage them to make as many deliveries and pick-ups as possible.

In my case, while some aspects of the traditional data infrastructure (the post) worked fine for this COVID-19 data collection research, they didn't necessarily all work together as they might. This meant that my test remained uncollected; therefore my data became 'missing data'. Thinking about the contexts in which data are collected (or not) can be both extraordinary and mundane, and we often don't hear of these stories—when they work, and the odd occasion when they don't, and what that might mean for the data.

We follow other case studies of data from mobile phone usage, social media data and tracking apps, for example. We, again, 'follow the data' and how they are used to interpret whether these data projects are primarily concerned with improving human well-being, or with refining data practice. It is crucial to problematise the ethics of Big Data for well-being, particularly their commercial aspects, rooting these in the larger questions of what data can do more generally and the limits of data for understanding well-being or improving well-being.

Half Time

The data we look at in the first half of this book are either all collected to better understand people or society, or have been analysed to do so to enable a government or a company to make better decisions. There is a sense that these data are all neutral—they are not affected by bias and can all be treated as fact. These chapters reveal the fragilities in the assumptions behind these kinds of data. When you consider the hypothetical and real-world examples, you can see lots of humans mainly doing their best to work with data. We can also see mistakes in the systems and analysis, and therefore, some of the data-driven decisions we live with are not the best decisions they are assumed to be.

The fact that data have real-world impacts and implications is not something that is often made clear by those who use data, or advocate data-driven decision-making. The impact of Big Data has seen an increase in those considering their social effects. Consequently, the negative aspects of data are an issue of government agendas with new emphases (DCMS 2020). However, the ways that data about people make the problems of society legible are not necessarily new, and neither are the problems. Data on residents, together with a map produced by the City Office of Statistics of Amsterdam, enabled the rounding up of the city's Jewish population under Nazi occupation in 1941 (Scott 1998, 77). Yet, the same techniques of mapping people and personal data about them also led epidemiologists to identify how the AIDS pandemic was spreading and of course the current COVID-19 crisis.

We need context to understand data practices and the possible ramifications of their social effects. They have their own 'social life' (Beer and Burrows 2013; Oman n.d.), meaning they might be thought of as living in that they act on the world as much as humans do. Data and numbers 'make up' people (Hacking [1983] 2002) and tese later theorists enable us to think. Decisions are made about our lives without asking us, but looking at how we are represented by data. Data decide whether you will get a commercial loan or access to financial support by the state. Postcode data in the UK will decide how you will receive medical treatment and what drugs you are entitled to. Data hold much power through metrics (Beer 2016) and algorithms (Kennedy 2015). But also, the very idea of data is powerful; it affects our day-to-day behaviour. Crucially, however, it is also in the desire for data where its power lies.

The Second Half

We 'switch ends' in the second half. The goal instead is thinking more about how society has increasingly required well-being data. So, while we do not entirely leave thinking about contexts of data collection, we think more about the contexts in which they are used. We continue to focus on how society works, its relationship to governance and decision-making, and the role of data in this. Given that data are social and cultural, we will, therefore, look at areas of social policy, focussing on cultural policy in particular to make comparisons more readily across some simple arguments about well-being that use data. To be truthful, it is also in looking at data in the cultural sector and in cultural policy that I came to understand data, and is my natural data habitat.

Chapter 6, 'Well-being, Values, Culture and Society', provides an overview of how cultural policy became a form of social policy, specifically looking at the role of well-being. The chapter historicises the idea that particular aspects of culture have a social role and are good for well-being using accessible interpretations of key philosophers from Aristotle to Kant. We reflect on the fact that much like population data, the arts have an honourable and dishonourable history (Belfiore and Bennett 2008), as both have been co-opted for political projects, such as fascism: that didn't just damage well-being, but were almost indescribably catastrophic for people and society. The chapter brings these empirical accounts of uses of culture into play with social theory from cultural studies scholars, including Raymond Williams ([1961] 1971, 1977, [1958] 1989a, [1968] 1989b). These later theorists enable us to think through some assumptions around the role of culture, even what gets to be called culture, and why that is a problem for cultural and social policy. In turn, we are in a position to contextualise how the institutions and historical assumptions that decide what is good culture, and manage cultural policy, are not so different from thinking about the institutions that manage data and the way we work with and understand data. These overlaps are rarely acknowledged.

We reflect on a genealogy of the idea that culture (broadly defined) is good for well-being (broadly defined); how that has been naturalised over time and then popularised. By this I mean, there is a generally accepted view that culture is good for well-being, and we look at the lineage of this idea as something that began with philosophers and is now common sense. We will then investigate how this relationship has been *instrumentalised* as a form of social policy. This involves looking at how culture is used as a means or 'instrument' for attaining goals in other areas of society. Examples of this can be found in policy documents, research agendas and in practitioner movements including 'arts in health' (ACE 2007; AHRC n.d.; AHSW 2019) or the use of culture in urban regeneration projects (DCMS 2004; LGA 2020; UNESCO 2018). The idea that the arts can be used to directly address societal problems has led to arguments that culture is—in fact—instrumental to these social policy areas.

The idea that arts are instrumental in delivering broader social projects and improving social infrastructure has been *operationalised* to advocate for funds for the arts. We have, therefore, witnessed changes in the value of culture from something belonging to everyone (Hall 1977; Keynes 1945), to how much social impact it can demonstrate, or indeed financial estimates of the creative industries (Campbell 2019; DCMS 2011). In return for advocating the value of culture, the sector is increasingly required to evaluate how much of this value it has generated in response to funding, or to argue for more funds.

This has also seen the slippery nature of culture and its definitions be instrumentalised in arguments, where one meaning of culture is used to justify another aspect of it. The benefits of culture as something more everyday (Williams [1958] 1989a) are used to justify the funding of art-forms which are considered the opposite of commonplace in that they are elitist, with often small numbers of people interested in participating (opera being the default perpetrator in this argument). This slippery effect is also used when it comes to 'creativity' and arguments surrounding the economic impact of the arts, where 'the arts' become 'the creative industries', including some professions in IT, which in many cases do not seem to be very creative at all—in the way we would normally use the word.

We have, therefore, seen a process in which the culture–well-being relationship is theorised (through philosophers) and become naturalised in people's day-to-day thinking: making it common sense. Figure 1.1 shows the full journey of processes described in the chapter. The common-sense nature of the relationship is operationalised in policy and instrumentalised

Theorised -> naturalised -> operationalised -> instrumentalised -> metricised -> capitalised

Fig. 1.1   The culture–well-being relationship

to argue the value of the arts and culture to other areas of social policy. This process, however, has led to the cultural sector finding itself in a bind to the burden of proof. It has to evidence the social impact of the work it does, which is a costly exercise of data production and analysis.

These shifts in the culture–well-being relationship have seen the value of data increase and become *capitalised* on (Oman and Taylor 2018). The increase in funding saw an upturn in evaluations required to report back to funders. With this came demand for data and data practices that are often outside of the skills and confidence of many working in the cultural sector, and broader areas of social policy. These skills therefore often need buying in from elsewhere. With the newer forms of well-being data introduced in the first half of this book, come new metrics and valuation tools, which are presented as a solution to issues of advocacy and proof in the sector. They also perpetuate this cycle of funding and evaluation, which preserve this process of instrumentalising, operationalising and capitalising on the culture–well-being relationship. We will therefore look at some examples of how well-being data are used to make arguments about culture—and we will follow the data in different ways to see *how* they work.

Chapters 7 and 8 draw from the framing in Chap. 6 to look at how the culture–well-being relationship has been operationalised in research to provide proof. Chapter 7 is called 'Evidencing Culture for Policy'. It takes three fundamental arguments about the culture–well-being relationship that are used in advocacy and looks at them more closely. The first is that culture warrants funding, because it is good for well-being. We look at a number of different examples of data to establish if a relationship between public funding and well-being can be found. Again, through investigating the contexts of data collection and analyses, we are able to think about the limits of what can be known using these data.

Why are well-being data in demand to understand some relationships and not others? Despite the naturalised belief that we should invest in culture for its well-being benefits? There is little research which explores whether a pattern can be established between increased funding and well-being. Why are some questions repeatedly asked and not others? Is this a matter of the data (what can be known) or the limits of what people want to know?

We look at the question of 'how much is culture good for well-being' in more detail. The chapter considers two pieces of research which investigate the well-being of cultural practitioners and creative professionals who are often presented as similar, even the same, population. The two studies ostensibly use the same approach to analyse survey data to understand this culture–well-being relationship. In comparing these two cases, we unpack differing findings and look at limitations of data, in categories, populations and analyses, and question how they help us understand well-being in this instance. Crucially, this is not necessarily a case of comparing studies to see if one is better than the other. Instead, we look at how asking (at least superficially) the same question using similar data about similar people at comparable points in time does not present the same results. So what does this mean for ideas of evidence?

The final section looks at a piece of research that is found in important and high-profile reports as evidence that culture is good for well-being. The article uses what it calls 'data mining' to understand 'cultural access'. We look under the bonnet of this idea of cultural access and the data that have been used to measure it. We also follow the authors' data mining practices and analyses to find combined variables which change the meaning of the category 'cultural access', resulting in an inflated outcome.

Unpacking the different ways that culture has been packaged as something that is good for people and society is important. In this chapter we discover how particular findings become popularised as 'common knowledge' and how they then become operationalised in reports, the media and policy documents. This is crucial to grasping the idea that the relationship between data and evidence is cultural, and relies on practices, understandings and meanings.

Once we begin to question the social value of generating evidence in this way, the economic value of contracting in well-being data and research practices warrants investigation. In Chap. 8, 'Talking Different Languages of Value', we follow a piece of research that was commissioned to help with advocacy for the arts. The commissioners were an organisation called the Happy Museum, and the research was funded by Arts Council England. Building on the work we have done in previous chapters to understand how data *work* in contexts (see also Oman n.d.), we look at how culture and well-being are operationalised in this study, and walk through the processes, step by step.

The chapter opens with this idea that this book seeks to challenge: that the arts and data speak different languages. Breaking down what is happening, we follow the data in various ways. There is a description of how the data were collected in a national-level survey. We look at the questions, as they appear in a survey, because it can be hard to imagine the mundane contexts that data originate from, when you are looking at the complex results. We follow the data forward, to see how key findings are interpreted by the world. This allows us to ask questions like: what does research do? How does it affect the world or change things?

We follow the conceptual work behind what is being measured before reflecting on some of the steps in the analysis. There was another way that these data were followed, as I was part of a research project to reproduce findings, using details on the processes and the data available. Crucially, the second piece of research arrived at different conclusions from the first. What does that mean for the very idea of 'evidence'?

How does commissioning well-being data analysis to support the arguments people want to make change the nature and role of evidence in different social policy areas? How does this affect overall knowledge of 'what works for well-being' in terms of social policy? Importantly, how does 'capitalising' on well-being data affect their capacity to do social good or to be good data? Do the economic value of data and their analysis change the relationship between well-being data and a good society? We have found indications that this is the case with COVID-19, but is this more generalisable?

Chapters 7 and 8 break down various aspects of how data are used in cultural policy to communicate quantitative expressions of well-being to people who lack confidence in these areas. Crucially, this will enable readers to think about how something that is described as culture or cultural is said to impact on well-being, whilst also looking at the limits of the data we have to make such claims. These chapters aim to encourage you to make your own mind up (with a little help) as to whether everything adds up (not just the numbers). Do the arguments make logical sense based on the evidence we actually have, rather than what we are told we have? How can considering the contexts of data help those working in data and working in social policy do more *good* with data? History tells us the dangers of ignoring the good and the bad that can be done with data, and that how it is used is a matter of culture.

The final chapter is simply called 'Understanding'. Here we will reflect on different ways of understanding well-being and different ways of interpreting data. We will look back on how well-being and data are related by way of policy and politics. We consider the relationship between evidence and policy, and the politics of data. How do these conflicting ideas work together when the aim of the game is well-being?

We reflect on how understanding contexts of data helps us better understand the politics of data and evidence for policy. We look at the limitations of well-being data that we have explored in terms of claims that can be made and we look at their limitations when it comes to calling data objective. The huge amounts of decisions involved in establishing the well-being measures in Chaps. 3 and 4 show these are not neutral decisions. Furthermore, Chaps. 7 and 8 reveal the decisions made in modelling: what data to clean, weights and adaptations to valuation techniques when well-being data are used to make arguments about value.

We think about what understanding means. It means understanding as knowledge, *shared understanding* of how something works and *being* understanding, or having empathy. Well-being data promise information that leads to knowledge and wisdom, but these do not currently lead to a shared understanding. Research is commissioned for the cultural sector and presented in ways preoccupied with proof, rather than communicating findings with those who work in the sector.

The concluding chapter presents a case study of how people crave understanding of why they are being asked certain questions on equality monitoring forms, what will happen to and with the data they offer. Yet, it is not common practice to share understanding of how and why different data are valuable. There is much room for understanding and empathy in approaches to inequality and well-being data, and this is currently overlooked in most projects that work with these data in the name of social justice.

The 'social life of methods' is a body of research proposing that methods are not neutral ways of capturing an objective reality, but have their own social effects; in fact, changing the reality they claim to capture. Data: how it is collected, shared, analysed and where the results are published are a fundamental part of this. We have looked at how data are cultural, in that they change culture, making new cultures, and we look at the implications of these social effects. Those who are campaigning for data rights are very focussed on what can be known about people from data. However, this is often framed as an issue of privacy as an abstract human right or as an issue of social justice, as the effects of data-driven decision-making disproportionately affect marginalised groups. This, of course, is an important ethical question.

A broader question, however, is what can these data *actually* tell us about people? There are limitations to most data when it comes to what we can actually understand about society that are not always taken into consideration. Crucially, the question we must ask ourselves at this moment is how can we also rethink questions of what can be known about people from data to incorporate data's limits, as well as their power? How might well-being data improve well-being? Can we be better at moving from understanding people as units of analysis to becoming more understanding in the way we collect and use data?

These are the provocations this book leaves us with and I hope to continue to do work that not only tries to answer these questions, but which goes about changing things. This book is set up so that we can look at the work that well-being *does* in policy and practice contexts for social and cultural policy, for third sector organisations and arts managers, for charities. Most of all this book is meant to help us all have a better grasp of ideas of well-being and ideas of data, how they work in different contexts and how they are used and manipulated for different ends. Neither are neutral. They are imposed by historical traditions which say what works and what doesn't. They are imbued with values—and I hope this book will help you value your own judgement to decide what they mean for you.

NOTES

1. Of course, you can use alternate search engines and change settings to have some control over this to some extent.
2. Although, it must be noted that the analyst on the BBC's *More or Less* programme did state that this was only a possibility—Boris Johnson's numbers were—in fact—far more generous than using the index that would give the best results, and within the best timeframe.
3. A recently formed network of practitioners, the Cultural Data and Research network, is tackling these issues in various ways. See: www.cdrn.uk for more information.
4. For further discussion of ideas of well-being: Sara Ahmed compellingly explains how the ideals of happiness are not available to all: they are reliant on race, class, gender and sexuality (2010). I have tested this using a Google search over different years (see Oman 2015b as an example). I found that when I searched for the word 'well-being', the majority of images comprised stock images of white people who were able-bodied and doing yoga or jumping, or they were a middle-class family sitting down to a healthy dinner together with perfect teeth. These very ideas of what well-being looks like,

who has well-being and who doesn't are reinforced by government health messaging. This changes what we think well-being means. See Ryan (2021) for some alternative messages.

5. See Airoldi (2021) for the most recent example of research on recommendations and YouTube.
6. Data, information, knowledge and wisdom are sometimes thought of in terms of a DIKW Pyramid. This pyramid helps imagine and visualise the relationships between them. Each is thought to be a step towards a higher level—first come data, then is information, next is knowledge and finally comes wisdom. Each step answers different questions about the initial data and adds value to it. This idea suits one way of thinking about the relationship between data and wisdom. This book explains how this process is more complicated. See also Frické (2009) for why it's more complicated than this.
7. We look at the idea of eudaimonia in greater detail in Chaps. 2 and 4. Most simply, eudaimonia means feeling purpose, or flourishing.
8. Mass Observation is a project that has long aimed to record everyday life in Britain. More detail can be found on the different phases of the overall project and its smaller projects, here: http://www.massobs.org.uk, and in Chap. 6.
9. There were a number of iterations of Mass Observation (n.d.), with different people initiating them, but the original founding members were anthropologist Tom Harrisson, poet Charles Madge and filmmaker Humphrey Jennings.

References

ACE. 2007. *Strategy for the Arts Health and Wellbeing*, 52. London: Arts Council England. https://www.artshealthresources.org.uk/wp-content/uploads/2017/01/2007-ACE-Strategy-for-the-arts-health-and-wellbeing.pdf. Accessed 29 April 2021.

Ahmed, S. 2010. *The Promise of Happiness*. Durham: Duke University Press.

AHRC. n.d. *Arts and Health, Health and Wellbeing Research Portfolio*. https://ahrc.ukri.org/innovation/health-and-wellbeing-research-portfolio/arts-and-health/. Accessed 29 March 2021.

AHSW. 2019. *Arts & Health South West, Arts & Health South West – Home*. https://www.ahsw.org.uk/. Accessed 29 March 2021.

Airoldi, M. 2021. The Techno-Social Reproduction of Taste Boundaries on Digital Platforms: The Case of Music on YouTube. *Poetics*: 101563. https://doi.org/10.1016/j.poetic.2021.101563.

Batchelor, T. 2017. Donald Trump Says All Negative Polls About Him Are Fake News. *The Independent*. https://www.independent.co.uk/news/world/americas/donald-trump-negative-polls-fake-news-twitter-cnn-abc-nbc-a7564951.html. Accessed 29 March 2021.

BBC. 2020. Child Poverty, School Inequality and a Second Wave. *BBC Radio 4: More or Less*. https://www.bbc.co.uk/programmes/m000kf82. Accessed 29 March 2021.

Beer, D. 2016. *Metric Power*. London: Palgrave Macmillan.

Beer, D., and R. Burrows. 2013. Popular Culture, Digital Archives and the New Social Life of Data. *Theory, Culture & Society* 30 (4): 47–71. https://doi.org/10.1177/0263276413476542.

Belfiore, E., and O. Bennett. 2008. *The Social Impact of the Arts: An Intellectual History*. Basingstoke; New York: Palgrave Macmillan.

Campbell, P. 2019. *Persistent Creativity: Making the Case for Art, Culture and the Creative Industries*. Palgrave Macmillan (Sociology of the Arts). https://doi.org/10.1007/978-3-030-03119-0.

Coughlin, T. 2018. 175 Zettabytes By 2025. *Forbes*. https://www.forbes.com/sites/tomcoughlin/2018/11/27/175-zettabytes-by-2025/. Accessed 29 March 2021.

DC Research. 2017. *Mapping-Museum Data in England: Arts Council England Final Report*. UK: Arts Council England. https://www.artscouncil.org.uk/sites/default/files/download-file/Mapping%20Museum%20Data%20-%20Final%20Report.pdf. Accessed 29 March 2021.

DCMS. 2004. *Culture at the Heart of Regeneration*. Department for Culture, Media and Sport.

———. 2011. *Creative Industries Economic Estimates*. Department for Digital, Culture, Media & Sport. https://www.gov.uk/government/collections/creative-industries-economic-estimates.

———. 2020. *Policy Paper: National Data Strategy*. Department for Digital, Culture, Media & Sport. https://www.gov.uk/government/publications/uk-national-data-strategy/national-data-strategy. Accessed 29 March 2021.

Devlin, H. 2020. Randomised Test of 100,000 to Help Decide End of UK Lockdown. *The Guardian*. http://www.theguardian.com/world/2020/apr/30/randomised-coronavirus-test-of-100000-will-determine-end-date-of-uk-lockdown. Accessed 2 May 2021.

Francis-Devine, B. 2020. Poverty in the UK: Statistics. *House of Commons Library* (7096). https://commonslibrary.parliament.uk/research-briefings/sn07096/. Accessed 29 March 2021.

Frické, M. 2009. The Knowledge Pyramid: A Critique of the DIKW Hierarchy. *Journal of Information Science* 35 (2): 131–142. https://doi.org/10.1177/0165551508094050.

Gove, M. 2016. *Gove: Britons 'Have Had Enough of Experts'*. https://www.youtube.com/watch?v=GGgiGtJk7MA. Accessed 29 March 2021.

GSS. n.d. *Glossary, Government Statistical Service*. https://gss.civilservice.gov.uk/about-us/glossary/. Accessed 29 March 2021.

Hacking, I. 1990. *The Taming of Chance*. Cambridge: Cambridge University Press.

———. 1991. How Should We Do the History of Statistics? In *The Foucault Effect: Studies in Governmentality*, ed. G. Burchell, C. Gordon, and P. Miller. Chicago: The University of Chicago Press.

———. [1983]2002. Making up People. In *Historical Ontology*. Cambridge, MA: Harvard University Press.

Hall, S. 1977. Culture, the Media, and the "Ideological Effect". In *Essential Essays*. Durham: Duke University Press.

Harford, T. 2017. How the World's First Accountants Counted on Cuneiform. *BBC News*. https://www.bbc.co.uk/news/business-39870485. Accessed 28 April 2021.

Ipsos Mori. 2020. Largest Testing Study for Coronavirus Publishes Latest Findings. *Ipsos MORI*. https://www.ipsos.com/ipsos-mori/en-uk/largest-testing-study-coronavirus-publishes-latest-findings. Accessed 2 May 2021.

Kennedy, H. 2015. Is Data Culture? Data Analytics and the Cultural Industries. In *The Routledge Companion to the Cultural Industries*, ed. K. Oakley and J. O'Connor. London; New York: Routledge.

———. 2016. *Post, Mine, Repeat: Social Media Data Mining Becomes Ordinary*. New York; Secaucus: Palgrave Macmillan. https://doi.org/10.1057/978-1-137-35398-6.

Kennedy, H., Oman, S., Taylor, M., Bates, J. and Steedman, R. 2020. *Public Understanding and Perceptions of Data Practices: A Review of Existing Research*. Sheffield: The University of Sheffield. https://livingwithdata.org/project/wp-content/uploads/2020/05/living-with-data-2020-review-of-existing-research.pdf.

Keynes, J.M. 1945. The Arts Council: Its Policy and Hopes. In *The Collected Writings of John Maynard Keynes*, ed. D. Maggridge, 367–372. London: Macmillan.

LGA. 2020. *Cultural Strategy in a Box*. Local Government Association.

Mass Observation. n.d. *Mass Observation*. http://www.massobs.org.uk.

Noble, S.U. 2018. *Algorithms of Oppression: Data Discrimination in the Age of Google*. New York: New York University Press.

Oman, S. 2013. Review of "Counting What Counts: What Big Data Can Do for the Cultural Sector". *Cultural Value Initiative*. http://culturalvalueinitiative.org/2013/06/08/review-of-nestas-counting-what-counts-what-big-data-can-do-for-the-cultural-sector-by-susan-oman/. Accessed 16 October 2017.

———. 2015a. Culture and Well-being – A Happy Marriage of Inconvenience?, presentation at Breaking into the Temples of Culture: Exploring Arts, Health and Well-being Initiatives in the Community, 27 November 2015, Tate Liverpool. Available at: http://www.everydayparticipation.org/breaking-the-temple-of-the-culture-well-being-relationship/. Accessed 29 March 2021.

———. 2015b. The Well-being – Culture Relationship: A Long and Happy Marriage of Convenience?, presentation at *Understanding Everyday*

Participation: Histories Symposium, 24 April 2015. Available at: http://www.everydayparticipation.org/wp-content/uploads/2015/07/Susan-Oman-Culture-Wellbeing-relationship.compressed.pdf.

———. 2019a. *Improving Data Practices to Monitor Inequality and Introduce Social Mobility Measures: A Working Paper*. The University of Sheffield. https://www.sheffield.ac.uk/polopoly_fs/1.867756!/file/MetricsWorkingPaper.pdf. Accessed 29 March 2021.

———. 2019b. *Measuring Social Mobility in The Creative and Cultural Industries: The Importance of Working in Partnership to Improve Data Practices and Address Inequality*. Sheffield: The University of Sheffield. https://www.sheffield.ac.uk/polopoly_fs/1.867754!/file/MetricsPolicyBriefing.pdf. Accessed 29 March 2021.

———. 2020. *The Management and Measurement of Inequality in the Cultural Sector*. The University of Leeds, February 27. https://ahc.leeds.ac.uk/performance/events/event/1821/the-management-and-measurement-of-inequality-in-the-cultural-sector. Accessed 29 March 2021.

———. n.d. How Data Work in Context. *Living with Data*. https://livingwithdata.org/previous-research/how-data-work-in-contexts/. Accessed 30 March 2021.

Oman, S., and M. Taylor. 2018. Subjective Well-being in Cultural Advocacy: A Politics of Research Between the Market and the Academy. *Journal of Cultural Economy* 11 (3): 225–243. https://doi.org/10.1080/17530350.2018.1435422.

ONS. 2016. *Early Census-Taking in England and Wales*. Office for National Statistics. https://www.ons.gov.uk/census/2011census/howourcensusworks/aboutcensuses/censushistory/earlycensustakinginenglandandwales. Accessed 28 April 2021.

Porter, T.M. 1986. *The Rise of Statistical Thinking 1820–1900*. Princeton: Princeton University Press.

———. 1996. *Trust in Numbers the Pursuit of Objectivity in Science and Public Life*. Princeton: Princeton University Press.

Ram, A., and M. Murgia. 2019. Data Brokers: Regulators Try to Rein in the 'Privacy Deathstars'. *Financial Times*. https://www.ft.com/content/f1590694-fe68-11e8-aebf-99e208d3e521. Accessed 29 March 2021.

Ryan, F. 2021. Cake and Inner Calm: 10 Ways to Improve Your Mood – Without Exercising. *The Guardian*. http://www.theguardian.com/lifeandstyle/2021/feb/23/cake-and-inner-calm-10-ways-to-improve-your-mood-without-exercising. Accessed 29 March 2021.

Scott, J.C. 1998. *Seeing Like a State: How Certain Schemes to Improve the Human Condition Have Failed*. New Haven: Yale University Press (The Yale ISPS Series).

The Economist. 2017. The World's Most Valuable Resource Is No Longer Oil, but Data. *The Economist*, May 6. https://www.economist.com/leaders/2017/05/06/the-worlds-most-valuable-resource-is-no-longer-oil-but-data. Accessed 29 March 2021.

UK Parliament. 2020. Engagements, Volume 677: Debated on Wednesday 17 June 2020. *House of Commons Hansard*. https://hansard.parliament.uk/Commons/2020-06-17/debates/D91FE96D-8668-4B3C-AC27-A9CE9E961015/Engagements. Accessed 29 March 2021.

UNESCO. 2018. RURITAGE: Rural Regeneration Through Systemic Heritage-led Strategies. *UNESCO*. https://en.unesco.org/ruritage. Accessed 28 April 2021.

Williams, R. [1961]1971. *The Long Revolution*. London: Pelican. https://doi.org/10.7312/will93760. Accessed 29 March 2021.

———. 1977. *Marxism and Literature*. Oxford: Oxford University Press.

———. [1958]1989a. Culture Is Ordinary. In *Resources of Hope: Culture, Democracy, Socialism*, ed. R. Gable. London; New York: Verso.

———. [1968]1989b. The Idea of a Common Culture. In *Resources of Hope: Culture, Democracy, Socialism*, ed. R. Gable. London; New York: Verso.

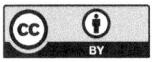

CHAPTER 2

Knowing Well-being: A History of Data

2.1   WHAT IS WELL-BEING?

> Centuries of philosophical inquiry have failed to result in agreement about
> what the 'good life' is. (Veenhoven 1984, 18)

How do we know what well-being is? The term 'well-being' is familiar and
widespread and yet there is ambiguity around its definition. There are
even disagreements in whether it is spelt 'well-being' or wellbeing. 'Health
and well-being' or 'mental health and well-being' are common expressions in public services and formal reports, from housing to arts councils
(i.e. ACE 2018). While well-being is key to social policy-making (Wolf
2019), it is increasingly distinguished from 'welfare' (Scott 2012, 37) and
instead linked to what we now call 'the wellness industry', which, at its
extreme is seen as a hybrid of clean eating, yoga and meditation
(Cederström and Spicer 2014; Davies 2015). So, well-being can therefore
be used to describe health, but more than health; it is key to public services, but is not used to describe welfare, as such—and the very idea of
well-being has been co-opted by big business who want to sell us what
they want us to believe is good for us.

   This chapter asks the question: 'knowing well-being, how did we get
here?' Its main aim is to present the historical and policy context of well-
being as an agenda. 'The well-being agenda' has emerged as a consequence
of people and organisations considering it a priority: as a problem that

© The Author(s) 2021   35
S. Oman, *Understanding Well-being Data*,
New Directions in Cultural Policy Research,
https://doi.org/10.1007/978-3-030-72937-0_2

needs solving, or an aim that warrants achieving. You might be familiar with the idea of a policy agenda: the well-being agenda is bigger than policy, with more individuals and associations involved and with an interest. We will establish how well-being is used, including definitions and traditions of well-being, beginning to see how well-being data[1] emerge as useful for measurement, and how measurement is used to *know* about well-being in certain ways. Well-being measures have two main uses: to track the health and wealth of nations and to make policy decisions. These involve either evaluating previous interventions or predicting how a future decision might have positive impact. The chapter reflects on well-being as a tool of policy that emerged as a result of an agenda across academic, technical, commercial and political interests. The story of the well-being agenda is important to understanding contemporary society, and the role of data, vital to it.

Some see well-being as synonymous with happiness,[2] and therefore arguably only a part of the human experience, and others as an all-encompassing concept to describe the quality of people's lives (Dodge et al. 2012). We will explore these aspects in Chaps. 3 and 4. As Veenhoven (1984) suggests, well-being as a concept can also encompass broader ideas about what a good life might be; which others, such as the Greek philosopher Aristotle saw as connected to how we might envisage a good society (Aristotle 1976).[3] It can therefore describe how humans experience the world as individuals, or as society.

Well-being is also used to describe things which aren't really about people or life at all, such as 'the well-being of the sector' when talking about the arts and culture (UK Parliament 2018) and 'the well-being of the economy'. We have seen this used recently to justify releasing of lockdown laws which were in place to protect the vulnerable, following peaks of coronavirus infections in the UK (John 2020). This linguistic trick can lead someone to connect the economy to well-being, when they would not necessarily have done before.

The well-being of the economy is not 'well-being economics', however, which aims to re-focus away from economic policy to account for the negative effects of growth on people and the planet. Think of the links between McDonald's and the destruction of the Amazon rainforest, for example (Vidal 2006), and calls for a 'local economy'. Thus, well-being economics is often ideologically opposite to concerns that we must safeguard the economy, instead directing attention to protecting community infrastructures and interests, while being sensitive to impacts on the planet in a move 'towards sustainability' (see Scott 2012).

Box 2.1   Ideology
When this book talks about **ideology**, it means a set of ideas that go together, as is common in a political ideology, like socialism, fascism or democracy, for example. The well-being of the economy might be thought to ideologically put the economy first, whereas well-being economics wants to foreground protecting people and the planet over economic growth.

Some economists and psychologists, however, might refer to 'happiness economics' when thinking about well-being. Rooted in positive psychology and behavioural psychology, happiness economics is based on the premise that what we do affects our well-being, and that people can make better decisions for themselves (Dolan 2014; Layard 2006). The approach has been adopted in policy-making as it offers rationales for decision-making and has also been capitalised on. For example, the digital mental health market was valued at $1.4 billion (£1.1 billion) in 2017 and is projected to reach $4.6 billion in 2026 (Morris 2020). This industry commercialises a solution for people's desire to improve themselves or make themselves feel better. If you take a moment to think about how making people feel more responsible for their own well-being is attractive to those in government who want to be *less* accountable for our well-being, this may make you feel suspicious of the links across the business of well-being and the governance of our welfare.

The well-being agenda has, therefore, manifested in different camps with different agendas—which have different relationships with data. As a result, we have different kinds of well-being data that are produced and generated for different purposes. They are also *used* differently: various parts of society use well-being data to manage themselves—and others— in different ways.[4] This makes it difficult to navigate well-being data and how it is used, or how *we* should use it—both in our own work, and when reading about others' work in our everyday lives or when watching the news.

While this book's primary concern is not to define well-being, nor is it to re-document the histories of ideas around well-being (there are many other excellent books which have done these things e.g. Davies 2015; Layard 2006; McMahon 2006; Schoch 2007), the fact that there is no single use of the term makes it complicated. It is also what makes it *so* valuable for those who use well-being data to suit their aims, needs and communicate their beliefs.

This book is designed to help navigate the complexities of well-being data: to reveal the roots of the well-being data you encounter profession- ally or in everyday life. So, in order to do that let's first outline how differ- ent aspects of well-being have been imagined historically, how they have been defined. We will also need to account for different moments in time that have resulted in the varieties and uses of well-being data. These politi- cal histories contextualise why certain data are generated, how they are generated—and how they may not represent what you may imagine. With this background knowledge and understanding, you should find it easier to navigate 'well-being' as an intellectual field; a social, cultural and per- sonal aspiration; and a policy agenda. This helps understand different forms of well-being data—and how they are used.

Traditions of Well-being Thought

There are two overarching ideas of well-being which emerge from two main traditions. These are found in the way well-being data are most often used to inform policy-making or evaluate decisions made in organisations. These two traditions have been described as 'Benthamite-subjective- hedonic-individualistic' or 'Aristotelian-objective-eudaimonic-rational' (Bruni and Porta 2005, 20). This way of describing these two traditions is a bit of a mouthful and can be broken down.

Hedonia: Most Simply Understood as Pleasure or Positive Feeling
The first account of well-being is based on *hedonia*: most simply under- stood as pleasure. The easiest way to remember its meaning is through the words: hedonism and hedonistic, as meaning 'a bit of a party animal' or as a good friend used to say: 'a pleasure monster'. This is a recent adaptation, however. Historically, it was grounded in peoples' subjective experience of their own lives. Hedonia is philosophically rooted in the Epicureans' (c. 300 BC) belief that pleasure is good—and morally virtuous to aspire towards. This was later adapted by the Utilitarians: Bentham asserted that an act was good based upon the outcome of the act, specifically, if it pro- vided more happiness for more people than harm. As a result, he believed that the maximisation of pleasure, and reduction of suffering, was the role of government (1996 [1789]).

Jeremy Bentham's 'hedonic calculus', also known as the 'felicific calculus', was a theoretical algorithm. We tend to think of algorithms as a recent invention, but instead it is a term from the late seventeenth century referring to a series of rules for problem solving, particularly in calculations.[5] Bentham proposed to understand the moral worth of an act as its value. By which he meant, that he wanted to be able to come up with a valuation mechanism to understand how people's actions were moral, based on their contribution to happiness. The economist Francis Edgeworth, some 100 years later, argued that utility was directly measurable. Utility is a term in economics that does not refer to the cost of your water bill, but instead captures the idea that when people consume a good or service, they do so to gain satisfaction. We will come to this in greater detail later, but much economics works on the proviso that humans make rational choices that will *maximise* the utility and the experience. Edgeworth believed that new developments in 'physio-psychology' made a 'hedonimeter' possible. The hedonimeter was imagined to measure pleasure through reading bodily responses. This, he argued, would allow economists a physiological underpinning of utility, based on the natural sciences (Colander 2007). In other words, it would *prove* the existence of rational choice and satisfaction, rather than this only being a theory. Improving knowledge of how we experience the world: our pleasure and pain is one of the motivations behind wanting to understand well-being. Making this seem more scientific is one of the drivers behind measuring it and using data, as is the idea of living a good life.

Eudaimonia: Most Often Understood as Purpose or Flourishing
The second account is not based on a mental state, as such, but on the process involved in human flourishing, as living our best possible life. This Aristotelian account of well-being, *eudaimonia*, is formed by what we do across all the aspects of our lives and is more aligned to purpose, rather than pleasure (Aristotle c. 330 BC). These days, many worry that Aristotle's ideas of living a best life (1976) go too far: they are too idealistic and purist. In order to live a good life, a person had to separate themselves from the mundane to consider the theoretical and the scientific. This not only is exclusionary, by today's standards, but depends on others to undertake these mundane activities. Despite the societal issues of slavery and elitism of Aristotle's Athens,[6] much of his thinking of Eudaimonia remains in use.

The binary of pleasure versus purpose grounds much of the well-being discourse. It manifests in proposals of how to achieve both in self-help literature (e.g. see Dolan 2014), or the role of government in reducing suffering or maximising people's opportunities to flourish (Sen 1999). The two traditions have been described as 'Benthamite-subjective-hedonic-individualistic' and 'Aristotelian-objective-eudaimonic-rational' (Bruni and Porta 2005, 20). As we have briefly covered these concepts separately, with any luck, they now mean more than a string of words. I'll now break down the last of those differences (individual vs rational), although, as will become clear later, the positions are not as much in opposition to each other as implied.

Individualism, as you might expect, foregrounds the individual. This position sees the moral right to autonomy, and the importance that people make their own decisions. It involves understanding how individual people live and appreciate things differently, which is why it has been aligned with the subjective and centres on experience. However, this should not necessarily mean that people can only care for themselves. Bentham, for example, believed the role of government was to enable the most happiness for the largest number of people[7] (Bentham (1996 [1789])).

Rationalism, on the other hand, does not necessarily seek empirical truth of experience, by which we mean concrete evidence of what someone else is feeling. Instead it favours what can be deduced via logical intellectual engagement. Rationalist thinking therefore seeks objective ways of understanding the world: meaning those who aspire to rationalism, also aspire towards facts which can be neutrally observed. In other words, how they feel or what they expect should not affect judgement. It is, as we shall discover, more difficult to be a neutral thinker, than you may imagine; similarly, the methods and tools used to capture objective data are not able to capture 'raw data',[8] but all data are contextual and shaped by decisions made on how they are collected and interpreted.

In general, the data that comprise objective indicators are considered more reliable than those in subjective indicators. If we think on a smaller, more everyday scale: in healthcare, objective data include X-rays, and subjective data include the reporting of symptoms. If you were to make a diagnosis of a broken rib, you would use a combination of these data, but the X-rays would be considered more reliable than someone saying they feel like they have broken a rib. However, if someone said they felt as if they'd broken a rib, and the X-ray said otherwise, you would undertake another test to collect more objective data. Statistics doesn't *quite* work like that as you very rarely go to the individual level to see how one bit of objective data corresponds to a subjective one. This, however, might be tested using qualitative research like interviews, which we'll discuss in the .

next chapter. Having briefly summarised the theoretical background to ideas of well-being and their uses, we will begin to look more at data and how they can be used by the well-being agenda.

Common Definitions Used with Well-being Data

There is no single definition of wellbeing. The terms wellbeing, quality of life, happiness, life satisfaction and welfare are often used interchangeably (although some disciplines draw distinctions between them). (Allin 2007, 46)

Paul Allin became Director of the UK's Office for National Statistics' (ONS') Measuring National Well-being programme. As he acknowledges above, there are a number of terms used as if they are substitutable in disciplines associated with measuring well-being. In addition to happiness, life satisfaction and quality of life are also synonymous with well-being. As we shall find out throughout the book, when it comes to data, although these ideas are linked in a common-sense way, life satisfaction metrics are largely from different sorts of data than quality-of-life metrics. Life satisfaction measures aim to capture how people feel and so they are from subjective evaluations. Quality-of-life measures are used to understand various *qualities* of life, such as health and relationships; the endgame is understanding how these work together, to then assess overall well-being. They are made from objective lists and measures.

Objective Well-being
This approach examines what are thought to be the components of the good life, using *objective* data which include resources (income, food, housing) and social attributes (education and health). Objective well-being data are then added up (aggregated) to become society-wide descriptions that imply concrete conditions, such as employment rate or life expectancy. They are objective because they measure material conditions, and are considered impartial. They are well-being data as they are used to understand how something like housing or income might impact our lives. In other words, they can be used as a proxy measure for well-being. By proxy we mean an indirect measure. For example, someone's income does not necessarily directly tell you about their quality of life, but because the relationship has been long-studied, assumptions can be made about well-being using what we know about how income relates to well-being—so the theory goes.

Objective well-being data predominantly come from what we call administrative data. These data are collected in the processes of our everyday lives, like taxation or the registration of births, marriages and deaths. Objective data are also collected from people using surveys. Questions that ask for details on salary and how many people live in someone's home (like in the census), for example, are objective. Chapter 3 looks at objective lists and measures in much greater detail.

Subjective Well-being

As with health diagnoses, subjective well-being data are generated by asking people questions about how they are doing and/or how they are feeling. This can be about their material conditions: how they feel about their local area; is it clean; is it safe? It can also be how they are feeling in and of themselves. One example is the UK's ONS' four questions to understand personal well-being. We will return to 'the ONS4' often in this book. They ask:

1. Overall, how happy did you feel yesterday?
2. Overall, how satisfied are you with your life nowadays?
3. Overall, to what extent do you feel the things you do in your life are worthwhile?
4. Overall, how anxious did you feel yesterday?

People score themselves out of ten, with most scoring around a seven out of ten for life satisfaction. These scores are aggregated to become the well-being data of a population who answered these questions. These aggregated data are used in a number of ways which can be tracked over time. Subjective measures are also used against objective measures, so if a measure of poverty spikes, we can see if this appears to be linked to anxiety using data produced by question 3. More recently, subjective well-being questions have been used to track impacts of the COVID-19 pandemic on different samples of different populations all across the world.

As we have touched on, understanding the human experience in a more scientific way is one of the key drivers of the well-being agenda. Chapter 4 looks in greater detail at the study of subjective well-being as 'a new science' (Layard 2006). Interestingly, this 'new science of happiness' is one of the academic and intellectual developments that saw a resurgence in interest in well-being measurement more generally, especially in policy. Somewhat confusingly, the well-being agenda—as the measurement of well-being—tends to be discussed in terms of objective indicators to replace Gross Domestic Product (GDP), rather than subjective well-being. As we discover in the next section, this is a more complex history than is ordinarily accounted for.

2.2   MEASURING WELL-BEING TO IMPROVE HUMAN WELFARE: A BRIEF HISTORY

The measurement of well-being and quality of life for policy-making has recently been described as 'an idea whose time has come' (Bache and Reardon 2013). Articles on happiness and well-being averaged less than five a year in the journals covered by the EconLit database[9] in the 1990s. By 2008 this had risen to over 50 each year (Fleche et al. 2012, 8). Bache and Reardon (2013) historicise this surge in interest as a political phenomenon that they term 'the second wave of well-being'.

The first wave of well-being evolved as a project of redistribution after World War II. Prior to this, in the 1920s, Gross Domestic Product was developed as a broad quantitative measure of a nation's total economic activity. It was treated as a proxy for increases in individual wealth, and fluctuations in unemployment, thereby tracking material quality of life at national level. A recent history of national accounts in different countries indicates that the well-being of citizens, not their bank accounts, was considered to be the end goal of government (Perlman and Marietta 2005). The goal of collecting information on income distribution, growth and productivity was to examine how those indicators influence the welfare of the nation, according to economist Simon Kuznets, one of the originators of GDP. Although Kuznets also acknowledged that economic indicators were only one piece of the puzzle of citizens' well-being, and that 'the welfare of a nation can 'scarcely be inferred from a measurement of national income' (Kuznets 1934, report to congress, cited in OECD 2007). He was, therefore, arguing for the value of GDP as an instrument, but aware of its limitations, crucially stating:

Goals for more growth should specify more growth of what and for what. (Kuznets in Croly 1962)

GDP and national accounts data were not only generated to go about understanding individual nations, but also meant that countries could be compared in these terms, reflecting a broader trend towards comparable data across nations at this time. In 1924, the League of Nations Health Organisation created the Permanent Commission on Biological Standardisation to monitor drug tests. This increasing momentum to share information on populations, including unemployment, wages and migration led to the new International Statistical Commission in 1947. The modern term 'statistics' was, in fact, coined with the invention of new system of accounting for national governance to ascertain 'the quantum of happiness' with a view to using these data to govern the nation better (Sinclair 1798, vol. 20, xiii).

Growing concerns evolved in the 1950s that personal prosperity created social costs which manifested as public poverty[10] (Noll 2002). There was also growing recognition that these social costs could not be captured by GDP. It was decided that this needed to be addressed through the development of new measurement tools that could help track whether life was *actually* getting better. These were hoped to be able to compensate for some of the shortcomings of GDP as a measure of human progress.

This is what came to be known as 'the social indicators movement', which emerged in the spirit of redistribution and an aspiration for new levels of knowledge of everyday life, birthing new surveys, such as the Level of Living Survey (The Swedish Institute for Social Research 1968; ONS 1970). These alternative but 'objective' benchmarks of progress grew in relevance on the international political agenda (Scott 2012; McGillvray 2007 in Bache 2012). The economic collapse of the 1970s is believed to have compromised the impact of these new indicators. The fact that economics had failed to avert economic crisis (Bache 2012), alongside a growing distrust of government, prevented the social indicator movement from toppling GDP as the primary measure of prosperity, and thus the focus on progress as growth remained.

The 'second wave' of well-being began in the comparative prosperity of the late 1990s (Bache and Reardon 2013) and was cemented in the high-profile commission of leading international economists.[11] This responded to ongoing work of the OECD and concerns that material growth was impacting negatively on the planet (Bache 2012). It also responded to what has become known as the Easterlin paradox (1973): the discovery that rising wealth was not—in fact—improving people's life satisfaction. The commission recommended, with considerable influence, that an alternative benchmark of progress should be found that was able to measure more than GDP and that all nations find a way to measure their own well-being. This task was taken on by most OECD countries, in different ways, and its timing in the UK resulted in its branding as Conservative Prime Minister of the Coalition Government, 'Cameron's happiness index', when it was a far bigger movement that started a decade earlier.

The second wave also coincided with recent developments in subjective well-being data collection. The ONS example which they called Personal Well-being was introduced in April 2011.[12] The measurement of subjective well-being for policy emerges from 'happiness economics' (Layard 2006), which builds on work in the positive psychology movement (e.g. Seligman and Csikszentmihalyi 2000) and which we explore in Chap. 4. Richard Layard (2006) used the term 'hedonic treadmill'[13] in response to the Easterlin paradox. It describes how we adapt to increasing wealth, resulting in a need for *more* income to maintain the levels of life satisfaction we are accustomed to. This results in greater consumption, which causes material growth and negative planetary impacts. Around the same time, other research was beginning to note the positive impacts of more social aspects of life on subjective well-being: social interaction, faith, intimate relationships, government spending and different political-institutional frameworks (Bache and Reardon 2013).

The demise of the social indicators movement in the 1970s was arguably not only the result of economic downturn (Scott 2012). Instead weaknesses in the objective indicators and data themselves made them unsustainable. Described as a 'bewildering array', these metrics were not linked to a robust theoretical or ideological analysis of what quality of life was exactly. The metrics and their analysis did not answer what needed to be achieved for whom and how (Scott 2012, 36). Thus, the second wave appealed to these proclaimed deficiencies.

The history of well-being measurement raises important questions regarding what measures are suitable for policy. Experts argue that the science behind measuring well-being is becoming more robust (O'Donnell et al. 2014; Helliwell et al. 2015; Cameron 2010; ONS 2015), but do the indices address the fundamental question of what 'quality of life' *is*? Do they accommodate how people will find different qualities more valuable in various circumstances? Also, if wealth remains a proxy for well-being for some, and addressing well-being inequality[14] is a new policy focus, has it been decided how redistribution of well-being would be undertaken in practice?

The very essence of well-being, as it is generally understood (particularly subjective well-being), not only is attached to the lived experience, but should encompass it. Instead, well-being is often discussed in a detached way as an object of politics that changes over time. Some argue that this is as a consequence of it becoming measurable (Beer 2016; Davies 2015; Doria 2013; White 2014) which means well-being assumed its own agency, and in ways which are not necessarily understood by the general public. Others argue that this is the very consequence of attributing value to values (Doria 2013; Kaszynska 2021). This obscures the political motivations, and the power of those creating and operationalising the measures and models, for policy evaluation. Remember when we were thinking about the idea of facts being neutrally observed, as objective and neutral, without factors which can affect judgement? Power is one reason why neutrality is harder to prove or argue than is always recognised.

These are the politics of data. It is imperative to consider these issues if we are to respond to the well-being agenda, including calls to move from 'national well-being measurement to a national well-being strategy' in a report by the All-Party Parliamentary Group (APPG) on Wellbeing Economics (Berry 2014, 4). Furthermore, different policy domains take different positions in a national well-being strategy. A well-being strategy might imply working towards a better social infrastructure, thus improving welfare provision overall, but it may actually be about foregrounding any one of a number of issues attached to the well-being agenda: social care, mental health resources, more NHS nurses, decarbonisation or increasing the minimum wage.

To understand how well-being data might enable a well-being strategy, we need to side-track briefly into some other historical contexts. We have mainly talked about national indicators: the social indicators' movement as an international imperative to change the way progress was measured (in the 1960s) as a project of redistribution, or the more recent second wave (of the 1990s and 2000s) encouraging individual nations and international bodies to devise more complex indices of objective and subjective well-being. The same kinds of data can be collected to evaluate policy decisions, actions and investments, and there are numerous techniques used in policy evaluation. These were generated to value the non-economic in the audit society, but 'they are too liable to be co-opted, in support of some broader notion of efficiency' (Davies 2014, 193). The following sections explore how we arrived at what has been called 'the cult of the measurable' (Belfiore and Bennett 2007, 137) and what that means for well-being data and what we value.

2.3   Audit Culture, Value and Public Management

[T]he 'fact of audit' reduces anxiety, or more positively, produces comfort. (Power 1994, 307)

One of the effects of developing better measures of well-being and human progress is that we are measuring more things. More than this, we are measuring things for *more* reasons. Some argue that this is just because we can, or a more cynical description might be to ask whether this is just because some people say we can (whether or not we can being still up for debate in some areas of society). Increasing the ways we measure and what we measure has been diagnosed as 'audit culture' (Strathern 2000) and living in 'the audit society' (Power 1994). This has been linked to the idea of a 'Thatcherite revolution' in UK politics[15] (named by Power 1994), which refers to UK Prime Minister Margaret Thatcher's reforms of how the public sector is managed, as well as how the public sector manages society.

Again, we must deviate into the task of defining some of these key terms. The public sector is responsible for public services in the UK, from the emergency services and healthcare, education and social care, to housing and refuse collection. It is, therefore, inextricably linked to delivery of social policy in a way that results in public managers having to ensure 'a cost effective and friendly service but with the need to defend the involvement of government in the delivery of such a service' (Halachmi and Bouckaert 1995, 324). This process was called 'new public management' (NPM) (Hood 1991).

Box 2.2   The Characteristics of New Public Management
NPM and has been summarised as:

1. the adoption of private sector management practices in the public sector;
2. an emphasis on efficiency;
3. a movement away from input controls, rules, and procedures toward output measurement and performance targets;
4. a preference for private ownership, contestable provision, and contracting out of public services; and
5. the devolution of management control with improved reporting and monitoring mechanisms. (Hope 2001, 120)

The NPM processes are inspired by the ways that commercial firms used financial auditing to demonstrate efficiency, with the idea that these should be applied to the public sector. NPM replaced existing aspects of account- ability, such as quality control, with 'auditabilty' (Power 1994, 302–303). Many analysts of NPM (and it has many critics) point out that what is bizarre about NPM is that it does not matter what the audit practices are, as it is the idea of having them which is their most effective property.

In other words, in appearance, it doesn't matter which value system (and here I mean moral and political values, rather than numbers) and which kind of valuation tool you use. For example, you might rank items by order of importance or working out the ratio of their value in compari- son to other items. It also doesn't matter whether you are deciding the social value of, say, someone choosing books over cigarettes (as George Orwell did), or saving local libraries open versus building new 'super- libraries' as 'palazzos of human thought',[16] the point is that the technique was used, and so the policy decision can be justified.

Data which enable auditing, therefore, appear to reassure that things are being done correctly, but 'the audit society is the anxious society', accord- ing to Power (1994, 307). Power argues that the system is set up so that the only way to deal with this anxiety is in the further commissioning of more auditing. Audit for audit's sake does not improve things, but 'audit success or failure is never a public fact' and the 'criteria of success are with- drawn from public discourse' (Power 1994, 308). Think of the recent rise in well-being at work surveys that you may have seen discussed on social media or which sit unanswered in our inboxes. At the time of writing this book, there was not much discussion of how the data these surveys gener- ated had done anything to improve well-being, yet there was much discus- sion on Twitter (in my bubble, at least) of how they exacerbate ill-being. They can make us feel watched and give us additional administrative tasks in the service of an employer who is compelled to audit well-being.

Consequently, the logic of NPM and its use of data to audit how policy decisions have performed (or how successful they were at achieving their aims efficiently) has trickled into all kinds of management and sizes of company. As we have recently seen, it has also trickled into apps and watches that help us manage ourselves and our own efficiency (which we discuss in greater detail in Chap. 5). The processes of 'audit culture' were initially argued to make policy-making more transparent to 'the public', but how data are used to make decisions, or monitor the effectiveness of such decisions, is not made clear. Arguably, this has resulted in the mecha- nisms of policy—and the accountability of politicians, civil servants and their decisions—becoming even more obscure to the general public.

We should remember the point that the first wave of well-being came to an end—in part—as a result of the mistrust of experts in the economic crash of the 1970s (Bache 2012). What is interesting is that the audit culture approach to efficiency which followed this crash has become naturalised as the way that policy is done. It has also become the way our working lives are managed; some of us even audit our efficiency by way of how many steps we walk a day or how many hours we sleep. In audit culture, well-being metrics replace, reinforce and underwrite expertise. We are therefore trusting metrics more than experts, rather than distrusting experts and their metrics, as was the case in the 1970s.

Social Policy

Just as policy decisions became less fathomable to people, NPM also changed the relationship between people and policy in other ways. Members of the public were increasingly regarded as customers, and compulsory competitive tendering (CCT) was introduced. CCT requires local council services to be tendered out, and the winning contract going to the most 'efficient' tender. The political relevance of this Thatcherite *evolution* lies in the fact that this government aimed to reduce 'dependency' on the state and encourage citizens to take responsibility for their own welfare.

A social policy-specific example might be the Right to Buy Scheme in the UK. This saw national government encourage local councils to offer up its social housing 'stock' (housing it was responsible for) to buy, for those people living in it. On face value, a policy that enabled more people to own their own home seemed a good one. Over time, people moved from the houses they had bought; consequently, housing that was looked after by the local council became private housing. However, many, many people cannot afford to buy, even rent this new private housing stock. Therefore, the welfare state has to step in to support this new rental market with private landlords and inflated rents for people to rent houses that may have belonged to the public sector 30 years ago, and which are now often left in unhealthy disrepair by private landlords.

In this instance, objective well-being indicators of home ownership, rental prices or homelessness enable researchers, journalists and policy-makers to piece together a retrospectively objective view of whether this policy was efficient and good for people's quality of life. In short, it was great for some people, but not for more people over time, and contributes to inequalities (Murie 2015). As we will continue to see, just because measuring well-being claims to improve how we monitor progress, and these ideas were born from belief in both redistribution and efficiency, does not mean they will improve welfare or are even value for money. In fact, the issue of value is—in and of itself—also complex and contradictory.

So, What Is Value?

To complicate the issue further, 'value' not only refers to what counts (what is valuable, or of value), but *how* to count. It can also be used to describe our *values*—as the moral codes we live by in terms of what is right and wrong. In this sense the word and meanings of value are incredibly important when thinking about well-being data, especially what it might mean for social and cultural policy.

To assess the value (or worth) of something, people can go about their own personal estimation, perhaps on a scale, for example: 'in a fire I would save my family photos over my TV'. This is a hypothetical ranking system, where you state you value photos more than television. Or people can use (or invent) a measuring device: a tool, which might include systems of rankings or ratings, for example. Crucially, no matter how neutral and scientific these tools and devices are (or claim to be), they perform an act of calculation that assigns value on behalf of the person who invented or is applying the scale (Espeland and Sauder 2007). As Sociologist Bev Skeggs explains, 'values will always haunt value' (Skeggs 2014, 1). Metrification— as the process of converting aspects of life into metrics for measurement— does represent existing inequalities, so that they can be addressed. However, it can also reproduce inequalities set out by demographics, such as class and race. This is a broader and bigger argument that we will return to, but let me begin to explain with the example of the photographs versus the TV.

What's interesting about the idea that you would save old family photos over your television is that this is an expression of your values, as a sort of moral value—or the kind of person you see yourself as—as much as it is scale of values (that you could translate into numbers). So, like any rankings scale, or well-being index, they express the values of the person who designed them. Sometimes a well-being index that is a ranking system might want to appear as if it cares about one thing, when in fact it cares about something else entirely. This is also true of people, and when you ask them about themselves, they may feel like they might be being judged in some way (asking people questions can have that effect, see Chap. 9). For example, many people may want to look like the sort of person who would save photos of their family, rather than a surround sound TV, because they think that will make them appear a better person. Sociologists have long been interested in the way we judge our own actions and compare them to the actions of others.

Sociologists often call this a process of 'distinction', after Pierre Bourdieu (1984). Bourdieu has proved very influential in how people understand class (working class, middle class, etc.). This includes how we classify and categorise each other in day-to-day life, as well as how society is ordered unequally. This means—as Skeggs (afore-cited) tells us—judgements about how we classify ourselves and each other affect how we also come to value things.[17] This is also wrapped up in how we want our 'taste' to be understood by others—what we like and dislike, or what we think is good and bad. So, how we want to express our taste, through music, for example, relates to other people's perceptions, values and how we wish to be seen by them. Likewise, taste can indicate social position or privilege. People judge people's class based on the beer they drink, the clothes they wear and what they say they watch on TV. It is a cultural cliché to joke that 'the middle classes just don't understand the importance of a giant telly' (Moran 2019), but that also they pretend they don't watch telly at all. This trope is an attempt to understand how a group of people value things in relation to their values.

Taste: how it is expressed and how we show our taste are very much embedded in cultural life, helping people to feel equal to their peers, or demonstrate superiority over others. For example, you might say, 'Lauren has a good taste in music', but what you decide is 'good' is different from what I decide is good. It is all caught up in this process of distinction, of how we classify people, and this is influenced by class. It also allows people to undermine perceived norms (what the majority does). For example, people in UK sub-cultures (whether rave, punk or Grime) might like similar things, products and clothing that are deliberately distasteful to many. How people 'use' this to navigate or succeed in social groups is called cultural capital (Bourdieu 1984; Bennett et al. 2009). Cultural capital means that how people connect to particular culture (e.g. knowledge of music, food, travel and history) can give them a particular privilege, but that the more privilege you have to start, the easier it is to gain. Evidence suggests that people's cultural capital changes how they value things and what they say are valuable.

So, how people answer a question on how they value one thing over another might change from a socially controlled situation (such as answering a questionnaire or social survey) to a real-life situation for many reasons and what people value differs quite a lot. In fact, in any mundane moment, any subjective valuing system might appear. Someone may wish to disguise the fact that they actually value the financial worth of their TV more than the priceless photographs, because this may be seen as crass or shallow. They might use another value system, for example: 'well, I would spend more time in the future watching TV than I would spend looking at photographs, therefore the TV would bring me more joy' (were they to use the Marie Kondo[18] value system of which objects to keep). We might argue they are protecting their future well-being here? Or they might think, what would I pay to replace these items? These are all examples where a rational value is applied to one object over another using a ranking system where the value of one thing is based on its relationship to another.

In cultural policy terms, the TV and the photo album might be considered relative: they could be categorised as cultural objects. For the UK's 'Happiness Tsar', Lord Layard, these two items could symbolise two aspects of culture he has pitted against each other: watching television is responsible for depreciating well-being in the country of Bhutan, because it reduced family relations (see Layard 2006, 77–78; and further discussion in Oman 2020 and Chap. 6). Couched in these terms, the TV has a proxy value that is bad for family relations, while the photo album represents a positive, symbolic value of the family; thus, one is good for well-being and one is bad.

The photo album and the TV could also be seen as incommensurable, meaning that they do not share enough in common to enable comparison. For example, the photos may have emotional value and are unlikely to hold much economic value (for most families, at least); the TV, perhaps, the other way around. But who is to assume that someone's TV isn't a family heirloom, when their photo album may be one where those that houses all the photos which have been rejected because they were badly taken? So we assume and judge how people value things over other things as making them a better person when we don't know about them: their rationales of value, or

---

Box 2.3   Intrinsic and Extrinsic Value
Extrinsic Value is value from external factors.

- Also known as Utilitarian Value.
- Placing a value on something, say, a park, based on what we can get out of it or get from it.

Intrinsic Value is something's own inherent qualities.

- Can be moral, ethical, emotional or spiritual value.
- Do animal species have value even if we can't 'use' them?

whether an object holds intrinsic or extrinsic value for them. Indeed, we are in no position to decide what *should* be valuable to them and why.

The problem with categories and ranking systems is that they have to assume all TVs are the same and all photographs are the same on at least one dimension. Also, how we judge people's behaviour using these categories is based on assumptions which are organised by class and race and disability, by gender and place and time; the tendency to judge people for watching TV is very *classed*, for example, and may not consider how able-bodied they may be, or indeed the quality of their relationships with people who may be in a family album. Value systems and tools also, therefore, tend to generalise who people are in order to make them 'commensurate' which is a process of making different things understandable in relation to each other.

Economics, Value and Human Behaviours

As observed by the historians of the hedonimeter (Colander 2007), economics has trends: periods of time where ideas, approaches and aspirations for what should be possible ebb and flow. This is not unlike any discipline or, to be honest, act of human effort. Following Edgeworth's failed dreams of a hedonimeter in the nineteenth century, economics largely lost interest in understanding the motives behind human behaviour in this way.

Instead of wanting to know how people felt about something, it was deemed sufficient to observe behaviour through consumption as a proxy for feeling. When someone buys a widescreen TV, a photo album, a frozen pizza or an avocado, the implicit assumption is that they make this purchase because it offers them satisfaction or makes them happy somehow. This presumes that people's preferences are revealed in such choices. In fact, it was thought that everything outside of the observable was beyond the realm of economists' study (i.e. Scitovsky 1976).

So, understandably, people tend to think of economics as being about the economy, but the discipline is far more than that. Some popular economists call economics 'the logic of life' (Harford 2008) while others dispute the 'hype' and 'megalomania' of some popular economists (Chang 2014, 19). Crucially, economics aims to understand the value of things to different people, and how much of any resource is estimated to be needed for particular populations in different domains (aspects) of their lives. Therefore, the discipline of economics is used for insights into how investment or resources should be distributed across a population. Or, to make the policy decision between, say, saving older, smaller community libraries, or investing in new 'super-libraries'.

Box 2.4   Positive and Normative Economics

It can be helpful to know **the difference between positive and normative economics.**

Positive economics attempts to explain **what** *is* **happening or what has happened thus far**. This might include the relationship between investment in super-libraries and how that has changed library usage. Although other changing societal factors will affect how you can measure this over time. For example, confounders will include digitisation, the rise of the audio book and of course the market forces of Amazon. A confounder *confounds* (or confuses) the possibilities of measuring a direct relationship, as such, economists try and 'control for' these effects. We shall get to this later with examples in Chaps. 7 and 8.

Normative economics aims to evaluate what *should* **happen**. This branch of economics draws heavily on philosophical or theoretical arguments to think about what is 'fair' and 'just'. It is, therefore, based on value judgements. This means that the policy decision to direct limited resources towards saving older, smaller community libraries because of the social benefits in local communities are weighed up against building new, super-libraries, for example, which update technology and perhaps encourage different groups to use them.

Both positive and normative economics have roles in evaluating the kinds of policy interventions described in audit culture and throughout the book. Economics forms the foundations of what is called the HM Treasury Green Book in the UK—and of how most OECD member countries evaluate their policy decisions. While the flaws of 'audit culture' have been presented briefly above, it is also important that evaluation of policy decisions happens: that policy-makers are accountable and that resources are handled with care and with a view towards social justice. What is called consequentialist welfarism dictates that actions should be evaluated by their outcomes and that the outcome which matters most is welfare.

Welfare in this instance does not only refer to the welfare state, but 'how people are doing'. So, economists have been trying to find the best ways to evaluate how a policy intervention impacts on how people are doing. Box 2.5 holds four key ideas of valuation that will help understand approaches that will appear throughout the book.

Box 2.5 Four Key Approaches to Valuation

Revealed preference was introduced by the American economist Paul Samuelson in 1938. Samuelson decided that consumers' **preferences** are **revealed** by what they purchase. The implications of this idea are that we can look at how people purchased one thing over another and assess the circumstances in which these purchases were made. This context may consider other things they may have purchased, how much these things might have cost and the limits people may have in their income.

Even the economists don't all believe that all preferences can be revealed in this way, by proxy. **Stated preference** techniques involve asking people what they would be willing to pay for something. Or, in public policy terms, sometimes this involves the hypothetical example of asking whether they would be prepared to pay more taxes to reduce hospital waiting times, for example. Because these approaches involve asking people their opinion, they are expensive to administer and, as we now know, there are doubts that what people state or declare is their preference is their actual preference.

Quality Adjusted Life Years (QALYs) is a form of economic evaluation of policy interventions that is particularly useful in health policy decisions. It involves estimating the value of quality and quantity in years of human life remaining for a patient following a particular treatment or intervention. It is often measured on a scale in terms of the person's ability to carry out the activities of daily life, and freedom from pain and mental disturbance. This is then translated into an economic analysis of cost-effectiveness for often very different health interventions. This process makes different things commensurate for easy comparison.

In the last ten years, **Well-being Valuation** has increasingly appeared across domains of social policy. This takes well-being data, say life satisfaction data, to calculate the impact of something which has no market value, or for which market value is not its primary value, as is common in much of social and cultural policy. There are many years of research on the relationship between income and well-being, and, although this is not fixed, some of the estimates are considered robust. Three data points can be taken from a survey. Let's say access to parks, life satisfaction and income. The Well-being Valuation approach works on the basis that you can not only find the relationship between parks and life satisfaction, but that you can take what you also 'know' about income and life satisfaction to estimate the value of this relationship in economic terms. We shall come back to this step by step in Chap. 9.

What Is Social *Value?*

> There is no single authoritative definition of 'social value'. Nevertheless, several leading organisations in this field do provide similar explanations of it. These explanations are almost always within the context of measuring social value. (New Economics Foundation 2016)

> The debate around value, its definition and its measurement will never be one on which consensus can easily be reached (if ever), but one which will require on-going negotiations of values, pressures, interests and power. (Belfiore 2015, 107)

One of the earliest uses of the term 'social value' on record dates from 1872, advocating 'the Scientific and Social Value of the British Medical Association' (Shettle 1872). What is particularly interesting in our ongoing discussions in the book is that the term emerged as a compulsion to assert the importance of an organisation that is both an intellectual and a practical endeavour to improve human well-being. Welfare economics—that is how the government can improve social welfare or well-being, is referred to in the UK Government's guidance on the appraisal and evaluation of policies, projects and programmes (the Green Book) as social value.

While the term 'social value' is widespread, there is little discussion of what it means in practice—and, again, when there is, there is much disagreement (Mulgan 2010; Barman 2016). More recently, the idea of social value has been used to describe the distinctive contributions of commercial companies and third sector organisations, such as charities or community groups, or a domain of society. Social values and value are also expressed via Corporate Social Responsibility, where, as Bill Gates said in the 2008 World Economic Forum, 'more people can make a profit, or gain recognition, doing work that eases the world's inequities' (Gates 2008). Such 'good work' is often incentivised by governments via tax breaks (McGoey 2019). Thus, the value to these companies of 'good work' exceeds the social value, instead being very much about private and corporate value which is, of course, ultimately about wealth generation for those already most wealthy.

In social policy terms, examples could include the social value of housing (HACT 2020; IPPR 2019) or the arts. The latter is touched on in Chap. 6 when we reflect on cultural policy as social policy. In the UK, the Public Services (Social Value) Act 2012 (UK Parliament 2012) builds on some of the principles of NPM described in the last section. It legally requires public bodies to consider how the services they commission and procure might improve economic, social and environmental well-being.

The idea of the Social Value Act is that calculating the potential social value created by public and voluntary services helps to ensure value for money. This also acts as an impetus to create additional value. In other words, the aim is for the impact of any public service to exceed the activity or programme being delivered. An example of this can be found in the domain of social housing. The argument for this is that in building new housing that is better quality than that which preceded it, it is not only housing which is improved, but the quality of life of those who live in these houses. It is also argued that this 'regeneration' will improve the quality of life of those people who live near this housing, as it will develop the area in various ways.[19] Your value-added could be the addition of a public park (where before it was brown land or wasteland, for instance, and thus unusable) and perhaps commission some form of public art with the development.

The Minister for Civil Society announced a review of the act (February 2017), emphasising that a commitment to social value ensures that public sector bodies are able to maximise the benefits of 'tax-payers' money'. This was after the collapse of Carillion, a private company, that specialised in public sector contracts across defence, transport, education and health. Contemporary critics said that 'the preoccupation with costs had hit the quality of public services because the outsourcing companies were sent a clear signal that cost, rather than quality, was the government's consistent priority' (Reuters 2018). The changes were intended to help restore public trust and confidence in outsourcing, by renewing focus on wider social values and increasing transparency (Reuters 2018). In other words, NPM and auditing had resulted in large private companies that not only delivered poor public services, but which went bust because 'efficient' meant cheap, thus costing more than was saved.

There is increasing evidence that the preoccupation with social value results in promises that are not kept. One example is with the promises of affordable housing in regeneration projects. These emerge from a commitment to contribute to social justice and well-being by improving infrastructure and retaining aspects of welfare redistribution. In other words, rather than just building more luxury flats for more 'lucky' and privileged people to move into, and the 'value' of the project going to the developers through economic rewards, the rationale is that affordable housing enables key workers to live in the centre of cities with housing issues, such as

Manchester and London. As part of audit culture, councils have targets to address the housing shortage in such cities, but the economic value of the homes built are at odds with, and arguably get in the way of, the social value of new houses for people who need them. This state of affairs can be dangerous and at its very worst, cost the lives of many, as in the Grenfell tragedy, 4 June 2017.[20]

Therefore, when we talk of social value, well-being metrics and efficiency, it is vital to ask: whose value is added when we mean 'social' value? We might also ask, who is the social of social policy? Who does it benefit?

2.4   CONCLUSION: WELL-BEING AS A TOOL OF POLICY

There are rising numbers of well-being metrics, which are increasingly used by those who want to *know* more about people and populations. These data influence national policies and international initiatives. The use of well-being data to make policy decisions is said to be premised on Jeremy Bentham's Greatest Happiness principle: that 'the right moral action is the one that produces the greatest happiness', and therefore, 'the best public policy is the one that produces the greatest happiness'.[21] As the introduction outlines, for some years there have been hopes to understand the well-being of a population at any given moment, which can then be traced over time. New models have been developed with the aspiration to appraise the impact of particular policy interventions by assessing their impact on specific measures of well-being.

An evaluation of how a particular action has impacted on the well-being of people or populations allows for predictions as to how similar choices will impact in the future. We may not *know* what will happen, but people in power like to make educated guesses. Governments and other agencies use this information to judge which policies are thought to 'maximise' well-being. According to the rationales of NPM, it is considered possible to estimate the most efficient way of increasing well-being by making decisions using econometric models and subjective well-being data to estimate impact valuations.

The supposedly neutral frameworks and technologies used to decide which lives benefit, and which do not, are, of course, never truly impartial (Williamson 2015; Oman 2015). Choices are made at all junctures when evaluating a policy action, and in the 'science' which informs the evidence: what is measured: what is included and excluded from the models and what proxies will be used. In times of increasing inequality, improving the well-being of the majority, a little bit, is potentially all the more dangerous for those with the least well-being, especially as it is 'easier to improve the quality of life of people who have relatively high levels of well-being to start with' (Oakley et al. 2013). This opens up questions for how knowledge about well-being is used, and in turn, affects well-being?

This naturalised belief that progress is about striving for well-being is engrained in society, becoming a central logic of policy-making and in our everyday lives. Yet, well-being is not a fixed concept; it shifts depending on who is using it when, and in what context. As we have seen, it has different levels of influence and impact and can be dangerous if used neglectfully. As a tool of policy, well-being is a concept that is applied in various ways which can be implicitly or explicitly guided by valuation. These definitions, histories and contexts are important and come to guide our knowledge of, understandings, measurements and policy implementations of well-being. Thus, reviewing how they all work together, as this chapter has done, is a useful exercise in introducing how we *know* well-being through data. Crucially, this background forms what well-being data *are*, where well-being data come from and how they are analysed, as we shall discover in the next chapter.

NOTES

1. You may be used to thinking of data as one thing. In this book, we will use data in the plural, as data are made up of many things. This also acknowledges that well-being data or data about well-being are so varied, as we shall discover.
2. For example, the OECD Guidelines on Measuring Subjective (2013, 10) say: 'The measurement of subjective well-being is often assumed to be restricted to measuring "happiness". In fact, subjective well-being covers a wider range of concepts than just happiness.'
3. Aristotle's ideas of the good society are not without flaws. In order for Athenians to have the time to engage in the activities of a good society, slaves performed duties that were manual and thought less skilled. They were considered and treated as an underclass. Arguably, these are not the conditions of a 'good society'.
4. Data about well-being have different units of analysis. In other words, some well-being data are analysed about individuals, and some about whole countries. Chapter 3 expands on these differences in more detail.
5. Algorithm still means any form of automated instruction. The majority of algorithms are simpler than most people think and can be a single 'if something is X, then do this' statement. Contemporary algorithms are long sequences of these instructions.
6. Aristotle has even been called 'the father of racism'; Sears 2018.

7. While this is a nice idea, we know that actions which focus on improving the material living standards of the largest part of population can lead to minorities being extremely unhappy through neglect and maltreatment.

8. Geoff Bowker says that 'raw data is both an oxymoron and a bad idea; to the contrary, data should be cooked with care' (Bowker 2005, 184).

9. The EconLit database is considered the authority on economic research citations and abstracts. It is managed by American Economic Association and contains more than 1.4 million records, indexed from 74 countries, with citations and abstracts dating back to 1886.

10. Similar to contemporary inequality arguments, such as Piketty 2013.

11. The Commission on the Measurement of Economic Performance and Social Progress (CMEPSP) is also referred to as the Stiglitz-Sen-Fitoussi Commission after the surnames of those who led it. It was a commission of inquiry created by the French Government in 2008 and so is also referred to by the name of Sarkozy, as France's president.

12. The ONS began measuring personal well-being in April 2011 to provide the indicator that the ONS call 'Personal Wellbeing' (see e.g. ONS 2015 for more detail).

13. The term was in fact coined by Brickman and Campbell in 1971.

14. See, for example, the What Works for Wellbeing website (2016) on addressing well-being inequalities.

15. Although this change in management of the public sector was also seen in the US, Australia and other countries (Hood 1991).

16. In the early 2010s, there was a wave of building 'super-libraries' in poorer communities, such as Peckham and Canada Water, as well as major city libraries elsewhere. Birmingham city council's leader, Mike Whitby, said of its £193 million Library of Birmingham, 'It will be much more than just a library. Perhaps we should call it a palazzo of human thought', cited in Jeffries (2010).

17. There is much work which addresses these issues of class, geopolitics and stigma, that there is no room to repeat here. Key texts include Skeggs and Loveday (2012); Bennett et al. (2009). See also Tyler and Slater's 2018 special issue of *The Sociological Review*.

18. Marie Kondo, a Netflix sensation, has encouraged people to go through their belongings to de-clutter by way of a value system that asks people to anticipate future joy.

19. 'Regeneration' may seem a good well-being solution. However, resulting 'gentrification' means that poorer and more vulnerable residents are pushed off social housing estates, and priced out of their local communities. A high-profile example of this is London's Heygate estate which was demolished and replaced by luxury flats, rather than replacement social housing. As the rental value of the area increased through gentrification,

the rental values of surrounding areas are further inflated. Therefore, the displaced residents have to move far from the community in which they had been living and the housing and social conditions to which they move are sometimes worse; hence their life chances and well-being are diminished, not enhanced.

20. Notably, the dangerous cladding which accelerated the fire remains on many buildings some years later (Kennedy 2019).

21. This description of 'the Greatest Happiness principle' is taken from Layard's introduction to Bentham, in his book, *Happiness: Lessons from the New Science* (2006, 5). Although a footnote later in the book points to the fact that Bentham corrected this phrase later, saying that he meant the greatest total sum of happiness (2006, 262). This is further discussed in Chap. 4 in the section on the Greatest Happiness principle.

References

ACE. 2018. *Arts and Culture in Health and Wellbeing and in the Criminal Justice System: A Summary of Evidence*. Arts Council England. https://www.artscouncil.org.uk/publication/arts-and-culture-health-and-wellbeing-and-criminal-justice-system-summary-evidence.

Allin, P. 2007. Measuring Societal Wellbeing. *Economic & Labour Market Review* 1 (10): 46–52. https://doi.org/10.1057/palgrave.elmr.1410157.

Aristotle. 1976. *The Ethics of Aristotle: The Nicomachean Ethics*. New York: Penguin Classics.

Bache, I. 2012. Measuring Quality of Life for Public Policy: An Idea Whose Time Has Come? Agenda-Setting Dynamics in the European Union. *Journal of European Public Policy* 20 (1): 21–38. https://doi.org/10.1080/1350176 3.2012.699658.

Bache, I., and L. Reardon. 2013. An Idea Whose Time Has Come? Explaining the Rise of Well-Being in British Politics. *Political Studies* 61 (4): 898–914. https://doi.org/10.1111/1467-9248.12001.

Barman, E. 2016. *Caring Capitalism: The Meaning and Measure of Social Value*, 266. New York: Cambridge University Press.

Beer, D. 2016. *Metric Power*. London: Palgrave Macmillan.

Belfiore, E. 2015. "Impact", "Value" And "Bad Economics": Making Sense of the Problem of Value in the Arts and Humanities. *Arts and Humanities in Higher Education* 14 (1): 95–110. https://doi.org/10.1177/1474022214531503.

Belfiore, E., and O. Bennett. 2007. Rethinking the Social Impacts of the Arts. *International Journal of Cultural Policy* 13 (2): 135–151. https://doi.org/10.1080/10286630701342741.

Bennett, T., et al. 2009. *Culture, Class, Distinction*. London: Routledge.

Bentham, J. 1996 [1789]. *An Introduction to the Principles of Morals and Legislation*. Oxford: Clarendon Press.

Berry, C. 2014. *Wellbeing in Four Policy Areas: Report by the All-Party Parliamentary Group on Wellbeing Economics*. London: New Economics Foundation.

Bourdieu, P. 1984. *Distinction: A Social Critique of the Judgment of Taste*. Cambridge, MA: Harvard University Press.

Bowker, G.C. 2005. *Memory Practices in the Sciences*. Ed. G.C. Bowker. Cambridge, MA: MIT Press.

Brickman, P., and D.T. Campbell. 1971. Hedonic Relativism and Planning the Good Society. In *Adaptation Level Theory: A Symposium*, ed. M.H. Appley, 287–302. New York: Academic Press.

Bruni, L., and P.L. Porta. 2005. Introduction. In *Economics and Happiness: Framing the Analysis*, 1–28. Oxford: Oxford University Press.

Cameron, D. 2010. *Prime Minister's Speech on Wellbeing*. Cabinet Office, Prime Minister's Office. https://www.gov.uk/government/speeches/pm-speech-on-wellbeing.

Cederström, C., and A. Spicer. 2014. *The Wellness Syndrome*. Cambridge: Polity Press.

Chang, H.-J. 2014. *Economics: The User's Guide*. London: Pelican.

Colander, D. 2007. Retrospectives: Edgeworth's Hedonimeter and the Quest to Measure Utility. *Journal of Economic Perspectives* 21 (2): 215–226. https://doi.org/10.1257/jep.21.2.215.

Croly, H. D. 1962. 'About rethinking the system of national accounting', *The New Republic*, vol. 147, p. 29.

Davies, W. 2014. *The Limits of Neoliberalism: Authority, Sovereignty and the Logic of Competition*. London: SAGE. https://sk.sagepub.com/books/the-limits-of-neoliberalism. Accessed 31 March 2021.

———. 2015. *The Happiness Industry: How the Government and Big Business Sold Us Well-Being*. London: Verso.

Dodge, R., et al. 2012. The Challenge of Defining Wellbeing. *International Journal of Wellbeing*, 2 (3). https://www.internationaljournalofwellbeing.org/index.php/ijow/article/view/89. Accessed 30 March 2021.

Dolan, P. 2014. *Happiness by Design: Finding Pleasure and Purpose in Everyday Life*. London: Penguin Books.

Doria, L. 2013. *Calculating the Human: Universal Calculability in the Age of Quality Assurance*. Basingstoke: Palgrave Macmillan.

Easterlin, R. 1973. Does Money Buy Happiness? *The Public Interest* 30 (3): 3–10.

Espeland, W.N., and M. Sauder. 2007. Rankings and Reactivity: How Public Measures Recreate Social Worlds. *American Journal of Sociology* 113 (1): 1–40. https://doi.org/10.1086/517897.

Fleche, S., C. Smith, and P. Sorsa. 2012. *Exploring Determinants of Subjective Wellbeing in OECD Countries: Evidence from the World Value Survey*. No. 921. Paris: Organisation for Economic Cooperation and Development.

Gates, B. 2008. *2008 World Economic Forum – Bill & Melinda Gates Foundation.* Bill & Melinda Gates Foundation. https://www.gatesfoundation.org/ideas/speeches/2008/01/bill-gates-2008-world-economic-forum. Accessed 28 April 2021.

HACT. 2020. *The UK Social Value in Housing Taskforce.* HACT. Ideas and Innovation in Housing. https://www.hact.org.uk/news/uk-social-value-housing-taskforce. Accessed 30 March 2021.

Halachmi, A., and G. Bouckaert. 1995. Re-engineering in the Public Sector. *International Review of Administrative Sciences* 61 (3): 323–327. https://doi.org/10.1177/002085239506100301.

Harford, T. 2008. *The Logic of Life: The Rational Economics of an Irrational World.* Random House.

Helliwell, J., L. Richard, and J. Sachs. 2015. *World Happiness Report 2015.* New York: UN Sustainable Development Solutions Network.

Hood, C. 1991. A Public Management for All Seasons? *Public Administration* 69 (1): 3–19. https://doi.org/10.1111/j.1467-9299.1991.tb00779.x.

Hope, K.R. 2001. The New Public Management: Context and Practice in Africa. *International Public Management Journal* 4 (2): 119–134.

IPPR. 2019. *Valuing More Than Money: Social Value and the Housing Sector.* https://www.ippr.org/research/publications/valuing-more-than-money

Jeffries, S. 2010. The Battle of Britain's Libraries. *The Guardian.* https://www.theguardian.com/books/2010/mar/07/future-british-libraries-margaret-hodge

John, N. 2020. Coronavirus Lockdown: Why Sajjan Jindal Fears 'Awakening' Economy Will Be a Challenge. *Business Today.* https://www.businesstoday.in/current/economy-politics/coronavirus-lockdown-why-sajjan-jindal-fears-awakening-economy-challenge/story/402231.html

Kaszynska, P. 2021. Cultural Value as Practice: Seeing Future Directions, Looking Back at AHRC Cultural Value Project. In *Exploring Cultural Value: Contemporary Issues for Theory and Practice,* ed. K. Lehman, I. Fillis, and M. Wickham. Bingley: Emerald Publishing Limited.

Kennedy, S. 2019. Two Years After Grenfell, Why Are Thousands Still Not Safe in Their Homes? *The Guardian.* https://www.theguardian.com/commentisfree/2019/jun/13/two-years-grenfell-government-blocks-cladding

Layard, R. 2006. *Happiness: Lessons from a New Science.* London: Penguin.

McGoey, L. 2019. *The Unknowers: How Strategic Ignorance Rules the World.* London: Zed Books Ltd.

McMahon, D.M. 2006. *Happiness: A History.* New York: Grove Press.

Moran, C. 2019. Caitlin Moran: The Politics of Mega TVs. *The Times.* https://www.thetimes.co.uk/article/caitlin-moran-the-politics-of-mega-tvs-dpbr0vt2c. Accessed 30 March 2021.

Morris, S. 2020. Mindfulness Apps Are Booming in Lockdown – How to Stay Chilled Using Your Phone or on Your Own. *The Independent*. https://inews.co.uk/inews-lifestyle/wellbeing/mindfulness-apps-coronavirus-lockdown-explained-chilled-headspace-448667

Mulgan, G. 2010. Measuring Social Value. *SSIR*. https://ssir.org/articles/entry/measuring_social_value

Murie, A. 2015. The Right to Buy: History and Prospect. *History & Policy*. http://www.historyandpolicy.org/policy-papers/papers/the-right-to-buy-history-and-prospect.

New Economics Foundation. 2016. *Social Return on Investment*. New Economics Foundation. https://neweconomics.org/issues/entry/social-return-on-investment. Accessed 12 January 2016.

Noll, H. 2002. Social Indicators and Quality of Life Research: Background, Achievements and Current Trends. In *Advances in Sociological Knowledge Over Half a Century*, ed. N. Genov, 151–181. Paris: International Social Science Council.

O'Donnell, G., et al. 2014. *Wellbeing and Policy*. London: Legatum Institute.

Oakley, K., D. O'Brien, and D. Lee. 2013. Happy Now? Well-being and Cultural Policy. *Philosophy and Public Policy Quarterly* 31 (2): 18–26. https://doi.org/10.13021/G8pppq.312013.131.

OECD. 2007. *Beyond GDP: Measuring Progress, True Wealth, and the Well-being of Nations*. OECD. https://www.oecd.org/site/worldforum06/38433373.pdf.

———. 2013. *How's Life? 2013 Measuring Well-being*. OECD (OECD Better Life Initiative). http://www.oecd.org/sdd/3013071e.pdf.

Oman, S. 2015. Measuring National Well-being: What Matters to You? What Matters to Whom? In White, S. and Blackmore, C. (eds) *Cultures of Wellbeing: Method, Place, Policy*. London: Palgrave MacMillan.

Oman, S. 2020. Leisure Pursuits: Uncovering the "Selective Tradition" in Culture and Well-being Evidence for Policy. *Leisure Studies* 39 (1): 11–25. https://doi.org/10.1080/02614367.2019.1607536.

ONS. 1970. *Social Trends*. Office for National Statistics. https://data.gov.uk/dataset/f3ba77f8-d598-4db2-a3bc-b59a1578d410/social-trends. Accessed 28 April 2021.

———. 2015. *Measuring National Wellbeing: Personal Well-being in the UK, 2014 to 2015*. Newport: Office for National Statistics.

Perlman, M., and M. Marietta. 2005. The Politics of Social Accounting: Public Goals and the Evolution of the National Accounts in Germany, the United Kingdom and the United States. *Review of Political Economy* 17 (2): 211–230. https://doi.org/10.1080/09538250500067262.

Piketty, T. 2013. *Le Capital au XXIe siècle*. Éditions du Seuil: Belknap Press.

Power, M. 1994. The Audit Society. In *Accounting as Social and Institutional Practice*, ed. A. Hopwood and P. Miller, 299–316. Cambridge: Cambridge University Press.

Reuters. 2018. Carillion Collapse Exposed Flaws in UK Government Policy: Lawmakers. *Reuters.* https://www.reuters.com/article/us-carillion-collapse-idUSKBN1JZ1H7. Accessed 30 March 2021.

Schoch, R. 2007. *The Secrets of Happiness: Three Thousand Years of Searching for the Good Life.* London: Profile Books.

Scitovsky, T. 1976. *The Joyless Economy: An Inquiry into Human Satisfaction and Consumer Dissatisfaction.* Oxford: Oxford University Press.

Scott, K. 2012. *Measuring Wellbeing: Towards Sustainability?* London: Routledge. https://www.taylorfrancis.com/https://www.taylorfrancis.com/books/mono/10.4324/9780203113622/measuring-wellbeing-towards-sustainability-karen-scott.

Sears, M. 2018. Aristotle, Father of Scientific Racism. *The Washington Post.* https://www.washingtonpost.com/news/made-by-history/wp/2018/04/06/aristotle-father-of-scientific-racism/

Seligman, M.E.P., and M. Csikszentmihalyi. 2000. Positive Psychology: An Introduction. *American Psychologist* 55 (1): 5–14. https://doi.org/10.1037/0003-066X.55.1.5.

Sen, A. 1999. *Commodities and Capabilities.* 2nd ed. Delhi and New York: Oxford University Press.

Shettle, R.C. 1872. An Address on the Scientific and Social Value of the British Medical Association. *British Medical Journal* 2 (625): 677–679.

Sinclair, J. 1798. *Statistical Accounts of Scotland.* https://stataccscot.edina.ac.uk/static/statacc/dist/home. Accessed 15 June 2015.

Skeggs, B. 2014. Values Beyond Value? Is Anything Beyond the Logic of Capital? *The British Journal of Sociology* 65 (1): 1–20. https://doi.org/10.1111/1468-4446.12072.

Skeggs, B., and V. Loveday. 2012. Struggles for Value: Value Practices, Injustice, Judgment, Affect and the Idea of Class. *The British Journal of Sociology* 63 (3): 472–490. https://doi.org/10.1111/j.1468-4446.2012.01420.x.

Strathern, M. 2000. *Audit Cultures: Anthropological Studies in Accountability, Ethics and the Academy.* London: Routledge.

The Swedish Institute for Social Research. 1968. *The Swedish Level-of-Living Survey (LNU).* The Swedish Institute for Social Research. https://www.sofi.su.se/english/2.17851/research/three-research-units/lnu-level-of-living/the-swedish-level-of-living-survey-lnu-1.65112. Accessed 28 April 2021.

Tyler, I., and T. Slater. 2018. Rethinking the Sociology of Stigma. *The Sociological Review* 66 (4): 721–743. https://doi.org/10.1177/0038026118777425.

UK Parliament. 2012. *Public Services (Social Value) Act 2012.* London: The Parliamentary Book Shop. https://www.gov.uk/government/publications/social-value-act-information-and-resources/social-value-act-information-and-resources.

————. 2018. *Arts: Impact of Brexit.* Thursday 11 October 2018, Hansard, UK Parliament, House of Lords Hansard. https://hansard.parliament.uk/Lords/2018-10-11/debates/64E52F7D-D698-40DD-8A11-9F50F94E542C/ArtsImpactOfBrexit. Accessed 30 March 2021.

Veenhoven, R. 1984. *Conditions of Happiness.* Boston and Lancaster: D Reidel Publishing Company.

Vidal, J. 2006. The 7,000 km Journey that Links Amazon Destruction to Fast Food. *The Guardian.* https://www.theguardian.com/business/2006/apr/06/brazil.food

What Works for Wellbeing. 2016. *What Wellbeing Inequalities Tell Us About the EU Referendum Result.* What Works Wellbeing. https://whatworkswellbeing.org/blog/what-wellbeing-inequalities-tell-us-about-the-eu-referendum-result/. Accessed 30 March 2021.

White, M.D. 2014. *The Illusion of Well-Being: Economic Policymaking Based on Respect and Responsiveness.* Palgrave Macmillan.

Williamson, B. 2015. *Testing Governance: The Laboratory Lives and Methods of Policy Innovation Labs.* University of Stirling. https://dspace.stir.ac.uk/bitstream/1893/22500/1/WilliamsonB_Testing%20governance_2015.pdf. Accessed 28 April 2021.

Wolf, M. 2019. The Case for Making Wellbeing the Goal of Public Policy. *Financial Times.* https://www.ft.com/content/d4bb3e42-823b-11e9-9935-ad75bb96c849

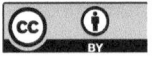

CHAPTER 3

Looking at Well-being Data in Context

3.1 Well-being Measurement (Other Data Are Available)

It measures neither our wit nor our courage, neither our wisdom nor our learning, neither our compassion nor our devotion to our country, it measures everything in short, except that which makes life worthwhile. And it can tell us everything about America except why we are proud that we are Americans. (Robert F. Kennedy 1968)

These remarks from Robert F. Kennedy are often found in arguments for measuring well-being,[1] as an alternative to gross national product (GNP, and what Kennedy calls 'it').[2] As touched on in the previous chapter, GNP (and GDP) are 'national accounts' and are administrative data that capture the economic activity of a country. Data on economic activity are used to measure financial success, compare countries against each other, and track progress over time.

Robert F. Kennedy's comments are from a speech at the University of Kansas on 18 March 1968, forming part of his campaign for nomination for the US presidency.[3] Fondly called 'Bobby', he is remembered for his advocacy for the civil rights movement. In this speech, he also declares support for student protests as good for society, and against the Vietnam War happening at the time (Kennedy 1968). Interestingly, his questioning of the value of GDP to measure human flourishing did not make much of

© The Author(s) 2021   67
S. Oman, *Understanding Well-being Data*,
New Directions in Cultural Policy Research,
https://doi.org/10.1007/978-3-030-72937-0_3

an impact at the time. It is only retrospectively, and with hindsight, that this quote has gained notoriety, thus implying that it resonates more now than it perhaps did to American citizens in 1968.

Why is this speech important? Kennedy advocates changing priorities of public policy-making in line with altering values (both *how* we value and *what* we value). It indicates that it was politically prudent for a politician like Robert F. Kennedy to argue for replacing GDP as the main indicator of human progress at that time; it also suggests that believing in measuring well-being, rather than GDP, was ideologically aligned with supporting student protests and problematising the Vietnam War. Likewise, it tells us that there is an alternative to GDP or GNP to measure at that time. With the previous chapter, we can historicise this speech as coinciding with the social indicators movement that characterised what Bache and Reardon (2013) called the 'first wave of well-being'. This means we can contextualise this political speech as from a time when different measures were called for—by people with particular values—to understand human flourishing, or how a nation was progressing. We are acknowledging that these comments were little repeated at that moment in time, but were later revisited to justify another 'second wave of well-being' (Bache and Reardon 2013).

So why are these historical and political settings for measuring well-being valuable for this chapter? Because they help contextualise well-being data. Context is key to recognising the role of methods in generating well-being data, as this chapter will show. Exploring the stories that lie behind data, and looking under the bonnet of how they are generated, is important to understanding: what they measure; whether they measure what they say; and the reasons why they have been collected and analysed in particular ways.

This is all part of what I call 'data contexts', arguing it is important to know *how* data *work* in what contexts (Oman n.d.). What do I mean by this? Well, understanding where data come from, and why they were generated, is important. Were they generated in a lab or in a real-world setting? Why do they exist? Were they collected for one purpose and are being used in another? Who has analysed them and how may that affect how we view the data? We also need to think about how different techniques of analysis are applied and how they are operationalised in different contexts. What do they achieve? Do they monitor people's toilet breaks in a call centre or how many steps a day we take while working from home? Do people know these data are being collected and why? Do the data help to hold governments accountable for national poverty or are they used to decide welfare distribution?

Measuring well-being as a political and scientific project does not have a consistent historic arc. There are moments where various technical and intellectual disciplines, and people with differing political interests, gather around 'the well-being agenda' as a project. This results in different types of well-being data being foregrounded, even acting as the catalyst for political change, at different times. The UK's national well-being measures are often called 'Cameron's happiness index' (Clinton 2011; Mirror 2011) after the UK's Prime Minister contributed to the launch of the Measuring National Well-being (MNW) project (Cameron 2010). As we shall see, the next section of this chapter opens with evidence that the idea of well-being measures for the UK (to become the MNW project) developed under the previous New Labour administration. The history of these measures is, therefore, not always obvious.

Similarly, it is not always clear what might be well-being data, and what are not. Data about well-being have long been valuable because they could help to understand how well a population was doing. Sometimes the data collected were believed to capture a specific aspect of happiness; other times to understand a particular part of a population, or indeed, one person's quality of life. Therefore, data about well-being do not all look the same, do not have the same unit of analysis (individual people, nations or communities), are not used the same way and do not all exist for the same reason. Again, this is why context is important.

This chapter considers how well-being data is collected: the diversity of methods and the range of data that can be called well-being data. This includes background and context to the well-being statistics you might read in newspapers, online, or have seen in COVID-19 briefings and press conferences. It also begins to look at claims about what can possibly be concluded from different kinds of well-being research. We will continue to break down technical terms to show well-being data and measurement are complex, and their uses in policy are not universal. It aims to show that this language and these ideas can be more accessible when you know where they come from.[4]

Well-being data as a term most often describes well-being metrics or indicators. This chapter offers some examples of how many decisions are made when choosing an objective indicator of well-being. Despite the name 'objective', which implies they are not affected by feelings or opinions, they do not fall from the sky as facts. If truth be told, they are the product of a specific *methodology*, which means they must fulfil certain practical and theoretical criteria that satisfy often long-established opinions of what are the best methods to capture the most objective data, and then how to go about analysing them.

Objective well-being indicators predominantly originate from survey data (like the census) or administrative data (such as mortality rates). They also include some subjective data where people are asked about aspects of their lives, such as how satisfied they are with their health. We come to this later. These datasets will include enough of the population that it is sensible to analyse them numerically—as quantitative data. These quantitative analyses are not always conducted by the person or the organisation who collects these data. Similarly, secondary uses of data can make the data useful as well-being data, when it may not have been collected for such a purpose.

Whether objective or subjective, it is mostly agreed that:

1. all well-being measures must be theoretically grounded (Haybron 2008), meaning that there is a clear, agreed rationale as to what exactly is being measured, what for and how the data are collected and handled
2. the limited impact of previous attempts to measure well-being lies in deficient theoretical grounding, and therefore failed understanding of what the measures are for and who they benefit (Scott 2012)
3. assessing one's own well-being is a subjective and aesthetic[5,6] experience (Rapley 2003)
4. well-being survey questions should involve concepts which are readily understandable and easy to relate to, such as 'satisfaction' and 'happiness' (Fleche et al. 2012, 9)
5. well-being measures need to be subject to harmonisation (GSS), meaning that they should be able to work with other well-being measures

Not all well-being data are numbers, or the result of large-scale data collection, however. It can be easier than you may imagine to produce and use well-being data. To discover how accessible other methods are, we will explore other ways of collecting data, such as interviews and focus groups. We will also look at policy documents as data, like the speech above, finding that ideas of measurement and well-being are used together, and how that can reveal the all-important context to why data are used to make certain arguments. As with the quantitative data found in well-being indicators, it is also important to understand the limitations to what we can *claim to know* as a result of analysing qualitative data. Whether from a few policy documents or interviews with a community in a particular place (rather than a whole population), these data tell us a lot about a small number of people and may not describe how things work on a larger scale. These are matters of *methodology*.

Box 3.1   Methodology

Methodology is more than the methods used to collect data (e.g. a questionnaire or interview) or analyse data (i.e. statistical techniques or thematic analysis[7]). It is more than who is using methods, whether in academic research, in national-level surveys, or in evaluations of how much a policy decision or an individual project has impacted on well-being. It is the system behind methods: why people have decided to do these things in these ways. This is what makes data 'theoretically grounded' (see above).

As we go about our day-to-day activities, we don't tend to consider the theory of what we are doing and why, but odd moments might make us stop and think about why we have done something in a certain way and whether that is the best possible, or the one most suited to our situation (how much time we have and where we are, for instance). Think about when we hear how other people do something, their tips or techniques might be different from ours and can be about something quite mundane.

Think about a cup of tea (English tea to non-native Brits, or depending on dialect: 'a cuppa' or 'a brew'). It has different names, depending on where you come from, and there are often discussions about how to make tea the *right* way: milk first or second; let the bag stew or not; in a teapot, cup or mug, and for how long. There are also TikTok videos and Facebook posts on the issue, Reddit feeds exclaiming the crimes of others' tea-making methods, and reports in the national press, saying certain methods 'spark outrage' (Morris 2020). What works best, and in which order, is therefore not a universal truth and there are opinions on how these all work together.

Methodology, similarly, involves the theory behind how stages of working *with* data work together. Working with theory doesn't only mean reading philosophers, but more practically involves careful consideration of each process.

Some useful questions to ask about these stages include:

Was it appropriate to apply this particular approach to collecting and analysing data to the particular issue the researchers want or need to know more about?

Or would it have been more appropriate to analyse data already available or accessible in a different, perhaps easier, and less intrusive way?

(continued)

Box 3.1 (continued)

Would people have been easily able to answer the questions?—we've all answered plenty of surveys where we cannot answer the questions truthfully, because the questions are badly designed. Or, indeed, because we do not want to tell the truth, exactly.

Is it fair to ask people to answer this question about themselves in this context (on the street, in a room full of others, at work where their screens might be viewed by colleagues, etc.)?

Is this ethical?

Methodology is often described as bringing theory to method. It is not so different from debating how tea is made, and how that affects the result. Methodology discussions are also often tribal, with in-fighting and disciplinary arguments—even disagreements over namings and meanings. In the case of data, this more simply involves thinking through what we *do* with data and how we have thought about collecting them. What order certain processes go in and what are our approaches to each process, and why that is best suited to the situation at hand. It is the foundations of why research has been done in a particular way.

There is often a tendency in the social sciences to feel the need for academics to take a position on the value of quantitative data over qualitative data or vice versa. This is colloquially called the 'Quants-Quals debate', which I had never heard of until I became an academic, but it is rife.[8] Other academics have requested I make it clear where I stand in the past. So, I want to make it clear that in this chapter—and the whole book, in fact—I resist this assumption that any data is better than another because we read them as text or count them as numbers, or collect them differently. All well-being data might be valuable to understanding well-being. Whether they are qualitative or quantitative is not the issue at hand. Instead, context is the issue: where the data came from, are they used appropriately and how are they applied? Are their uses ethical and fair? What are the limitations to the data we have? What can we know as a result of the data? What happens next?

The chapter describes different sorts of data: a moment from my research, hypothetical examples, as well as case studies from international statistics agencies to reveal some of the contexts of data collection, interpretation and uses of well-being data. It does this to show that *all* data have origins of thought, process and practice and are therefore rarely completely neutral or objective. All methodologies have their limitations, which thereby limits the claims that can be made. These are not always fully recognised.

If limitations are acknowledged in one place, that place is often far removed from the headline findings[9] to make caveats clear when interpreting results. The de-contextualising of data removes how we understand their limits and appropriateness. It must, therefore, impact on how 'good' the data can be in understanding society and well-being. It also affects the capacity for data to *do good* and inform societal change in such a way as to improve social, personal or national well-being. We need to account for the data used and we need to heed different accounts of what well-being means, as well as how we might understand it better.

3.2   ACCOUNTS OF WELL-BEING

Example 1 Wellbeing is a positive state that people experience when they are able to meet their needs for strong social relationships, equality of opportunity, rewarding work, economic and physical security, health, and opportunities to participate in cultural activities and enjoy contact with nature. It is enhanced when an individual is able to fulfil personal goals and achieve a sense of purpose and fulfilment in society.

Example 2 Wellbeing is a positive physical, social and mental state; it is not just the absence of pain, discomfort and incapacity. It arises not only from the action of individuals, but from a host of collective goods and relationships with other people. It requires that basic needs are met, important personal goals are achieved and people are able to achieve a sense of purpose and fulfilment in society, and that they are satisfied with their lives. (Levett-Therivel Sustainability Consultants' Report to DEFRA 2007)

The above definitions are examples from a consultation across government and well-being experts, in response to the UK's 2005 Sustainable Development Strategy. Called Securing the Future, the new strategy (HM Government 2005) committed the UK government to working towards new well-being indicators and to work towards policies with an explicit well-being focus (Levett-Therivel 2007).

The final definition that is often assumed as *the* working definition for the UK's Measuring National Well-being programme combines these two examples (DEFRA 2007), also drawing heavily on the World Health Organization's definition of health:

> Health is a state of complete physical, mental and social well-being and not merely the absence of disease or infirmity. The enjoyment of the highest attainable standard of health is one of the fundamental rights of every human being without distinction of race, religion, political belief, economic or social condition. (WHO 1946, 1)

When the UK's Office for National Statistics (ONS) started to produce working papers on well-being, they began with DEFRA's final statement:

> Wellbeing is a positive, social and mental state; it is not just the absence of pain, discomfort and incapacity. It arises not only from the action of individuals, but from a host of collective goods and relationships with other people. It requires that basic needs are met, that individuals have a sense of purpose, and that they feel able to achieve important personal goals and participate in society. It is enhanced by conditions that include supportive personal relationships, involvement in empowered communities, good health, financial security, rewarding employment and a healthy and attractive environment. (DEFRA in ONS 2009, 6)

As the previous chapter indicated, there are many definitions of well-being from different parts of the world and philosophical traditions. These different accounts of what well-being *is* have lineages: they are cumulative; learning from and adapting previous versions to suit who is using it, and for what: to suit its context. The same is true with policy.

Here we have traced the lineage of definitions across policy documents over a number of years, which can be a useful methodology to help understand how meanings adapt in policy documents to suit the context. In other words, we have 'followed the data' in a very different way, those data being textual. They are still important data about well-being, however, as they help us understand how well-being is understood and why.

The quotation immediately above is an example of the ONS establishing the lineage of their working definitions. They account for their categories before explaining how they might go about using them to measure well-being. In 2007, Paul Allin, who was to become Head of the ONS' MNW programme, explained that well-being 'can best be viewed as a multidimensional, shifting concept' (Allin 2007, 49). Despite indications that the self-named new sciences of happiness (Layard 2006) were evolving (O'Donnell et al. 2014; Helliwell et al. 2015; ONS 2015; Dolan et al. 2011b), as we explore in the next chapter, some academics fear that the concept of well-being itself has lacked attention, as the 'empirically-oriented field' needs more theoretical input (Jugureanu 2016, 68). The lack of consensus on how to conceptualise well-being for policy and measurement is a concern, however, when policy-making (OECD 2013, 11). As is deciding on what the best methods might be for measuring well-being effects and outcomes (Dolan et al. 2011a). So, as you can see 'objective well-being data' involve many decisions: what to measure and how to measure it are key to understanding what are the best well-being data.

Before the UK started collecting well-being data to form its well-being national accounts, the MNW programme took a novel approach to making the decision on what to measure. The methodology chosen to inform this decision became a national well-being debate that was launched by then Prime Minister David Cameron (2010) and administered by the ONS. This large-scale exercise collected different kinds of data, using different methods, asking people what mattered to them about well-being; what to measure and how to measure. The UK's 'What Matters to You?' debate received 34,000 responses and has been applauded for its democratic approach to meaning and measurement (Kroll 2011, 6), which we shall come to later.

So, GDP and GNP were 'national accounts'[10] that used economic activity to measure progress and the international well-being agenda was keen to replace these with new national accounts of well-being.[11] The UK's MNW debate was to inform this work in the UK, alongside expert consultations, such as the one that wrote the report quoted at the opening of this section. In this context, national accounts are called this because they ordinarily track economic transactions, like an organisation's accounts. The ONS still do not formally include well-being in its national accounts, a label they still reserve for transactional data.[12] Somewhat confusingly, the economists informing the MNW programme also talk of accounts of well-being too. Their meaning is slightly different. We encountered the two main traditions in the previous chapter: 'Benthamite-subjective-hedonic-individualistic' or 'Aristotelian-objective-eudaimonic-rational'. The shorthand versions of these being pleasure (or feeling) and purpose (or flourishing). In addition to these traditions are three different 'accounts' of well-being that are used to understand well-being and inform policy (Dolan et al. 2011a). These are:

1. Objective lists
2. Preference satisfaction
3. Mental states (or what has come to be known as subjective well-being)[13]

Different ways that well-being might be captured and measured are therefore 'accounts' of well-being. These have informed the programme to devise 'the national accounts of well-being'. We cover the ways that well-being is captured as an account below.

Objective Lists

Objective lists of well-being involve a list of assumptions regarding basic human needs, rights and conditions that are believed to impact on well-being. A simplified example is the Human Development Index (HDI), which is a composite index of three separate indicators: life expectancy, education and gross national income per capita. A composite index means a single number is calculated from these three indicators to make the data easier to use and visualise. This enables the HDI to rank countries into 'tiers of human development' (Human Development Reports 2020; United Nations n.d.). The key aspect of the HDI's design is its simplicity. Rather than intending to capture all aspects of well-being, the idea is that it is simplified and made easy for a broad audience to read and understand.

The use of indices like the HDI to understand international development has been criticised. One source of criticism is that the dimensions that contribute to these indices are those things that are considered important in the richer countries in the global North, rather than those things that are considered important in the countries where these indices are being used.[14] Another source of criticism is to do with what happens when these dimensions are combined. In the case of the HDI, the three dimensions are treated equally: for example, the income dimension is treated as holding the same importance as the two social dimensions (education and life expectancy). This assumes that all human beings value the three dimensions equally (United Nations 2020). However, this is not always the case and the representations of these various 'achievements' are sometimes criticised as being arbitrary, subjective or depending on a priori value judgements (OECD 2011b). In particular, because wealthier countries will always appear higher up the scale as a consequence of the importance placed on income.

Box 3.2   A Composite Index

A more familiar type of index might be from hearing or seeing things about the stock market on the news. The Dow Jones Industrial Average is a composite index. Ordinarily called the Dow or the Dow Jones, the index is made up of financial data from 30 large companies listed on US stock exchanges. Composite indexes are used to conduct investment analyses, measure economic trends, and forecast market activity in a way that is easy to read. 'The Dow' is criticised because it only includes 30 companies, as it was designed in the 1880s to represent the main markets at the time. Markets are, of course, now more complex. It is also criticised because it is weighted by price, when other indexes use alternative weights that capture more of the intricacy of the market.

As you can see, there is even methodological disagreement on how to best represent stock market data so they capture the most important aspects of the market (change) while remaining understandable. Interestingly, both in spite of and because of its age, the Dow is still the most used.

The objective list approach (or establishing a list of objective indicators) is mainly used by national and international statistics offices, with the aim of generating a complete list of what is necessary to satisfy a good life or ensure a good society. The OECD and ONS examples of well-being indexes are more comprehensive examples of these lists and have closer to 50 indicators (rather than the HDI's three).

Preference Satisfaction

Preference satisfaction accounts work on the premise that 'what is best for someone is what would best fulfil all of his[15] desires' (Parfit 1984, 494). This is how economists have long approached understanding well-being (Dolan and Peasgood 2008). The rationale behind expressing well-being like this for economists is that people's preferences are revealed by what they purchase (see Chap. 2, Box 2.4 for a description). By extension, this means that the higher a person's income, the more they are able to gain access to what they want. Also, the greater the choice available, the more able people are to satisfy their desires. The idea that choice is better is also a driving principle of new public management we also encountered in

Chap. 2: the rationale being that people should be free to purchase from a wide variety of market providers, rather than public services being delivered by the public sector.

It is this account which has historically informed policy decisions at a monitoring level, using GDP as a proxy for well-being.[16] It is also this account of well-being that the Easterlin paradox (1973) found wanting, as Easterlin's analysis found that improved material living standards had not improved measured happiness in wealthy countries over time. This is largely assumed to be as a result of adaptation, in that as one preference becomes satisfied, we adapt and want more.[17] This is ultimately seen as benefiting the economy, but bad for people and societies. Alongside empirical issues are concerns that 'making preference satisfaction the measure of political health completely cuts out the possibility of public deliberation about the ends we should pursue as a self-governing people' (Williamson 2010, 171). This latter issue was, of course, what the UK's MNW debate aimed to overcome.

Mental States (or Subjective Well-being)

Subjective well-being is 'an umbrella term' (Hicks 2011, 3) which covers three strands of a person's self-assessment of their happiness levels: life satisfaction, mood and meaning. The whole of Chap. 4 is about subjective well-being, so we only cover it briefly here. The term can also, confusingly, be used to just describe mood or happiness, rather than necessarily encompassing all ´concepts. Subjective well-being can be measured in various ways, like asking people about their happiness in any given moment, or about how satisfied they feel with their life overall. Along with preference satisfaction, subjective well-being measures have been thought to be more democratic than objective lists (Graham 2010), because they allow people to decide how well they are doing, without someone else assigning a level of well-being to them on their behalf. We will come to people deciding their own well-being later.

The above 'accounts' of well-being have been formulated with quantitative data in mind, collected through large samples and national-level surveys. It is these data that are used most in decision-making, especially in policy. However, other kinds of data allow you to derive preference satisfaction, subjective well-being—even objective lists. These methods collect people's own accounts of well-being from them on a smaller scale. Various methods can be used, like interviews or diaries, and are designed to understand how people's lives work in more detail. Owing to the smaller scale of these projects, they are more available to the researcher who does not have the resources of the United Nations (UN) or a national statistics office to understand well-being at national or regional levels. These methods also tend to present more detail about specific people and contexts, and so are often better for a project that wants to understand the well-being of the staff of an organisation or, perhaps, how one thing affects a small group of people in great depth. It is also especially useful for understanding people's lives and experiences in the everyday.

As we touched on earlier in the chapter, there is a history of researchers gathering around their own preference for qualitative or quantitative approaches. This can result in habitual silos of research and a history of squabbling over the value of one kind of data over another. The tradition of a divide tends to obscure the fact you can make the most of both worlds. It is possible to take a mixed methods approach to research, using both qualitative and quantitative data generated by various methods. There are also ways of collecting data that can result in both sorts of data. Many surveys offer a chance to answer using tick boxes and text. What should be at the forefront of any research is what is most appropriate to the context of collection and the question at hand. We shall think a little bit more about everyday contexts of data in the next section.

3.3   Everyday Well-being Data: Asking People Questions About Their Lives

Well-being data are not only for policy-makers or international economic development agencies. They can be collected in various ways available to us in everyday situations. Many of us have seen an increase in emails popping into our inboxes or Facebook timelines asking us to complete some kind of questionnaire about our well-being. COVID-19 has seen collection of these kinds of data increase.

These are well-being data collected through a questionnaire not so different from a national-level survey, but on a smaller scale. Although most require good planning and ethical consideration of how the questions you ask people may have some negative impact on them. In short, could your research negatively impact on people's well-being?

The following section offers a brief overview of methods that can collect 'smaller data' for different ends. Vignettes from my own research, a hypothetical questionnaire scenario, and the ethics of ethnography are presented to help you consider the different contexts and considerations of well-being data. Table 3.1 shows the advantages and challenges of different

Table 3.1 Data sources and their uses

Type	How generated/collected	Examples	Well-being example	What kind of questions	How used?	Some opportunities and challenges
Existing administrative and monitoring data	Data gathered as part of operations, routine surveys.	Equality monitoring data (organisation level) Births (national level)	Firms increasingly asking well-being questions as part of monitoring.	Closed multiple-choice Qs, for example, nationality, gender identity.	To monitor or understand whole populations (i.e. of countries or organisations). Can help understand how specific demographics experience ill-being, for example.	Data access issues (e.g. legal issues, internal procedures, identifying the target group(s), collecting comparator data)
Existing large-scale survey data	Long-term, large-scale survey data, administered by international bodies (i.e. OECD), central governments, the ONS (in the UK).	Labour Force Survey (LFS, ONS)	'ONS4' Personal well-being Qs are now in LFS.	Closed multiple-choice Qs. e.g., Do you do shift work in your (main) job?	Nationally representative sample, claims can be made of the whole nation. One example might be understanding if shift work is linked to anxiety at population level.	Quantitative modelling most likely required. Access can be difficult for some kinds of data and individual researchers.

Type	How generated/collected	Examples	Well-being example	What kind of questions	How used?	Some opportunities and challenges
Existing qualitative data	Previous research projects may archive their qualitative data for re-use. This could be from a survey, interviews, diary submissions or free text from surveys.	1938, Mass Observation project: 'what is happiness?'[18]	This example is a project about happiness, but one well-being-related question could be added to a questionnaire on something else.	Open Question, 'what is happiness?' Participants answer with short or long descriptions.	Can be used to understand one or many people's depths of experience of well-being at a particular moment in time. For example, asking people to keep mental health diaries in COVID-19.	Permissions required. Not all open access/available to all. Long descriptions are often time-consuming to analyse and may require specialist knowledge.
New data collected with a specific purpose (quantitative)	Small-scale or one-off surveys	'BBC Loneliness Experiment'	This example is a one-off loneliness survey, but one or more well-being-related questions could be added to a questionnaire on something else.	How would you define loneliness? Options included: having no one to talk to; feeling disconnected from the world; feeling left out; sadness; feeling misunderstood.	This survey was used to interrogate how whole populations experience and define loneliness. It addressed a gap in knowledge, which is what a large-scale one-off survey would be for.	Surveys are expensive and harder to design properly than people imagine. Small-scale surveys in organisations are notoriously poorly designed, compromising the data collected.

(continued)

Table 3.1 (continued)

Type	How generated/ collected	Examples	Well-being example	What kind of questions	How used?	Some opportunities and challenges
New data collected with a specific purpose (qualitative)	Qualitative methods (interviews, observation, focus groups)	Measuring National Well-being debate		What matters to you? What things make life worthwhile?	The MNW Debate also used quantitative data from an online questionnaire. Qualitative data were collected via group discussions and free text in the online questionnaire.	This was incredibly resource-heavy to collect the data, costing millions of pounds, and took months to analyse. Analysing focus groups correctly is more complicated than sometimes imagined.
Social media data	Web-scraping.	Tweets	Analysing geo-located tweets using sentiment analysis could help begin to understand how people feel in: (1) parks, or (2) public transport.[19]	People aren't asked questions. In fact they often don't know their tweet could be used in research.	Social media data are mainly used as qualitative data where you ask research questions of the large dataset.	Ethics of data use. Not everyone can use scraping software or sentiment analysis software. As with all qualitative data, you can analyse by hand, which is resource-heavy.

kinds of data for understanding well-being. While this section might help you design your own research, there are countless exhaustive textbooks out there that devote more space to that. Here the goal is to help you to imagine data contexts, and so better evaluate how other people have used data.

Questionnaire Data

If the idea of data collection is new to you, perhaps the easiest way to imagine well-being data being collected is by using a questionnaire that asks people how they feel about things related to their well-being. Questionnaires are easily distributed, and ask the same questions in the same way and can be repeated numerous times with the same or different people. This means their data are easily comparable, providing insights into well-being across a group or sub-population. If you ask the same people, you can understand their well-being over time. Online questionnaires distributed by organisations that have some responsibility for our well-being are increasingly familiar, for example, universities surveying their students and employers, their staff.[20] These tend to ask us questions about our well-being that are useful to the running of the organisation in some way. The data can be used 'by management' to decide if it is allocating resources well, or if HR needs to make an intervention, in the same way that policy-makers can use well-being data.

Another way to imagine the context of questionnaire data collection might be the market researchers who used to be on the streets with clipboards (that my mum would always desperately avoid at the shops). In our increasingly online world, people's opinions are still sought using questionnaires in person (although, along with everything else, COVID-19 has compromised this, and we are yet to see how social research will find its new normal). Questionnaires could involve asking whether people would buy a product in the case of market research, but can also include questions about something they have just seen, an experience they just had, or how they feel about a particular place, like the park they are in. Some have had questionnaires after their COVID-19 vaccine, asking about their healthcare experiences. People can fill in the questionnaires themselves, or the researcher could complete the questionnaire on their behalf. If the research wanted to understand how people feel about a local, publicly subsidised event, the questions answered could look something like:

Q1 Have you just seen [specific subsidised concert]?	Y/N
Q2 Is this your local park?	Y/N
Q3 How are you feeling right now—out of 10, with 10 being the best you've ever felt, and 0 the worst?	0, 1, 2, 3, 4, 5, 6, 7, 8, 9, 10

These questions would generate binary data (yes/no) that can be aggregated (totalled) alongside numeric data from the scale. These sorts of data are easy to work with quantitatively, as you can categorise easily across the binary questions. Q3 uses a Likert[21] rating scale that presents a series of answers to choose from, ranging from one extreme attitude to another. It's sometimes referred to as a satisfaction scale as it is ideal for measuring satisfaction, and is therefore often used to measure well-being. The numbers from the scale are used to establish trends or averages.

Say, a researcher was lucky enough to get 100 people to speak to them on their way home from a concert in a park, they would have a sample of 100 people, and would know that they saw the event (is that the same as attended, you may ask? We will see what to do about that shortly). The researchers could establish what percentage of those spoken with were local residents (although, note, that what is meant by 'local' is not specified, which is not ideal). They could then look for trends in how people felt having attended the concert using the numeric data.

Or, they could ask the question,

Having seen this subsidised concert in your local park, how are you feeling right now?

Yeah, good, ta. There was a great atmosphere.

This box, called a free text field or open text, allows people to answer a question in their own words. Whilst this is less easy to process and compare at scale, it can sometimes provide valuable information. In each case, the majority of the data collected would be subjective, as the numeric or textual answers would reflect the reported experience of the individual. Therefore, the answers collected—the data—may be considered a valuable reflection of how they are feeling.

However, not all textual or verbal responses are succinct. In fact, when you ask people how they feel in themselves or about something to do with well-being, their responses can contain much rich detail (Oman 2015, 2017, 2019). So they might say, something like:

I feel great! It was great to have the opportunity to go to a gig close by. Because I only earn £6000 a year, I don't get to go to concerts any more. I think that because I never get to go, that made this all the more special Yeah, good. There was a great atmosphere.

These qualitative data contain: objective data in the salary disclosure, an example of preference (in that they chose to spend their limited income on the subsidised concert), as well as what they think this means for their well-being and concert attendance.

However, there are confounders, too: their limited income = limited concert attendance, which means that they think their enjoyment of this concert was heightened. How does this compare to other people who attended, etc.? How could it compare? How might a valid argument be made for the impact of this concert (as a cultural product, or an arts event) rather than capturing 'the social value' (which we covered in the previous chapter) of going to an event in the local park? How could claims made be generalisable? Meaning how could what is learnt from 100 people in one context be used to understand different people who attend different kinds of concerts with different life circumstances in different places at different times? Also, the fact that this person lives locally to the concert is probably a factor impacting on their decision to go. How might we isolate the relationship between concert attendance and happiness from these confounders? Here we mean how much of an effect did proximity to the concert have on attendance versus wanting to go to the concert for another reason? How do you know they weren't caught in a very limited moment of elation that meant they said they felt great, but which didn't last? How do you know the people spoken to could possibly represent diverse opinions? Perhaps they were all picked because they were all wearing band T-shirts for those on the line-up? It may be that people who are more likely to stop and answer questions will also have more time to go to concerts? How do you know if you need to know these things, or indeed, which of them you need to know?

Perhaps, more importantly, how sure can we be that what people say is an accurate representation of their feelings and opinion more generally? There is evidence that people who are approached will say nice things to people because, despite popular belief, people are generally nice, and they don't want to offend people. This may mean giving an answer they think the interviewer wants and is called the 'interviewer effect'.[22] In our case this would mean that people are inclined to say that something has improved their mood or happiness or well-being because they think that is what the person posing the question wants to hear. Asking the question, did you see the concert? followed by how do you feel right now? will suggest to the person asked that the researcher wants to understand if the concert has positively impacted on how they are feeling and is a leading question.

There are other aspects of situations like this which will affect people's answers: can they be overheard, for example? Do they want to look like they like the music played, or do they want to suggest they have 'better' taste? Sometimes people answer for the benefit of others, rather than truthfully.

It is not only how truthful someone is in the moment, but also a question of how long that moment lasts. If you ask someone directly after the concert how they feel, are you able to argue for a longer-term effect on well-being? We don't know how long such an effect will last. Can feeling great for five minutes be argued as a positive impact on well-being? These are contextual issues with data: often the context in which data have been collected compromises the claims which can be made through analysing them. These are issues of validity (see Box 3.3). Yet, when you read a local council's report about an event like a park concert, it will rarely acknowledge the limits to what can be known.

Similarly, how do you also account for negative effects on well-being and social impacts that are less positive? What of the park being shut for the concert take down and put up? What of the noise pollution affecting older people, pets or babies sleeping? All of these are examples of confounders on the claims that what might seem a simple initiative, such as the local council subsiding a concert in a local park, can have social impact in a way that is simple to express. The negative impacts are not often accommodated in research which asserts social impact, yet is clearly important to account for these issues in any claims made for any positive effects.

It is not often acknowledged that good questionnaires that collect 'good data' are not easy to design or execute well. Questionnaire data therefore may be useful for many purposes and relatively easy to access, but need testing. One way of feeling more secure in the quality of questions, even on a small scale, as with our concert scenario, can involve the same questions and techniques as questionnaires used in large surveys. Of course, the claims cannot be generalisable, as you are less likely to speak to a range of people, but you can then compare your data with a representative sample.[23] Researchers should, therefore, think very carefully about the

> **Box 3.3 Validity**
> Researchers need to think in terms of validity to understand the limits of what can be known by what they are asking. There are two main types of validity.
>
> **Internal validity** is concerned with how capable a research tool (say a survey question) is in enabling a researcher to answer their research question. For example, when you ask someone 'how are you feeling right now' without asking them to connect the feeling to the concert, you are unable to know that the feeling is linked to attending a concert. This will limit the claims you can make with validity.
>
> **External validity** is concerned with how generalisable the results of a piece of research are outside of the study; by which we mean 'can the findings of this study (speaking to 100 people outside X park) explain how people that we didn't speak to feel about concerts?'
>
> Limits to validity are not always bad, it depends on the context, but they should be accounted for.

context of where they want to use the questionnaire, who and what they want to know about, and the limits of what can be known from specific questions asked of the people they are able to speak to. They also need to think about their impact: will they ruin the experience of the concert? Will they offend people in some way, or indeed, will the simple act of asking them if they enjoyed something affect their desire to say yes or no, and to communicate how much they enjoyed it? How much can be known from such a short-lived interaction with a hundred people? What use are these 'snapshot' data in answering bigger questions?

Interview Data

Interviewers are able to ask people what they think well-being means and what things are important in their life. We have already noted that questionnaires are used in national-level survey data collection; these usually use closed questions which can easily be added up quantitatively. The questions are asked by 'interviewers', whose job is to ask closed questions and make the experience of the questionnaire as similar as possible for all respondents.

Contrarily, interviews are a common feature of smaller data collection projects, where the questions can be more open-ended and may have very few questions at all. It is also common for an interviewer to develop a rapport[24] with an interviewee: something which you might hear talked about in positive terms when journalists interview key figures. Having a connection with your interviewee can, therefore, make the interview better, because people trust the person they are speaking to—because the data (the information) are richer and more detailed.

We tend to think of interviews as one-to-one situations, but you can do group interviews, often called focus groups.[25] In my PhD research, I started my focus groups with a question from the ONS' MNW debate: 'What Matters to You?' They were designed as group discussions, where people had a lot of time to talk about a few questions at length, rather than asking lots of questions and people having less time to answer them. There are merits to both approaches, but I decided that it was more important to my research that people speak amongst themselves about what was important to them and think about how it related to well-being (Oman 2017). What we call 'a structured interview' has a strict set of questions which all interviewees answer, and these can be applied in a group setting. A 'semi-structured interview' is more fluid, allowing the interviewee to bring up whatever they want, which could be entirely unexpected, and so each discussion can take a completely different direction. Taking the former approach would have made my conversations as similar as possible for comparability; the latter allowed me to watch people chat away about anything they thought important.

The group discussions[26] I have organised in previous research projects have produced qualitative data that are largely subjective and about all different domains of people's lives and experiences. For my well-being focus groups, people talked about all sorts: redundancy, bereavement, suicidal thoughts, loneliness, parenthood, their sexuality, education, careers, disabilities, dwindling community resources and transport and their hobbies. To return to the concert example, in the kind of well-being data I collected with open questions, people might talk amongst themselves about local events, without being asked a question about concerts at all. As it was, although many people talked about the value of their leisure activities (Oman 2020), the only occasion people talked about concerts specifically was not to say how much they enjoyed one in particular. Instead, one young person barely noticed and the other (in the exchange below) was highly critical of a large-scale cultural event in Northern Ireland. Here's a snippet between a 17- and 18-year-old, who I've renamed James and Jack:

James: *During the summer when they had the big concerts and stuff, that was like the only time I noticed that town was different. It kind of seemed like it was all decorated and everyone was kind of buzzing.*

Jack: *Yeah but I just think was kind of a distraction purpose to turn everyone's heads away from the real issue. Like a home basically, we need a home to live, people die on the streets how many times a year? And they're dressing up the city as, oh we're a great city and people are lacking the basic human rights, that is not right.*

One thing about research which aims to evaluate how people feel about things is that the longer you allow them to talk, the more comfortable they feel, which can mean that they become more honest. It can also mean that they deviate from the topic, and may not say what you anticipate. Another example from this research was a community arts project where I expected people to mention the arts project in relation to their well-being—especially as it was the one thing they had in common and the reason we were meeting. Yet, they did not refer to it, not even once. Instead, they held a very political discussion about the lack of community services for their families in their area. This may be that they thought that was what I was there to listen to, so I could report back in some way to an authority that would do something about these aspects of their lives. It is not always possible to conclusively know why an open conversation has followed a particular path, and part of qualitative research is to reflect on the possibilities of why that may be.

Another thing to bear in mind with these sorts of data collection is that through discussion, people find themselves agreeing with others in the group. This may mean that opinions expressed independently at the beginning of a focus group[27] have evolved through discussion and group 'meaning-making' (Freeman 2013) or it can mean that they feel pressurised to assimilate to 'groupthink'. It can be hard to establish which of the two processes have provoked a changed opinion and how that affects your results. Again, aspects of the context can give you clues and are part of your methodology in group interviews and focus groups, as much as any other approach. Their limitations can be as much opportunity as confounder, as long as they are considered.

My PhD[28] focus groups enabled me to speak to over a hundred people and listen to them discuss what mattered to them about well-being. This was important to my research question which wanted to recreate a debate-like feel and therefore encourage people to talk—and debate—amongst themselves. But this can mean that quieter people's views are not as audible and that it is not possible to understand how many of a group feel one way over another. As you can see, all decisions have pros and cons to weigh up.

One-to-one interviews enable you to understand the perspective of one person in detail and then compare that with the views from another interview, if appropriate. They can be used in evaluations and impact studies, providing testimonials of experience. Also, much like with focus groups, these are often transcribed into long pieces of text. This turns audio qualitative data into textual qualitative data and can take considerable time to analyse and compare. Interviews offer incredibly rich data on a person's well-being, and with a well-thought-out strategy, can enable researchers to make some broader claims about how a particular group of people experience something like well-being, or indeed what is important to them about it. However, these claims must acknowledge the limits of context as discussed above.

Ethnographic Data

Another way that interview data might be useful for understanding well-being would be in the case of ethnographic research investigating the impact of a social policy. Ethnography involves a researcher spending a long time in their research site. This means they understand as much about the context in which they are collecting data as possible. For example, Kelly Bogue was embedded in her local community investigating the impact of 'the bedroom tax' (2019). 'The bedroom tax' was a nickname for an aspect of the Welfare Reform Act (DWP 2012) which meant that people living in social housing saw their benefits reduced by 14% if they have a spare room or 25% if they have two or more. The negative well-being implications of this policy on the community studied were multiple, with carers and those registered disabled being penalised for necessary home adaptations, alongside the anxiety and stress of people forced to leave the homes in the communities in which they had lived for decades (Bogue 2019). While this research was not seeking data to answer questions on well-being *per se*, the study produced much data that could inform well-being research for policy.

Some ways of doing ethnography allow you to participate in a context as a contributing member. This means practitioners, whether social workers, artists or people working in an office, might find it a useful way to examine well-being within their own work contexts. Overall, it's rich, meaning that there is much detail gathered to deepen understanding, but time-intensive and gaining permission can be difficult to negotiate unless the researcher is already embedded in the community. Crucially, this kind of ethnography writes you into the context, so you affect it to an even greater extent than time delimited interviews. This requires thinking through in terms of whether it is ethical, or too intrusive. It also needs to be considered in terms of the claims that can be made: how would the particular context have been different had you not been there?

Secondary Qualitative Data

Qualitative data are increasingly collected with a view to the data being used again. This means those collecting data must be mindful of this when designing the questions asked and ensuring interviewees give permissions for storage, secondary access (used by someone else) and re-use (in publications or otherwise). Secondary data usage involves analysing data collected by someone else, as opposed to analysing primary data that you collect yourself and is more common with quantitative data.

It is sometimes possible to ask permission to access qualitative data that were not collected with the same questions in mind. This would mean that the same data, collected for a different purpose, could possibly be reanalysed to answer the specific question: 'what were the impacts of X social policy on the well-being of a specific community between X and X date, for example?' However, much qualitative data are too specific, in that they contain too much data and information about issues that are too personal to the people involved. For instance, given the sensitive nature of Bogue's data on the bedroom tax, it would be unlikely that these data could be reanalysed to answer a broader question on well-being for ethical reasons, even if it were a practical possibility. It is unlikely that permissions for re-use would have been sought at the time of collection, and were people told the data might be placed in a repository, they may have not been as honest. These kinds of data are extremely difficult to anonymise in a way that completely protects participants and were one to try, perhaps there would be very little left to analyse. The benefits of qualitative data in capturing the specificities of people's experiences, therefore, mean there can be barriers to secondary qualitative research.

Data collected by international bodies, such as the International Monetary Fund (IMF) or the UN, and national statistics agencies, such as the ONS in the UK, make their data publicly available for secondary analysis. These are primarily quantitative data and in addition to the findings that these bodies publish themselves (often presented as tertiary data). The ONS have pages and pages of findings and data on their website under well-being now, and there are a lot of data available from the UN's HDI on its website.[29]

Sometimes large surveys managed by national and international agencies, and available for secondary analysis, contain free text data (as shown above). If qualitative data has been collected at a large enough scale, then there is sometimes value in coding these and then adding up (aggregating) the answers which are similar, and turning this qualitative data into quantitative data. In 2013, I requested permission from the ONS to access free text fields from the Measuring National Well-being debate. I had developed a hypothesis from reading a report which contained quotes from the debate that I wanted to investigate.

My research question for these data, related to the issue we found outside the imaginary concert (described earlier in this chapter). If the evidence we have about the well-being impact of particular leisure and cultural activities can be argued as circumstantial, and from leading questions, the credibility of data is called into question—most specifically, its collection (Selwood 2002; Belfiore 2002). This is an issue that plagues arguments over the quality of the evidence on the relationship between aspects of culture and well-being that we return to in the second half of this book. If the data can be dismissed as resulting from leading questions and years of research projects that are therefore not able to offer generalisable results, then how might this issue be addressed?

I proposed we turn this question on its head. How does that help us overcome some of these issues with the context in which these data are collected? What if the question was more like: 'When people describe well-being, how often do they talk about participating in different kinds of activities—and what might that tell us about aspects of social and cultural policy?' I coded 6787 free text fields on well-being that were collected by the ONS and collated them into themes of all the things they talked about. I then quantified the themes (Oman 2015, 2020) and then ordered them in terms of prevalence of response.

Table 3.2 shows the difference in order according to what the ONS said it found in the overall debate (34,000 responses) and what I had found in the free text fields. Again, people did not refer directly to

Table 3.2 'A re-ordering' of priorities in the Measuring National Wellbeing Debate Questionnaires

	ONS' ordering of tick box responses (most prevalent at the top)	A re-ordering of free text field responses (most prevalent at the top)	
1st	Health	Leisure and spare time	1st
2nd	Having good connections with friends and relatives	Quality of natural environment	2nd
3rd	Job satisfaction and economic security	Family	3rd
4th	Present and future conditions of the environment	Security	4th
5th	Education and training	Protect planet/nature	5th
6th	Personal and cultural activities, including caring and volunteering	Freedom/power	6
7th	Income and wealth	Access to leisure possibilities	7th
8th	Availability to have a say on local and national issues	Healthcare	8th
9th	Crime	Equality	9th
10th	Other	Happiness/well-being of others	10th
		Government	11th
		Fairness/social justice	12th
		Access to services	13th
		Politics	14th

Adapted from (Oman 2019, 2020)

concerts (using the word) in the national debate, and only once in a subsequent consultation (Beaumont 2011, 29), but people did refer to the importance of broader concepts of social and cultural participation (Oman 2015, 2019, 2020).

Well-being data include many sorts of data beyond those used in national indicators or the statistics we read in the media. They can all be extremely useful to inform work of many kinds from social work and policy, to arts administration, to the management of a particular company or understanding how to better care for students away from home at university. The data required, and how they are analysed, involve a balance of what needs or wants to be known (see Table 3.1). It is also a practical matter of preference of approach, skill and resource; all need to be balanced and there are various limits on different kinds of data to answer different questions. Table 3.3 offers an overview of how different data can help answer different questions for different reasons and/or audiences.

Table 3.3 Overview of data types and possibilities for answering well-being questions

What do we want to know?	About who/what?	For who/what?	How to find out?	What kind of data?	Does this answer our Q?
Did this concert improve people's well-being?	People attending a local event	To report to local council	Ask people after the event with questionnaire	Ask them to comment = qualitative Ask them to rate it on a scale = quantitative	Yes, but with many limits, such as people not understanding the question, interviewer effect, etc.
Does government funding in the arts improve social inclusion?	Social impact of government funding	Think tank or government evaluation	Secondary analysis of longitudinal data	National survey data and administrative or monitoring data (such as financial accounts)	Yes, but with many limits. Relationship between money spent and proxy indicator of social inclusion (access to further education is an example) can only tell so much.
What is the social value of public parks in London borough?	Residents and visitors to London borough	Local council	Public consultation	Online questionnaire	Access only to some users, if online, but also recruiting in person will have limits.
			Evidence review	Looking at findings and/or data from other reports and synthesising[viii]	Constrained by other people's findings and methods. Evidence synthesises often don't evaluate how well the methods of others answer the question.
Does money buy happiness?	Global population over time	Academic study	Secondary data analysis	Life satisfaction data and a proxy for wealth (GDP), tracked over time, per country	GDP is a limited understanding of the lived experience of wealth.

How does crime rate affect well-being?	Population of different countries	International well-being index, that is OECD Better Life Index	A combination of primary survey data collection, complemented by some secondary data	Online questionnaire (in this case the Gallup World Poll, but OECD mainly use data they collect itself)	Not exactly, it is a proxy indicator as risk of crime affects well-being, but it cannot tell you how one affects the other without modelling.
How did 'the bedroom tax' affect people's well-being?	A specific community identified as particularly affected	Academic research to inform policy decisions	Ethnographic approaches	Qualitative data from observations and interviews	This research may not be aiming to answer this question explicitly, but would be expected to show a relationship between the policy and well-being. The research answers the question about the people studied in one community in great depth. It may not be generalisable to a wider population.
What is important to people about well-being?	All people—within a specific population? (i.e. the UK)	To inform the national measures of well-being	Various methods, including survey and live events	Qualitative and quantitative data	Yes, but different methods may find different answers, so would then have to be looked at together.

Understanding whether data are 'good data', as in good at the job you need it to do, requires an appreciation of all the many aspects of the context, situation and/or population you want to understand. It requires an understanding of what you want to know about well-being, which we have discovered is contestable and varied in different contexts. Thus, for them to be data for good (and thus good for well-being) requires context and reflection. There is a tendency to view and to use certain kinds of data as if they are objective and unaffected by human decisions. The next sections look at objective data and their issues.

3.4   Objective Well-being Data and Measures

In terms of quantitative data, you might imagine that the key question is how should well-being be *measured*? Really, this is a much bigger question, or series of inter-related questions, which are how should well-being be conceptualised, operationalised and measured? Or before well-being can be measured, we need to decide what we mean by well-being (conceptualise) and find measurable dimensions of our concept (operationalise),[30] and *then* we can decide on a way of measuring it.

We have discussed some of the methods of collecting well-being data. Many decisions are involved that are not always made obvious, but are all important. The point here is that the conceptualisation of 'what is it we're actually trying to get at when we want to understand well-being' is distinct from its operationalisation. It is also worth noting that to operationalise a concept in research has a slightly different meaning than it does in everyday life. We come back to this in Chaps. 6, 7 and 8. If someone operationalises something, it generally means they put it to use, or bring it into use. In research, it is more a process of establishing how we can measure. So, conceptualisation is different from operationalisation, but connected. The operationalisation of 'here is the form of words we're using to ask the question' is different again from 'here are the options for the answers people can be provide (and if applicable, how we'll combine these answers from different questions to give people an overall well-being score)'.

As we have hopefully established in the introduction to this chapter, money is important in most contexts, but is far from everything. There are many more features that shape people's lives and that need to be understood if we aim to understand well-being as quality of life (Dodge et al. 2012). You could ask a population any number of questions to understand aspects of their quality of life. For example, is your housing adequate? How sanitary is your local environment?[31] Do you have public institutions that respond to your needs? Would you say have an active social life? Are quality healthcare and education services easily available to you? You may note that all of these questions are phrased in such a way that they ask for people's opinion on aspects that are thought to affect our quality of life. They are therefore going to produce data that are subjective.

All of these issues can also be measured using data that are objective indicators. For example, administrative data such as GP visits and hospital wait times could be used to generate a benchmark for 'fair access to health-care', and then community-level data could be measured against this benchmark. These are proxy indicators because they do not directly answer the question 'does this person have fair access to healthcare', but are used to stand in for data that could.

Proxy indicators have a number of pros. They are not biased by people's inaccurate memories of how long they waited in hospital, which, for obvious reasons, may be clouded with frustration. You do not have to worry about issues of sampling bias (see Box 3.4). Also, proxy data have often already been collected and cleaned by someone else, or a statistical organisation. So, while they can only partially answer the question of how many people have fair access to healthcare, the pros will have been thought to outweigh the cons. Similarly, being able to answer a research question on fair access to healthcare doesn't tell us everything we need to know about well-being: it is one aspect of well-being. It only partially *indicates* someone's quality of life, and so to understand quality of life more completely at population level, we need more indicators.

Objective measures of well-being are based on assumptions regarding human needs and rights, believed to impact on quality of life. Herein is the difference between quality of life and well-being. The academic literature tends to assume that quality of life involves material conditions, whereas well-being also involves life satisfaction, mood and meaning (although as we know from the previous chapter, this is not always clear-cut). It is the quality of life aspects of well-being that are measured with objective indicators using the objective list theory that most indexes are based on.

The existence of the list, of course, suggests that a person or people with expertise have decided what should go on the list: what is important and what standard measures should be used, or indeed to whose standard? There is even an 'objective list theory of well-being' (Rice 2013) that is pluralistic. This means that instead of identifying a single feature common to all states of well-being (think of an overarching argument for 'what is the meaning of the good life?'), it identifies a number of characteristics of what makes for a good life. This philosophical theory is applied to lists of objective indicators, of what would be all the qualities needed for a good life. The key is that the aim is to cover all the important domains in life, so unlike a simple index, like the HDI, these tend to have lots of indicators. In other words, the well-being data are about lots of aspects of life.

The previous chapter explained a brief history of the move away from a single measure of progress (GDP) towards multiple measures of well-being in the twentieth century. These tended to be an index of multiple objective indicators of quality of life, associated to different 'domains' of life. Some organisations and nations recognise the same six major objective and observable dimensions for the measurement of objective well-being. These include international organisations, such as the Organisation for Economic Co-operation and Development (OECD 2011a) and the United Nations Development Programme (UNDP 2015), as well as national statistics offices, such as the Italian Statistics Bureau (ISTAT 2015). Notably, within each dimension are multiple indicators (ordinarily two or three). Figure 3.1 shows just how many indicators there are within domains in the OECD's index and per member country. As we shall discover in the following chapter, these bodies all heavily influence each other by way of advisory groups and drawing on perceived best practice.

Given that the theory behind the objective list approach means you need to analyse data from across all these dimensions, this can make it difficult to interpret these data, even at headline level (see Fig. 3.1), but also to compare them. Changing the unit of analysis from each indicator, to per country, or domain, makes them more readable. This is the same as with the Dow Jones, where the index is designed to have a single measure for readability. With the HDI,[32] the three dimensions are combined into a single measure for easy comparison.

With more complex indexes than the HDI, such as the OECD's (Fig. 3.1), decisions need to be made on balancing the importance of the different domains. As we know, each of the three domains contributes equally to a country's overall HDI score (United Nations 2020), this is not the case with all indexes. If domains are not equally weighted, then decisions have to be made about the relative importance of each to overall well-being decisions. As Table 3.2 demonstrates, establishing the importance of different domains of well-being is not a neutral process.

To this end, these weights involve subjective decisions by experts on what is more important about the objective indicators. That is not to say it is not a rigorous process, that it is not based on much evidence, and that experts do not debate and review these processes to ensure robustness. Yet, the term objective can obscure what is going on behind the scenes, or underneath the hood, if you like, of what are called 'objective indicators' of well-being, or imply that they arrive at some sort of universal truth about well-being. As criticisms over the HDI surface, people do not value these aspects of life equally, or, indeed, the same as each other. Remember that there is a difference between measuring what is valuable and what is valuable to measure—to whom and why.

An attempt to counter criticisms of weights applied by experts, The OECD states that its 'Better Life Index is an interactive composite index that aggregates average measures of country's well-being outcomes through weights defined by users' (OECD 2018, 4). What does this mean, and why have the OECD attempted to do this? Let's break this down.

The OECD's Better Life Index website has an interactive dashboard, enabling people to use sliders to order and balance the importance of different aspects of well-being. When people use the sliders, they are effectively applying weights to the different aspects of well-being to construct an overall index that is personal to them.[33] In this instance, the index aims to avoid representing the experts' view of what is valuable, presenting those of the person interacting with the dashboard back at them.

This is all well and good, but how does this impact on change for social good? Are the OECD listening/watching/recording these interactions, and how might it change the way they value what is important? While some analysis has been done on people's interactions and values (OECD

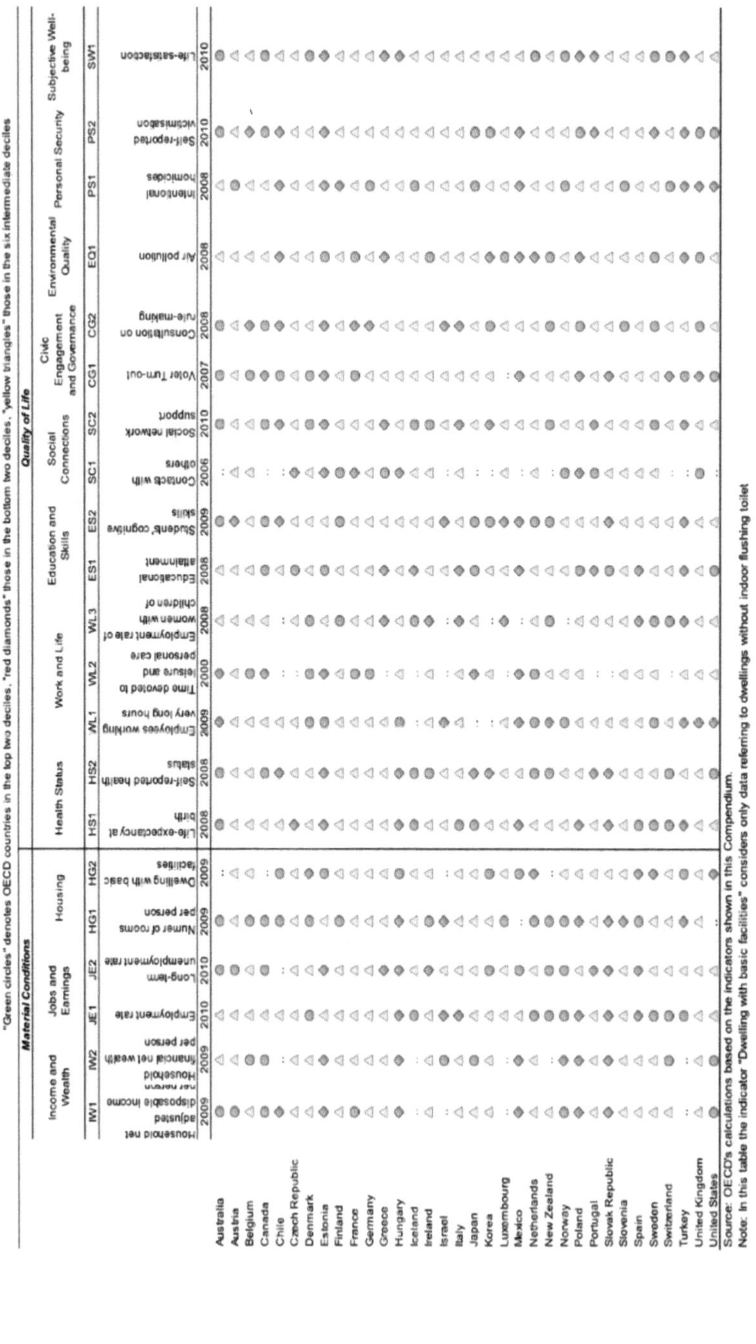

Source: OECD's calculations based on the indicators shown in this Compendium.

Note: In this table the indicator "Dwelling with basic facilities" considers only data referring to dwellings without indoor flushing toilet

Fig. 3.1   OECD well-being indicators. (Source: OECD Compendium of OECD Well-Being Indicators 2011)

Box 3.4   Weights and Sampling Bias

Weights

The term 'weighting' is used in several different ways in the analysis of quantitative data, and it's important to be clear about which way we're talking about.

In this section, we are concerned with how different bits of information about countries are combined to give an overall score for those countries. Or, how important money is, as opposed to education or health. The HDI applies an equal weight to these categories.

Weighting is also used to describe a technique when working with survey data to correct for **sampling bias**. As we have discussed, it is rare to achieve a whole population, and so most survey data are a sample. No matter how large that sample is, your sample is unlikely to look the same as the whole population, so you need to adjust for different proportions who answered the survey. For example, younger people are often less likely to respond to surveys, so estimates based on surveys often weight young people's responses more heavily to adjust for this difference.

These two different meanings of the term 'weighting' are applied in very different ways—in one case, to the questions that are being asked, and in another, to the people who are being asked the questions—and shouldn't be confused.

2018), and this dashboard implies democratic engagement or participatory decision-making to a degree, there is no commitment to this. People are also only able to interact with the pre-defined categories: were something of importance to you not there, there is no way to include this in the dashboard or tell anyone it should be included.

The terminology, processes and decisions behind what are used for objective well-being data, and how they are used together—as an objective list of indicators—are complex. I have tried to cover specific examples and drill down into the processes of why things happen in certain ways and to explain some of the terminology. We are going to look at one index in greater detail in the next section. This is to help those who wish to understand what goes on underneath the hood of a well-being index and to have a better understanding of what decisions are made about what good data practices might be for well-being data.

3.5   THE OECD AS A CASE STUDY OF WHAT LIES BEHIND OBJECTIVE WELL-BEING DATA

> Measuring well-being and progress has been and will continue to be a key priority for the OECD, in line with its founding tradition to promote policies designed to achieve the highest living standards for all. (OECD 2011a, 4)

The OECD have been key to the 'second wave' of framing well-being as important to measure (Bache and Reardon 2013). National well-being initiatives have tended to be in OECD or EU countries, and it is thought that the OECD had a hand in the process of the influential Sarkozy commission (Bache 2012, 26, 30). The OECD Framework for Measuring Well-Being and Progress is said to be based on the recommendations from the commission (OECD n.d.b). We are going to peer under the bonnet of how the OECD devised its well-being indicators to reveal the decisions and care that go into such a programme.

The OECD claim that:

> the ultimate objective of this work is not just measurement per se, but to strengthen the evidence-base for policy making. Better measures of well-being can improve our understanding of the factors driving societal progress. Better assessments of countries' comparative performance in various fields can lead to better strategies to tackle deficiencies. (OECD 2011a, 4)

The OECD wanted to understand well-being in a way that can both offer comparisons across nations and potentially inform policy evaluations. They decided the qualities that best represented well-being; made objective lists; researched appropriate proxy indicators using existing data that can answer the dimensions of well-being. They tested the indicators that they have used to meet the demands of their well-being framework and ensured that they meet additional quality criteria; they sought expert advice on these moving parts and then offered a caveat on the experimental and evolutionary nature of these metrics: they will change and they are not perfect. This level of detail is not always readily available when research is published. So, we are going to look at the decisions made in the devising of the index in order to understand what lies behind these well-being data.

The OECD devised a list of criteria of what would be good to measure. Crucially, they also undertook a review of the data available from member countries (who, of course, may not be measuring the same thing). Prior to finalising the index, a compendium was released, which contained the framework on which decisions were made regarding which well-being indicators they might use (OECD 2011a). This was the criteria they published in the compendium:

- *the well-being of **people** in each country, rather than on the macro-economic conditions of economies; hence, many standard indicators of macro-economic performance (e.g. GDP, productivity, innovation) are not included in this Compendium.*
- *the well-being of different groups of the population, in addition to average conditions. Measures of **inequalities** in people's conditions will figure prominently in the "How's Life?" report but are only discussed briefly in this Compendium.*
- *well-being achievements, measured by **outcome** indicators, as opposed to well-being drivers measured by input or output indicators.*
- ***objective** and **subjective** aspects of people's well-being as both living conditions and their appreciation by individuals are important to understand people's well-being.* (OECD 2011a, 5)

The OECD were also keen that their framework distinguished between current material living conditions and quality of life, on the one hand, and the conditions required to ensure their sustainability over time, on the other. Notably 'material living conditions' do not always mean economic, and often the term elsewhere incorporates quality of life dimensions, as discussed above.

- ***Material living conditions*** *(or 'economic well-being') determine people's consumption possibilities and their command over resources. While this is shaped by GDP, the latter also includes activities that do not contribute to people's well-being (e.g. activities aimed at offsetting some of the regrettable consequences of economic development) while it excludes non-market activities that expand people's consumption possibilities.*
- ***Quality of life***, *defined as the set of non-monetary attributes of individuals, shapes their opportunities and life chances, and has intrinsic value under different cultures and contexts.*

- *The **sustainability of the socio-economic and natural systems** where people live and work is critical for well-being to last over time. Sustainability depends on how current human activities impact on the stocks of different types of capital (natural, economic, human and social). However, suitable indicators for describing the evolution of these stocks are still lacking in many fields. For this reason, indicators of sustainability are not included in this Compendium, although some of them will feature in 'How's Life?'* (OECD 2011a, 5).

The OECD claim that the framework reproduced above 'underlies the selection of indicators in each dimension of well-being' that work within two additional quality criteria:

- *conceptual soundness (i.e. relevance in terms of measuring and monitoring well-being across the population in the perspective of informing policies)*
- *data of high quality (i.e. based on well-established standards and codes of practice). The selection of indicators has been made following extensive consultation with National Statistical Offices and experts from various OECD directorates.* (OECD 2011a, 5)

It is within the tension between conceptual soundness and the quality of data that the sustainability indicators sit: they would be what we would ideally be measuring if we want to capture well-being; remembering that the principle of an objective list is that the indicators included (BetterEvaluation 2012) are all vital to well-being. It is interesting that the OECD consulted with individual statistics offices on which indicators to select. The UK's ONS also state they consulted the OECD to decide their well-being metrics (Oman 2017).[34] Therefore, despite apparently separate investigations, the same experts were informing different indices. Sharing expertise is undoubtedly a good thing, especially when it comes to methodological rigour, but it might arguably limit the possibility for independence or innovation in how countries measure the well-being of their citizens. Notably, despite the fact that Bhutan's measures of Gross National Happiness are often cited as inspiring the OECD, Sarkozy commission, and so on, expertise from Bhutan is not very evident on these advisory groups. We return to this in Chap. 6, but who the experts are, are always important questions to ask.

Another important thing to note about the OECD's contribution to well-being data are the caveats that were presented alongside these domains, namely that the indicators are:

experimental, in that the proposed selection of indicators has not yet reached the stage of meeting all agreed standards;

evolutionary, as the indicators proposed in this Compendium are, in many cases, only proxies of a broader underlying outcomes, for which ideal measures are currently lacking. (OECD 2011a, 7)

The report also notes that the selection of indicators will change in the future as better measures are developed, and as member countries reach agreement on indicators that are more appropriate to summarising conditions in the various dimensions of people's lives (OECD 2011a). So, whilst these national indicators tend to be presented as absolute, or fixed, in some way, like other forms of science and social science, they are invented to respond to developments and improvements. This is rarely acknowledged when objective indicators are presented in official reports and briefings.

So, what might these indicators look like?

The description 'bewildering array' (Scott 2012, 36) may come to mind when looking at Fig. 3.1. As a result, Table 3.4 shows only the domains and indicators in 2010. There are 21 indicators across the 11 domains, with a row for each member country. This is how the indicators were presented in 2010. Some of these have now changed, perhaps imperceptibly to most. It can be difficult to establish *exactly* what is meant by or what has changed about an indicator, why, and when that change happened, because this information is not readily available.

To explain what I mean here, we are going to zone in on the 'domain' of 'Personal Security', in our case study. Personal Security has two indicators in our 2010 visualisation: intentional homicides and self-reported victimisation. So, one question might be, 'why not just say crime, if you mean crime?' If you look at all the domain names, they are all positive in their inflection: environmental quality might read as pollution, or litter, for example. What is also interesting about the idea of personal security is that it does not necessarily mean crime, really. It could possibly include financial security to most people: do you have a pension; do you own your own home, and so on?

Table 3.4   Summary of the OECD indicators in 2010

Domains	Indicators
Income and wealth	Household net adjusted disposable income per person
	Household financial net wealth per person
Jobs and earnings	Employment rate
	Long-term unemployment rate
Housing	Number of rooms per person
	Dwelling with basic facilities
Health status	Life expectancy at birth
	Self-reported health status
Work and life	Employees working very long hours
	Time devoted to leisure and personal care
	Employment rate of women with children of school-age
Education and skills	Educational attainment
	Students' cognitive skills
Social connections	Contacts with others
	Social network support
Civic engagement and governance	Voter turn out
	Consultation on rule-making
Environmental quality	Air pollution
Personal security	Intentional homicides
	Self-reported victimisation
Subjective well-being	Life satisfaction

Source: Adapted from Compendium of OECD Well-Being Indicators 2011

Another question is why, then, has the domain changed in the current 2020 version of the index? The Personal Security domain name is now called 'safety'. The OECD explain this domain as follows: 'Personal security is a core element for the well-being of individuals, and includes the risks of people being physically assaulted or falling victim to other types of crime' (OECD website/topics/safety). Therefore, the headline domain name has shifted from 'personal security' to 'safety', but has retained the credibility of the original measures.

Not only has the domain name changed. The indicators themselves have shifted: 'homicide rate' remains the same, but 'self-reported victimisation' has been replaced with 'feeling safe walking home at night'. Thus, an objective indicator has been replaced with a subjective indicator, as the data were collected by surveying how someone feels, rather than the administrative data from reporting crimes.

There are methodological reasons why this is a sensible change. In some places people do not report crimes, as they happen, so as a chosen proxy measure of a domain well-being, this is not necessarily the best indicator of the relationship between crime and quality of life. Secondly, it could be argued that it is in the 'feeling safe', rather than the reporting of crime that we experience well-being. This is why more subjective measures—even on an objective list—can be a better way of capturing what it is about well-being that we need to know.

In the previous section we encountered what objective indicators are, and this section has presented a lot of detail on one well-being index, as it is not always clear where such official-looking data come from. We focussed on some of the decision-making aspects of devising an index. This also revealed their methodological complexity—even without the quantitative modelling involved in statistics. We have also questioned the nature of the data assembled in objective lists and what is implied by their naming as objective. We have learnt that they are, in fact, shifting rather than fixed sets of measures. They evolve and respond to reflections on their limitations and how they could be done better. As we continue to use these sorts of data as objective facts, we lose these qualities, which are not considered important. Yet, the contexts of these data practices are both valuable and credible. It is a disservice to statistics and people who wish to understand them, that they remain obscured.

3.6 CONCLUSION

Understanding whether data are 'good data', as in good quality—or whether they are data for good (and thus good for well-being) requires us to look at context. We have to consider whether international indicators appeal to certain standards, and if so, how so, or to whose standard? Data are often used as if they are neutral and context-less, yet they have rich context that is rarely acknowledged. Understanding the expertise, reflections and decisions involved in these 'objective data' makes them appear richer and therefore could be argued to demonstrate, rather than decrease the appearance of rigour.

This chapter has aimed to offer an overview of different contexts that dictate both what and how *good* well-being data are. These environments have varied from local parks to international statistics forums; from a youth club in Derry five years ago, to a presidential candidacy speech in Kansas over half a century ago. Across qualitative and quantitative data; primary, secondary and tertiary data; proxy data, administrative data, survey data and ethnographic data. Data collected from talking to people can be harder to imagine as data, because we usually think of data as numbers. However, the contexts of these data—how they are collected and analysed—are also often easier for most people to imagine than those of international statistics. This is because it is easier for most people to picture themselves being the person speaking to people, either asking questions or answering them.

Most of us don't spend much time thinking about how data experts work. Why should we? But then how statisticians and data experts work are not transparent, or often discussed. This is, in fact, a barrier to understanding how their statistics and data work. This is not a textbook, and so looking at all these different types of data may not make you a statistician, but in reading this chapter, you may have improved your understanding of well-being data and their diversity. Looking at these data in context should also better enable you to better appreciate these data when you next see them in the media or in another government briefing (hopefully not about COVID-19).

We start this chapter by contextualising a political quote that is used a lot to justify why well-being data are good. We also look at a collection of attempts to define well-being for data across some policy documents over time that coincides with the recent rise of well-being data. The reflections on this political speech and policy documents treat these texts as data, enabling us to contextualise policy, politics and data with well-being.

The chapter then reflects on a number of different situations in which well-being data are generated, interpreted, analysed and applied. A hypothetical scenario of a well-being at work survey, a questionnaire outside a concert and real-life examples of well-being data that are relevant to social and cultural policy are shared to show the variety and accessibility of some approaches to well-being data collection, but the need for caution, consideration of others and the foregrounding of context in these matters. How you affect the data and the participants by collecting and using data is crucial to all research on society, especially that which supposedly improves it. This is not only a moral and ethical issue, but one that can limit the claims that can be made using these sorts of well-being data, should the wrong decisions be made, or should they not be explained. Therefore, the consequences of well-being data are crucial contexts, as well.

The HDI and the OECD well-being measures evolved from working within professional codes to innovate and generate the indices. It is not always obvious that this is a long process of organising and interpreting by experts before final decisions are made. In presenting good practice and contextualising how these things work, these sections hoped to improve your capability and confidence (which we identified as data issues in Chap. 1) if you are less familiar with these data. The objective lists that feature in these new well-being indices are often made of data that have been long collected. Once this context is understood, they seem less revolutionary than the politics sometimes implies. It is actually the newer subjective well-being measures that were being developed over the 2000s that were the more novel aspects of these well-being indicators, and we come to the limits of these claims in the next chapter.

The very name 'objective indicator' suggests it is that: objective, but often the data does not measure what they say it measures, instead being a proxy for what would ideally be measured, were there a measure for it. You may have found yourself reading the section on quality of life indicators, thinking how these indicators would pick up on the negative well-being impacts of the bedroom tax that Bogue's research uncovered. The answer is they are very unlikely to at national population or international population level, and were not designed to do that.

Well-being data are not all one thing. They have different purposes, pros and cons. Qualitative data are able to get closer to the meaning of well-being and the experiences of ill-being in some cases, but are often unable to generalise and are criticised for the subjective nature of the associated processes and the limits to claims of causation. We will look at how asking people how they really feel in surveys attempts to address some of these circumstantial issues of capturing the human experience in the next chapter where we put 'the new science' of happiness into context.

Notes

1. One example of this is that the UK's national newspaper, *The Guardian*, offered him his own blogpost to put the UK's Measuring National Well-being measures into context. See Rogers 2012.
2. Gross domestic product (GDP) and gross national product (GNP) are measures of a country's aggregate economic output. They are both widely used, differing in what exactly they measure: GDP is a measure of (national income = national output = national expenditure) produced in a particular country. GNP = GDP + net property income from abroad.
3. This speech was a few months before he was sadly assassinated.
4. These contexts of data can be notoriously difficult to find out about! It can be difficult to know where to begin looking. Even all the fact-checking,

and then re-checking, to finalise this book (and I have been doing this for years, now) required hours wrestling with broken links and inconclusive information on websites and in reports. I even emailed international statistics bodies for clarification. Most people probably don't even know that this is a thing you can do if you have questions. The ONS and the OECD have both replied extremely quickly to my general queries this last year, and they are mandated to answer queries. Hopefully this book offers a starting point to help answer some of your queries.

5. We tend to think of aesthetics as a sense of beauty, but more generally it means being actively engaged and conscious of the world's effect on us, whilst at the same time appreciative how we might affect the world. According to philosopher John Dewey ([1934] 1958), this enables us to appreciate how our experience is organised, making it coherent, and allowing us to appreciate the past, present and future—whether we are satisfied, or dissatisfied.

6. According to Rapley, 'asking about the quality of life amounts to a request for an aesthetic judgement', rather than a scientific one, from the person asked. You cannot take for granted that people have the same notion of quality of life, and therefore its assessment is a qualitative appraisal of how things stand. 'Aesthetic judgement', according to Kant ([1790] 1951), is dependent on discriminatory abilities at a sensory, emotional and intellectual level all at once.

7. Thematic analysis groups people's responses into themes to help a researcher understand commonalities and differences across their sample.

8. There is much written on this so-called debate, but Gary Goertz and James Mahoney are interesting on how it is *A Tale of Two Cultures* (2012).

9. Headline findings are provided in separate documents and executive summaries and are written to underpin messages that are the intended 'take away' findings from research. They are presented accessibly for the interested public, policy-makers and media with the intention that people will know what they need to know from reading a few bullet points, rather than looking at detailed results.

10. For more information on national accounts, the ONS website explains their national accounts here: https://www.ons.gov.uk/economy/nationalaccounts/uksectoraccounts/methodologies/nationalaccounts.

11. Some key figures in the well-being agenda, in particular The New Economics Foundation, foregrounded the term national accounts of well-being (New Economics Foundation 2009; Diener and Tov 2012).

12. The OECD also hold a useful repository of different country's national accounts, which is also useful to see similarities and differences (OECD website https://www.oecd-ilibrary.org/economics/data/oecd-national-accounts-statistics_na-data-en).

13. This section on the three accounts of well-being is largely influenced by Dolan et al. (2011a, b), who wrote a working paper for the UK's measures of national well-being. However, each country's index of well-being (collection of individual indicators or well-being) may be informed differently. Again, this is part of the lineage of the account.

14. The HDI has received critique (Kovacevic 2010) as has the use of any index in developing contexts. For example, anthropologically-informed well-being research tends to focus on how policy approaches overlook the specificities of culture: people, places and their histories (White 2006). Non-Euro-centric practices, which may be culturally different, are often categorised as deficient in some way: either bad for well-being or inefficient (Gough 2004). Work in this field extends that of Critical Development Studies, which state that imposing the agenda of the global north elsewhere is problematic (White 2015, 5).

15. *His* desires being all that were considered important in 1984, of course.

16. By proxy we mean it is an indirect measure, described in Chap. 2. Preference satisfaction has also been used widely in policy appraisal as a form of cost-benefit analysis (CBA) which values benefits according to people's willingness to pay (HM Treasury 2003), but these are contested (Dolan et al. 2011a).

17. Layard explains the principle of adaptation well in his book (2006, 48–49).

18. For more discussion on Mass Observation and two examples of their qualitative data on the meaning of happiness, please refer to Chap. 5.

19. For more information on these approaches, please see Chap. 5.

20. Elsewhere I have written that universities aren't necessarily that good at looking after the well-being of staff or students. See Oman and Bull 2021 and Oman et al. 2015, forthcoming.

21. The scale is named after its inventor, psychologist Rensis Likert. There can be confusion with Likert scales, when it comes to the middle of the scale and moderate or neutral options, as sometimes these will record 'don't knows', rather than my well-being is five.

22. Matarasso's (1997) 'now discredited' Use or Ornament report (Belfiore 2002; Merli 2002; Selwood 2002) was highly influential for its 'impressive sounding numbers' (Belfiore 2009, 348). It was described by the then Secretary of State as 'compelling', despite the 'paltry evidence' (Belfiore 2009, 348). One of the key methodological flaws highlighted by Belfiore are those relating to asking participants whether they were happier or healthier as a result of participation (2002, 99). The interview effect is an ongoing issue with qualitative research in the cultural sector, in which questions, such as Matarasso's: 'has the project changed your ideas about anything?' or 'since being involved I have been happier' lead the interviewee to respond positively—to appease the interviewer in some

way. These questions about the degree to which you can trust responses to these questions are a problem for evidence in a number of fields, particularly the cultural sector, that we will return to.

23. A representative sample is quite simply a sample that is representative of the population, in that it holds similar characteristics. It is useful when thinking about how different kinds of people will respond to questions, depending on their age, health, ethnicity, gender, and so on. If the characteristics of the sample are similar to that of the population studied, then they are more generalisable.

24. Qualitative researchers will often acknowledge how they affect the person being questioned. Interviews can be quite intimate meetings, where interviewers hear important details about someone's life. How that person relates to the interviewer will greatly affect what they say—the data. Also, qualitative researchers acknowledge their own relationship to the person being interviewed, the research questions or issues being discussed, even the 'research site'. This is called 'positionality' and in-depth qualitative research acknowledges how a researchers' position—be it race, gender or life experience, (e.g.) affects how they interpret qualitative data.

25. Focus group methodologists can often be very specific on the difference between a group interview and a focus group (see note 24 for great literature on how to do focus groups, and the limitations and benefits of different approaches).

26. As Table 3.1 acknowledges, resource is a big consideration. This is both in time processing data but also in compensating people to participate in data collection. If people give up their time for a focus group, it is important to consider compensation, at least in transport cost. This isn't a how-to guide but it may be relevant to factor this in to your thinking when designing your own research, or thinking about that of others.

27. For the benefits and complexities of focus groups, see Carey 1994; Crabtree et al. 1993; Hennink 2008; Kamberelis and Dimitriadis 2013; Kitzinger 1994; Liamputtong 2011.

28. Very briefly, my PhD looked at the Measuring National Well-being debate, conducted by the ONS in 2010 to establish what the UK should adopt as its measures of national well-being. My PhD reanalysed some of the debate data (described in this chapter), undertook policy analysis, observation of well-being experts, focus groups with people and interviews with key actors in the debate from the ONS.

29. See ONS n.d. and UN n.d. for more information.

30. Box 7.1 explains operationalisation in research in greater detail. Notably, Chap. 6 talks about operationalising an idea in policy, which is different from operationalising a concept for measurement in quantitative research. These are different applications of the same word, which can be confusing.

31. For additional detail, you may notice the first two questions will collect different kinds of data. Is your housing adequate? invites a yes/no answer (probably with a don't know option for best practice). How sanitary is your local environment? invites a scale, so you will probably offer someone a scale to mark. Perhaps a Likert scale, as described in note 18.

32. It is important to note that something being easier or more readily available for measurement does not necessarily mean it is accurate. Remember that the advice from the important, game-changing Sarkozy commission (see Chap. 2) was that each nation should devise its own measures. This is because each country has its own culture and priorities that may not be reflected in existing large-scale indices.

33. See the OECD Better Life Index website (OECD n.d.).

34. The politics of who were involved in well-being measurement are discussed by Bache (2012) in greater detail.

REFERENCES

Allin, P. 2007. Measuring Societal Wellbeing. *Economic & Labour Market Review* 1 (10): 46–52. https://doi.org/10.1057/palgrave.elmr.1410157.

Bache, I. 2012. Measuring Quality of Life for Public Policy: An Idea Whose Time Has Come? Agenda-setting Dynamics in the European Union. *Journal of European Public Policy* 20 (1): 21–38. https://doi.org/10.1080/1350176 3.2012.699658.

Bache, I., and L. Reardon. 2013. An Idea Whose Time Has Come? Explaining the Rise of Well-Being in British Politics. *Political Studies* 61 (4): 898–914. https://doi.org/10.1111/1467-9248.12001.

Beaumont, J. 2011. *Measuring National Well-being: A Discussion Paper on Domains and Measures*. Office for National Statistics. http://webarchive. nationalarchives.gov.uk/20160106195224/http://www.ons.gov.uk/ons/ dcp171766_240726.pdf.

Belfiore, E. 2002. Art as a Means of Alleviating Social Exclusion: Does It Really Work? A Critique of Instrumental Cultural Policies and Social Impact Studies in the UK. *International Journal of Cultural Policy* 8 (1): 91–106. https:// doi.org/10.1080/102866302900324658.

———. 2009. On Bullshit in Cultural Policy Practice and Research: Notes from the British Case. *International Journal of Cultural Policy* 15 (3): 343–359. https://doi.org/10.1080/10286630902806080.

BetterEvaluation. 2012. *Use Measures, Indicators or Metrics*. BetterEvaluation. https://www.betterevaluation.org/en/plan/describe/measures_indicators. Accessed 29 April 2021.

Bogue, K. 2019. *The Divisive State of Social Policy: The 'Bedroom Tax', Austerity and Housing Insecurity*. Bristol: Polity Press.

Cameron, D. 2010. Prime Minister's speech on wellbeing, Cabinet Office, *Prime Minister's Office*. https://www.gov.uk/government/speeches/pm-speech-on-wellbeing.

Carey, M.A. 1994. The Group Effect in Focus Groups: Planning, Implementing and Interpreting Focus Group Research. In *Critical Issues in Qualitative Research Methods*, ed. J. Morse, 225–241. California: SAGE Publications.

Clinton, J. 2011. Is David Cameron's Happiness Index Your Cup of Tea? *Express. co.uk*. https://www.express.co.uk/expressyourself/237065/Is-David-Cameron-s-happiness-index-your-cup-of-tea. Accessed 29 April 2021.

Crabtree, B., et al. 1993. Selecting Individual or Group Interviews. In *Successful Focus Groups: Advancing the State of the Art*, ed. D. Morgan, 137–149. California: SAGE Publications.

DEFRA. 2007. *Wellbeing: A Common Approach*. Working Conference Paper. DEFRA. Online. http://www.sdcommission.org.uk/sdc_images/commonapproachtowellbeing.pdf. Accessed 1 October 2016.

Dewey, J. [1934] 1958. *Art as Experience*. Capricorn Books.

Diener, E., and W. Tov. 2012. National Accounts of Well-Being. In *Handbook of Social Indicators and Quality of Life Research*, ed. K.C. Land, A.C. Michalos, and M.J. Sirgy, 137–157. Dordrecht: Springer Netherlands. https://doi.org/10.1007/978-94-007-2421-1_7.

Dodge, R., et al. 2012. The Challenge of Defining Wellbeing. *International Journal of Wellbeing* 2 (3) https://www.internationaljournalofwellbeing.org/index.php/ijow/article/view/89. Accessed 30 March 2021.

Dolan, P., and T. Peasgood. 2008. Measuring Well-Being for Public Policy: Preferences or Experiences? *The Journal of Legal Studies* 37 (S2): S5–S31. https://doi.org/10.1086/595676.

Dolan, P., R. Layard, and R. Metcalfe. 2011a. *Measuring Subjective Well-being for Public Policy*. Office for National Statistics.

———. 2011b. *Measuring Subjective Well-Being for Public Policy: Recommendations on Measures*. London School of Economics: Centre for Economic Performance.

DWP. 2012. *Welfare Reform Act 2012*. London: The Stationery Office. http://www.legislation.gov.uk/ukpga/2012/5/contents/enacted/data.htm.

Easterlin, R. 1973. Does Money Buy Happiness? *The Public Interest* 30 (3): 3–10.

Fleche, S., C. Smith, and P. Sorsa. 2012. *Exploring Determinants of Subjective Wellbeing in OECD Countries: Evidence from the World Value Survey*. 921. Paris: Organisation for Economic Cooperation and Development.

Freeman, M. 2013. Meaning Making and Understanding in Focus Groups: Affirming Social and Hermeneutic Dialogue. *Counterpoints* 354: 131–148.

Goertz, G., and J. Mahoney. 2012. *A Tale of Two Cultures: Qualitative and Quantitative Research in the Social Sciences*. Princeton University Press.

Gough, I. 2004. Human Well-Being and Social Structures: Relating the Universal and the Local. *Global Social Policy* 4 (3): 289–311. https://doi.org/10.1177/1468018104047489.

Graham, C. 2010. *The Challenges of Incorporating Empowerment into the HDI: Some Lessons from Happiness Economics and Quality of Life Research.* SSRN Scholarly Paper ID 2351536. Rochester, NY: Social Science Research Network. https://papers.ssrn.com/abstract=2351536 Accessed 30 March 2021.

Haybron, D.M. 2008. *The Pursuit of Unhappiness: The Elusive Psychology of Well-being.* Oxford: Oxford University Press.

Helliwell, J., L. Richard, and J. Sachs. 2015. *World Happiness Report 2015.* New York: UN Sustainable Development Solutions Network.

Hennink, M. 2008. Language and Communication in Cross-cultural Qualitative Research. In *Doing Cross-cultural Research*, ed. P. Liamputtong. Dordrecht: Springer.

Hicks, S. 2011. *Spotlight on Subjective Wellbeing.* ONS.

HM Government. 2005 *Securing the Future: Delivering UK Sustainable Development Strategy: Promises, Actions and Challenges.* Report. Sustainable Development Commission. https://research-repository.st-andrews.ac.uk/handle/10023/2301. Accessed 30 March 2021.

HM Treasury. 2003. *The Green Book: Appraisal and Evaluation in Central Government.* London: The Stationery Office. http://greenbook.treasury.gov.uk/.

Human Development Reports. 2020. *Human Development Data, United Nations Development Programme – Data Center.* http://hdr.undp.org/en/data.

ISTAT. 2015. *Il benessere equo e sostenibile in Italia.* ISTAT.

Jugureanu, A. 2016. A Short Introduction to Happiness in Social Sciences. *Belvedere Meridionale* 28 (1): 55–71.

Kamberelis, G., and G. Dimitriadis. 2013. *Focus Groups: From Structured Interviews to Collective Conversations.* New York: Taylor & Francis Group.

Kant, I. [1790] 1951. *Critique of Judgement.* Trans. J.H. Bernard. New York: Macmillan.

Kennedy, R.F. 1968. *Remarks at the University of Kansas,* March 18, 1968, John F. Kennedy Presidential Library and Museum. https://www.jfklibrary.org/learn/about-jfk/the-kennedy-family/robert-f-kennedy/robert-f-kennedy-speeches/remarks-at-the-university-of-kansas-march-18-1968. Accessed 30 March 2021.

Kitzinger, J. 1994. The Methodology of Focus Groups: The Importance of Interaction Between Research Participants. *Sociology of Health & Illness* 16 (1): 103–121. https://doi.org/10.1111/1467-9566.ep11347023.

Kovacevic, M. 2010. *Measurement of Inequality in Human Development – A Review.* UNDP.

Kroll, C. 2011. *Measuring Progress and Well-Being: Achievements and Challenges of a New Global Movement*. Berlin: Friedrich-Ebert-Stiftung.

Layard, R. 2006. *Happiness: Lessons from a New Science*. London: Penguin.

Levett-Therivel Sustainability Consultants. 2007. Wellbeing: A Common Approach. Working Conference Paper. *DEFRA*. http://www.sdcommission. org.uk/sdc_images/commonapproachtowellbeing.pdf.

Liamputtong, P. 2011. *Focus Group Methodology: Principle and Practice*. London: Sage Publications.

Matarasso, F. 1997. *Use or Ornament? The Social Impact of Participation in the Arts*. Stroud: Comedia.

Merli, P. 2002. Evaluating the Social Impact of Participation in Arts Activities. *International Journal of Cultural Policy* 8 (1): 107–118. https://doi. org/10.1080/10286630290032477.

Mirror. 2011. Guru Who Inspired David Cameron's Happiness Index Is Not Happy. *Mirror.co.uk*. https://www.mirror.co.uk/news/uk-news/guru-who-inspired-david-camerons-120819. Accessed 29 April 2021.

Morris, S. 2020. Mindfulness apps are booming in lockdown — how to stay chilled using your phone or on your own, *The Independent*. Available at: https://inews.co.uk/inews-lifestyle/wellbeing/mindfulness-apps-coronavirus-lockdown-explained-chilled-headspace-448667.

New Economics Foundation. 2009. *National Accounts of Well-being: Bringing Real Wealth onto the Balance Sheet*. New Economic Foundations. https://repository.uel.ac.uk/item/863zv.

O'Donnell, G., et al. 2014. *Wellbeing and Policy*. London: Legatum Institute.

OECD. 2011a. *Compendium of OECD Well-Being Indicators*. Paris: OECD.

———. 2011b. *How's Life? Measuring Well-being*. Paris: OECD.

———. 2013. How's life? 2013 Measuring well-being. *OECD (OECD Better Life Initiative)*. Available at: http://www.oecd.org/sdd/3013071e.pdf.

———. 2018. *Policy Use of Well-being Metrics: Describing Countries' Experiences*. No. 2018/07. Paris: OECD.

———. 2020. *Measuring Well-being and Progress*. OECD.

———. n.d. *OECD Better Life Index*. http://www.oecdbetterlifeindex.org. Accessed 27 September 2020.

Oman, S. 2015. Measuring National Well-being: What Matters to You? What Matters to Whom? In *Cultures of Wellbeing: Method, Place, Policy*, ed. S. White and C. Blackmore. London: Palgrave Macmillan.

———. 2017. *All Being Well: Cultures of Participation and the Cult of Measurement* [PhD Thesis]. The University of Manchester.

———. 2019. Re-ordering and Re-performing: Re-placing Cultural Participation and Re-viewing Wellbeing Measures. In *Cultures of Participation: Art, Digital Media and Cultural Institutions*, ed. B. Eriksson. Taylor and Francis.

———. 2020. Leisure Pursuits: Uncovering the "Selective Tradition" in Culture and Well-being Evidence for Policy. *Leisure Studies* 39 (1): 11–25. https://doi. org/10.1080/02614367.2019.1607536.

———. n.d. *How Data Works in Context*. Living with Data. https://livingwith-data.org/previous-research/how-data-work-in-contexts/. Accessed 30 March 2021.

Oman, S., and A. Bull. 2021, forthcoming. Joining up well-being and sexual misconduct data and policy in HE: 'to stand in the gap' as a feminist approach. *The Sociological Review*.

Oman, S., J. Rainford, and H. Stewart 2015. 'Stories of Access in Higher Education: A Triumph (or Failure) of Hope Over Experience? *Discover Society*, December 1. https://archive.discoversociety.org/2015/12/01/stories-of-access-in-higher-education-a-triumph-or-failure-of-hope-over-experience/. Accessed 28 April 2021.

ONS. 2009. *Measuring Societal Wellbeing in the UK: A Working Paper*. London: Office for National Statistics. http://www.ons.gov.uk/ons/guide-method/user-guidance/well-being/publications/working-paper%2D%2Dmeasuring-societal-well-being-in-the-uk.pdf.

———. 2015. *Measuring National Wellbeing: Personal Well-being in the UK, 2014 to 2015*. Newport: Office for National Statistics.

———. n.d. *Well-being*. Office for National Statistics. https://www.ons.gov.uk/peoplepopulationandcommunity/wellbeing. Accessed 30 March 2021.

Parfit, D. 1984. *Reasons and Persons*. Oxford University Press.

Rapley, M. 2003. *Quality of Life Research: A Critical Introduction*. London: SAGE Publications.

Rice, C.M. 2013. Defending the Objective List Theory of Well-Being. *Ratio* 26 (2): 196–211. https://doi.org/10.1111/rati.12007.

Rogers, S. 2012. Bobby Kennedy on GDP: 'Measures Everything Except that Which Is Worthwhile. *The Guardian*. http://www.theguardian.com/news/datablog/2012/may/24/robert-kennedy-gdp. Accessed 2 May 2021.

Scott, K. 2012. *Measuring Wellbeing: Towards Sustainability?* London: Routledge. https://www.taylorfrancis.com/https://www.taylorfrancis.com/books/mono/10.4324/9780203113622/measuring-wellbeing-towards-sustainability-karen-scott.

Selwood, S. 2002. Measuring Culture. *Spiked*. https://www.spiked-online.com/2002/12/30/measuring-culture/. Accessed 30 March 2021.

UNDP. 2015. *Sustainable Development Goals*. United Nations – Department of Economic and Social Affairs. https://sdgs.un.org/goals. Accessed 1 October 2019.

United Nations. 2020. *Are the HDI Dimensions Weighted Equally?* Human Development Reports. http://hdr.undp.org/en/content/are-hdi-dimensions-weighted-equally. Accessed 30 March 2021.

————. n.d. *Human Development Index.* Human Development Reports. http://hdr.undp.org/en/hdr-data. Accessed 29 April 2021.

White, S. 2006. *The Cultural Construction of Wellbeing: Seeking Healing in Bangladesh.* Number 15. http://www.welldev.org.uk/research/workingpaperpdf/wed15.pdf

————. 2015. *The Many Faces of Wellbeing.* In *Cultures of Wellbeing*, ed. S. White and C. Blackmore, 1–44. London: Palgrave Macmillan.

WHO. 1946. *Constitution of the World Health Organization.* World Health Organization. http://apps.who.int/gb/bd/PDF/bd47/EN/constitution-en.pdf?ua=1.

Williamson, T. 2010. Beyond Sprawl and Anti-sprawl. In *Critical Urban Studies: New Directions*, ed. J.S. Davies and D.L. Imbroscio. New York: SUNY Press.

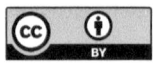

Discovering 'the New Science of Happiness' and Subjective Well-being

'The rise of well-being' in politics and policy-making emerges from developments across intellectual fields, including psychology, social policy, economics and social statistics (Bache and Reardon 2013, 908). In Chap. 2, we also discovered that happiness and well-being are linked, but different, and hard to define, while Chap. 3 offered a brief overview of how well-being data can be collected and analysed. We also discovered that questionnaires can be used in one-to-one interviews and national-level surveys, collecting qualitative and quantitative data.

Subjective well-being data are largely generated using questionnaires. These could be a paper form you may be asked to fill in before entering a weekly therapy session. These data would be looked at in isolation from data on others, are private and confidential, and will be used to track one person over time. Similar questions are increasingly used in national-level surveys, which can generate large-scale datasets to inform national indices. These won't be traceable back to the individual when analysed and are used to understand how populations and sub-groups are feeling, inviting comparisons between groups of people over time. The latter kind of subjective well-being data are then used to inform important decisions in policy development, monitoring and evaluation, and to promote behaviour change in populations. We are going to look at how these data gained popularity and standing in this chapter by looking at the rise of happiness economics and its impact on well-being data.

© The Author(s) 2021   119
S. Oman, *Understanding Well-being Data*,
New Directions in Cultural Policy Research,
https://doi.org/10.1007/978-3-030-72937-0_4

Chapter 2 explained that the discipline of economics also has trends over time and sub-disciplines. While people think of economics as primarily financial, it has far broader concerns and also tries to understand the value of things to people. For example, where the nineteenth-century hedonimeter project hoped to measure how people feel about things in a way that was 'more scientific', some economists have subsequently tended to focus on understanding what people do in the belief that this indicates what they value, and how they feel, whether subconsciously or consciously.

It is here that happiness plays a role for economics: to understand what makes people happy (in broad terms) at scale. Connectedly, to understand how to best go about measuring and modelling to establish this, and evaluate policy decisions of the past, in order to make better ones in future. This idea is based on the Greatest Happiness principle (Bentham 1996 [1789]), which you may recall from Chap. 2, and is elaborated here. We also spend more time thinking through what is meant by subjective well-being, and how it is defined in relation to happiness, before exploring categories of subjective well-being measures that are used, and what they do, or at least what they claim to. A key thing to keep in mind is that happiness economics measures more than happiness, using the broader (and more complicated) concept of subjective well-being.

We are going to look at the rise of happiness economics, for two main reasons: (1) it is acknowledged as one of the key drivers of the second wave of well-being, and (2) it positioned itself as a new science of happiness, advocating new measures, different data and analyses. This chapter, therefore, looks at how developments in psychology and economics come together to intervene in social statistics and social policy. The introduction argued that well-being data are used to (1) track the health and wealth of society using social statistics and (2) evaluate the success and progress of social projects and policies. Therefore, how all these interventions come together are key to understanding how well-being data *work*.

4.1   Happiness Economics

People down the ages have agreed that money can't buy happiness, though this exact form appeared only in the nineteenth century. (Cresswell 2010, 278)

Lord Richard Layard was called the UK's 'Happiness Tsar'[1] and his seminal book *Happiness: Lessons from a New Science* (Layard 2006) consolidates aspects of what Bache and Reardon call the second wave of well-being (Bache and Reardon 2013). The book presents the rationale behind 'happiness economics', which this chapter covers as the Greatest Happiness principle, combined with aspects of positive psychology, together with established well-being indicators and newer subjective well-being measures that we will come back to in greater depth throughout this Chapter.

The book *Happiness* is a call to action to do things differently, in a similar way to the politicians' statements and reports from international agencies we have already encountered. We are going to begin by looking at Layard's presentation of knowledge and understanding of well-being and data, as an example from the field of happiness economics. The book opens with the idea that money cannot buy happiness, explaining that this is 'no old wives' tale', but proven by 'many pieces of scientific research' (Layard 2006, 3).

The book opens with 'the Easterlin Paradox' (Layard 2006, 3) that we encountered in Chap. 2. In short, through looking at subjective well-being data, together with data on income, Easterlin found that while people with higher incomes tend to be happier than those with lower incomes, increased average income has not increased average happiness (Easterlin 1973, 1974). On this basis, Easterlin states that economic growth does not lead to an increase in happiness, at least in countries that are already relatively wealthy (Easterlin 2001). 'The Easterlin Paradox' remains a recurrent topic in discussions of well-being data and measurement, even though it has been challenged several times (most notably Stevenson and Wolfers 2008, 2012). Easterlin has nevertheless come out to defend the idea when it has been challenged (i.e. Easterlin et al. 2010) and much work continues to build on this thesis. For example, testing whether it is generalisable (i.e. Grimes and Reinhardt 2019), that is whether the theory works when tested in various ways across countries, contexts and wealth bands. The paradox therefore remains a compelling idea for economists.

The Easterlin paradox is a popular framing narrative to introduce the importance of well-being data and knowledge, especially when it comes to understanding society and policy. If he is not the opening gambit, he's near the top of the bill (e.g. see Adler 2013, 9; Alexandrova 2017, 4; Allin 2007, 47; Bache and Reardon 2013, 902; Benjamin et al. 2012, 18; Blanchflower 2008, 32). Or, more specifically, his findings published in 1973 are presented as the turning point in understanding the relationship between social progress and societal well-being. For if economic growth does little to improve social welfare, should it be a primary goal of government policy? Layard explains why not, as well as how economics can help us understand how not, with the help of philosophy.

The position taken is that 'much of the social progress that has occurred in the last two hundred years' has been driven by 'the Greatest Happiness principle' (Layard 2006, 5). The point of Jeremy Bentham's 'noble idea of utilitarianism' for Layard is that:

> it is fundamentally egalitarian, because everyone's happiness is to count equally. It is also fundamentally humane, because it says that what matters ultimately is what people feel.

The best society, therefore, is one where citizens are happiest and therefore the best policy produces the greatest happiness and the most moral action produces the most happiness for those affected (Layard 2006, 5). This is in tension with ideas of happiness maximisation, which is that people will, or should, have the right to pursue or consume or do whatever makes them happy, and they will always want more happiness. We touched on issues associated with individualism in Chap. 2, as fundamental ones of ideology and social justice.

Layard introduces eighteenth-century enlightenment philosopher Jeremy Bentham as a 'shy kindly man' who was a great thinker. He argues that Bentham's ideas had been difficult to apply in practice because 'so little was known about the nature and causes of happiness', which 'left it vulnerable to philosophies that questioned it' (Layard 2006, 5). The implication being, of course, that this has been resolved because 'the new science' means we now have this information. Indeed, the front cover of Layard's book proudly states using red block capitals in a golden sun-like graphic shape: 'INSIDE: THE SEVEN CAUSES OF HAPPINESS'.

It is actually rather brave for an academic to announce they know the causes of happiness; doing so asserts a degree of certainty that is infamously evasive. In fact, the influential Sarkozy commission report that also surveys the evidence, in particular from economics, notes:

> A general difficulty for the study of the determinants of subjective well-being is to distinguish between causes and correlates. (Stiglitz et al. 2009, 150)

Ironically, it is difficult to identify the 'seven causes' in the book, as they are not explicitly presented inside. Instead, on page 62, in a sub-section of a sub-section called Adult Life, and approximately half way through the chapter called 'So What Does Make Us Happy?' is a box, much like the ones in this book. Layard's is called 'The Big Seven factors affecting happiness'. The box lists family relationships; financial situation; work; community and friends; health; personal freedom; and personal values. It states the first five are in order of importance. Interestingly, they are able to be ordered by a sense of importance using data from the US General Social Survey. Freedom and values are added as 'two other key factors' and in a footnote, Layard explains: 'these last two factors cannot be ranked, but their relevance is shown in the table' (Layard 2006, 63; 255). It's not explicit why they cannot be ranked; it is also, therefore, not made clear why they were included to make seven, rather than five.

As you will see in the second half of this book, unequivocal claims that one thing 'causes' happiness, or improves well-being, rather than more modest claims, such as 'contributes to', 'is related to' or 'affects' are extremely difficult to substantiate. As with the Easterlin Paradox, which states that increased wealth does not [necessarily] cause increased happiness, it is difficult to claim something is a universal truth. Studies looking at similar relationships with similar data have not resulted in causal claims, and other evidence and theories that are drawn on are contested. Yet, as Chaps. 7 and 8 of this book demonstrate, we often find that useful insights with well-being data become repackaged to make causal claims, which when we look 'under the bonnet' should be a bit less assertive or emphatic.

Layard's 'big seven' may read a bit like an 'objective list'[2] of what is important to well-being, similar to those OECD and UK Office for National Statistics (ONS) examples from the last chapter. Coincidentally, Layard informed both of these organisations as an expert on the advisory panels. You will see that just as the categories differ slightly between the ONS and OECD lists, Layard's own list of categories as to what causes happiness differs slightly, again.

You may note that Layard's list does not explicitly include personal security and safety, as the domains discussed in the OECD example from Chap. 3. When you think about the concepts of safety and security, for you they may also sit in relationships, financial security or community. To re-cap briefly on Chap. 3, there are no perfect objective lists of the components of well-being, which tend to involve a subjective carving up of societal and personal concerns. In terms of data, objective lists of indicators tend to rely on 'proxies', by which we mean proxy measures where the thing we want to understand, say 'personal safety' or 'personal security' is measured by data that is seen to stand in for it, in some way, but is not exactly the same thing. The OECD example in Chap. 3 demonstrates how personal safety and/or security is difficult to measure directly and so 'self-reported victimisation' is used instead as a proxy. These are administrative data from crimes reported in individual countries (which of course is not the same as actual crime, risk or safety). The OECD replaced the proxy metric with 'feeling safe walking home at night'. Thus, an objective indicator has been replaced with subjective data, as it has come from surveying how someone feels, rather than the administrative data from reporting crimes. However, we can feel safe and secure because of different domains in our life, and we can feel unsafe and insecure across numerous domains as well.

Crucial to the story of data is the moment when well-being is acknowledged to be more than a list of objective indicators, such as crime rate per nation or in a local area. Instead, well-being is understood as how risk of crime is experienced. Even more crucial to this chapter is the delineation between subjective data about well-being and subjective well-being data. Somewhat confusingly, how people feel about crime is subjective data about an objective well-being indicator. Subjective well-being indicators are different again. They are about how we understand our own well-being and how we feel.

Replacing some proxies with subjective data about how people feel about an objective indicator, such as crime, still leaves many questions about personal well-being. To answer questions about personal well-being, we need more rigorous subjective well-being measures that tell us how people feel over time. This was the gap 'the new science' aimed to fill and the driving force of the new well-being indices.[3] This chapter goes on to unpack the development of subjective well-being measures: how they were decided on; what the different measures capture and what they do not, and so on. It looks under the bonnet of 'the science', its: history, theory, politics, data and its methods. First of all, we will return to the Greatest Happiness principle.

The Greatest Happiness? And Other Principles

It is said that Jeremy Bentham himself was not convinced that his political project would work, or indeed, could be proven, and he corrected the Greatest Happiness principle later in his life from 'the greatest happiness of the greatest number' to 'the greatest total sum of happiness'.[4] Let us briefly consider the limitations to the Greatest Happiness principle. There are pragmatic objections, which we shall deal with first. The principle assumes that happiness can be affected by what we do and what others do; therefore, happiness is a consequence of our own choices and behaviours, as well as those of others.

To apply the Greatest Happiness principle in policy, then, we need to be able to predict how different behaviours and actions affect happiness, so decisions can be made. In turn, this means we need to know what happiness is, and that behaviours, actions and happiness must be measurable. As we already know, agreeing on what either happiness or well-being is has long proved difficult for philosophers and more recently for measurers. We will also discover in Chaps. 6, 7 and 8, that measuring what we do at a large scale is also challenging. This makes it hard to be sure that one action (whether on a personal or policy level) has positively impacted on happiness, or if an alternative would have done better.

Of course, it is here that the new science is presented to best intervene. As Layard indicates, it generates data and the means to analyse them in order to address the pragmatic objections to the happiness principle. Yet, not all believe that happiness can actually really be influenced by targeted actions or changing an individual's behaviour. In contemporary society we see judgements regarding other's behaviours being demonised as bad for well-being (as discussed in Chap. 2), and in 'COVID-19 world', the endless recommendations that people go for a walk or a run have little consideration as to whether that is available to them (Ryan 2021). So, targeted actions are not universal.

Some argue that it is easier to improve those with better well-being first (Oakley et al. 2013, 23). Relatedly, 'the utility monster' was a thought experiment in ethics first developed in the 1970s. It presents a challenge to the Greatest Happiness principle, and to Utilitarianism, more generally. It asks what if a monster could accrue greater happiness from any given resource than anyone else? For example, imagine if being able to attend a concert in a park alone means that the utility monster is happier than all the other audience members in the local community put together. Following utilitarian principles, in order to maximise happiness overall, we'd have to ban everyone except from the utility monster from attending this concert, and potentially any future events ever again. More generally, if the way to maximise utility overall is to make the utility monster as happy as possible, even if this comes at the cost of everyone else's happiness, are we obliged to do so? While the designer of this thought experiment, Robert Nozick, was proving a point of his own, the issue remains, that achieving the Greatest Happiness principle is not unequivocally fair, or egalitarian.

As such, some argue that instead of focussing on happiness (or well-being), we should focus on social justice and equality. There is an uncomfortable tension in the well-being agenda and those of equality, diversity and inclusion.[5] We have previously touched on Aristotle's idea of a good life as dependent on a society supported by slaves. The question remains, at what or whose expense do the good lives of some, who make the 'good society' depend?

Returning to the Greatest Happiness principle, the main moral objection holds that it justifies a-moral means. This is owing to its consequentialist ethics: that if the aim is generating the most happiness for the most people, or the greatest total sum of happiness, then many actions *may* be justifiable. An easy way of imagining how this works is in the distribution of financial resources across a population. If you do something to improve the well-being of the largest number, it is highly possible that those who are marginalised (often the most vulnerable) in society will disproportionally suffer. We will return to this issue in the next chapter when we look at how Big Data and newer data practices disproportionately affect people of colour and the poor, for example. At the more dramatic end, such principles are argued against because they can be used to justify genetic manipulation, mind-control and dictatorship (Veenhoven 2010, 606). A useful example comes from science-fiction. Writer Ursula Le Guin's (2017) short story *The Ones Who Walk Away from Omelas* features a thriving, joyful city whose prosperous existence depends on the extreme misery of a single child that lives in a dungeon.

Another issue taken with the 'Greatest Happiness principle' emerges from questioning the value of happiness as a goal: is it too focussed on pleasure, or is it just an illusion? Some question whether happiness as a goal fosters irresponsible consumerism and that it makes us less sensitive to the suffering of others. In other words that 'happiness maximisation' leads people to pursue an idea of happiness that is fuelled by irresponsible consumption, or to do what makes them happy without considering the consequences. This never-ending pursuit of things 'to make us happy' is called 'the hedonic treadmill[6]' and never satisfies; people always want more happiness and have been encouraged to seek gratification in the wrong places, to the detriment of their well-being, social well-being and ecological well-being.

You may think this sounds a culturally specific idea of happiness that applies to Western consumerism and you may recall the example from Chap. 2 which points to the dangers of assuming *how* people value things, comparing a TV to a photo album. You may also be thinking of criticisms of economists' ideas of 'preference satisfaction' from Chap. 3, as well as those who disapprove of applying Western values, and valuation techniques to developing contexts, as we discussed was the case with the Human Development Index (HDI). You may also note that this idea of people as individual consumers seeking personal gratification is at odds with many societies that operate as collectives and, indeed, many of the values of societal well-being that the well-being agenda appeals to. These are not the only contradictions in the well-being agenda and we will continue to explore value judgements of what happiness is, and for who (especially if what we do, or are able to do is a driver of happiness) in further chapters.

John Stuart Mill was Bentham's godson and another key figure in the story of happiness and economics. He is said to have disagreed with the idea of general happiness as something universally experienced. He believed that happiness from a game of 'pushpin' was not comparable to that from poetry; that without the idea of higher and lower forms of happiness, we should have to believe that a dissatisfied Socrates was worse off than a satisfied fool (Layard 2006, 22; 118). These variations in values and value systems are some of the key tensions in the agenda, especially when they inform us of what is good for our well-being.

'The status race' between people is seen as a key contributor to unhappiness (Layard 2006, 7) and is one of the behaviours we are encouraged to adopt in our commercialised society. Yet, competition is considered a contributor to progress.[7] More than that, though, of course, there is competition between policy domains for resources and competition between academic fields to produce the method that gets used, the data that get used and the knowledge that gets used for policy.

There are several discussions surrounding how the well-being agenda addresses competition. On the one hand, it pretends to flatten competition, while on the other, it reinforces it. See OECD (2014) and concepts, such as 'sustainable competitiveness' (World Economic Forum 2013[8]). Other influential advocates for the well-being agenda naturalise a desire for 'success' and well-being measurements as tools for competition. For example, in a section entitled 'Why use wellbeing as a measure of progress in society?' in a report to a think tank, ex-Cabinet Secretary Lord O'Donnell explained:

> As individuals we all are keen to know how we are doing: Are we top of the class or in the middle of the pack? So how should we measure success? (O'Donnell et al. 2014, 10)

Layard's book both sells the Greatest Happiness principle, whilst also embracing some of the critiques, such as how the endless drive for happiness is bad for people and society, and how ideas of competition and success perpetuate this. There is a sense that some advocates of the movement cherry-pick, ignoring contradictions to tell a clear story, and this is familiar in criticism of the movement and its politics.[9] The focus on meaningful goals (Layard 2006, 197) will always lead to questions of meaningful for who and leading to happiness for who. The focus on individualising happiness as something we can (and should) address for ourselves is linked to prominent positive psychologist, Martin Seligman, and his ideas of 'authentic happiness' (2002). Here we move on to consider 'positive psychology' for its influence on happiness economists like Layard, and society more broadly.

4.2   Positive Psychology

> At this juncture, psychology can play an enormously important role. We can articulate a vision of the good life that is empirically sound and, at the same time, understandable and attractive. We can show the world what actions lead to well-being, to positive individuals, to flourishing communities, and to a just society. (Seligman 1998)

In his speech to the American Psychological Association (APA) in 1998, its new president outlined his hope for a 'positive psychology': a psychology which could help everyone as 'a new science of human strengths' (Seligman 1998). Positive psychology was more formally launched some two years later in a special issue of *the American Psychologist*. The editors: Seligman and Csikszentmihalyi framed it as a 'new science' for the new millennium (2000, 8).

The authors proposed a move away from psychology's pathologising tendencies, by which they meant that the academic discipline and practice of psychology typically concentrate on the negative and the abnormal, to instead focus on the 'positive features that make life worth living' (Seligman and Csikszentmihalyi 2000, 5). Subsequently, Peterson and Seligman developed a formal classification handbook,[10] *Character Strengths and Virtues* (2004). There were six virtues: wisdom and knowledge, courage, humanity, temperance, transcendence and a series of 'character strengths' (perhaps more traditionally called a trait) that fell under each category. Each of these character strengths is defined behaviourally, and it is recommended that it is measured using psychometric tests.

Having established a person's strengths, a range of 'empirically validated interventions' were proposed to make the most of their positive traits, rather than address their weaknesses (Seligman et al. 2005). This was seen to assist lasting happiness (Seligman et al. 2005). The authors attempted to 'present a measure of humanist ideals of virtue in an empirical, rigorously scientific manner' (Peterson and Seligman 2004, back cover). These claims were echoed in reviews at the time in publications such as the *American Journal of Psychiatry* (e.g. Cloninger 2005,[11] 821).

Positive psychology has been lauded (by Seligman and his co-authors) as uniting the dispersed and disparate lines of theory and research about what makes life most worth living (Seligman et al. 2005). In 2000, Seligman and Csikszentmihalyi recognised that 'positive psychology is not a new idea ... and [they] make no claim of originality' (Seligman and Csikszentmihalyi 2000, 13), instead arguing that they were able to present a 'cumulative, empirical body of research to ground' the ideas of 'distinguished ancestors'.

It is interesting that positive psychology is presented as a 'new science' and 'a cumulative body of research', as these are also Layard's claims in his book. These new, but linked, *sciences*, then, work on several levels as a valuable body of knowledge to claim that happiness can be a new science. The new science asserts that we now know the causes of happiness; that we now know the actions we have undertaken in the name of science, which are wrong; that these can now be measured; and that these measures can overcome philosophical queries via claims to science.

The happiness message here is that knowledge that is both policy-ready and accessible (popular, even 'pop') rests on clear and encouraging messaging (positive), innovation (new), authority (science) and morality (philosophy). It also, of course, must be measurable on an individual level that can be aggregated to population level.[12] It is, therefore, entirely dependent on well-being data, in particular the newer subjective well-being data that emerge from developments in positive psychology and economics' interest in happiness, as an idea that has appeal for policy-makers and the public.

4.3   Establishing a New Science of Happiness

Layard's (2006) book, *Happiness: Lessons from a New Science* emerged from a series of public lectures called 'Happiness: Has Social Science a Clue?' (Layard 2003). The LSE's well-being programme was founded as a result of Layard's public lectures. The website states:

Research from the programme has been devoted to understanding the causes of wellbeing and how wellbeing affects other outcomes that policy-makers care about (such as education and physical health). (LSE Centre for Economic Performance n.d.)

The LSE's well-being programme foregrounds making well-being knowledge popular by way of 'lessons', making knowledge 'that policy-makers care about'. These words might imply that the aspects of happiness that policy-makers don't care about fall outside of the remit of the centre. This is indicative of a general feeling amongst some social policy areas that the work that they do is 'invisible' to policy-makers (as with Holden 2012, in the case of culture). Such a feeling is corroborated by academic research (e.g. Stevenson et al. 2010; Gray 2004) and evidence that some domains of social policy hold more sway with policy-makers than others.

Knowledge that policy-makers care about is, therefore, very much a concern. Let's remember from Chap. 1 that the very idea of using well-being data to inform policy decisions (evidence-based policy) hangs on the idea that policy-makers *can* make neutral and objective decisions—if fed the right evidence. We have discovered already many indications to the contrary, as with the different interpretations of poverty data to suit political arguments in Chap. 1. We also know that 'facts' which reinforce established moral beliefs (or what we *feel* is right) are attractive to policy-makers and the public (Davies 2018) as confirmation biases. What we see here is the possibilities for the new 'science[s] of happiness' to become influential, with some believing the field is dominated by economics' adaptations of psychology's tools.[13] It is easy to see how this might be the case, as a result of their capacity for persuasive arguments that we come to later in this chapter.

Economics (and its sub-disciplines) tend to have much influence with governments and multi-lateral institutions (like the UN, where many countries are represented in the decision-making processes). However, economists have not necessarily presented ideas in accessible ways as a rule. Their relevance to decision-making institutions is also a matter of tradition: they have long-held sway and so are highly represented in the decision-making process. Similarly, decision-makers tend to be literate in the principles of economics and in the UK, there is a trope that all MPs attend the very same course at Oxford or Cambridge universities: PPE (Philosophy, Politics and Economics)—to the extent that it 'runs Britain' (Beckett 2017). Decision-making processes are reputedly controlled by Treasury's economic approaches, including the valuation techniques discussed in Chap. 2. Economics *for* well-being is an easier message to communicate than economics' more abstract ideas, and borrowing the language of positive psychology is useful in promoting ideas that governments are, and individuals should be, taking positive action themselves.[14]

What we can also see, therefore, is the appeal of happiness in making economics an applied and more relatable discipline. This attraction can be seen in the increase in journal articles on well-being in the EconLit database (EconLit (n.d.) and see Chap. 2). Yet, despite the increase in happiness economics papers and emphasis on the increasingly robust 'science' of well-being (O'Donnell et al. 2014; Helliwell et al. 2015; ONS 2015a and 2015b), the lack of conceptual consensus outlined in Chap. 2, and expanded on in Chap. 3, has remained a concern for policy-making (Fleche et al. 2012, 11). Layard himself told a journalist (Rustin 2012) a decade ago that we were a decade away from well-being measures that are good enough for policy to be made using them. Yet numerous policy recommendations have been made on account of these measures over the last decade, as this book can attest to.

In their advisory paper to the ONS' MNW Programme, Dolan, Metcalfe and Layard explain that any measure of well-being must be 'empirically rigorous', by which they mean 'that the account of wellbeing can be measured in a quantitative way that suggests that it is reliable and valid as an account of wellbeing' (Dolan and Metcalfe 2012, 411). Although the insistence that any empirically robust account must always be quantitative is preferred practice for certain disciplines, that does not mean it should not be questioned. Measurement of well-being basically wants to understand either change over time or difference between people or groups of people. These data can be captured by qualitative approaches, such as diaries or photographs, as described in Chap. 3, and do not *need* to actually be quantitative, therefore.

The authors continue by making an important point regarding any measure of well-being: that it should 'be sensitive to important changes in well-being and insensitive to spurious ones. In practice, distinguishing between the two is quite a challenge and often relies on judgement based on a priori expectations' (Dolan and Metcalfe 2012, 411). Returning to the well-being data examples we have already come across in Chap. 3, whether the OECD indicators or a small-scale questionnaire, understanding someone's well-being using data gathered from any questions will have limits.

Recalling our hypothetical example of understanding whether a concert in a local park might improve well-being, how do we understand which aspects of the experience were the contributing factors? How can you dis-aggregate the contribution of the park, from the music itself, the people you were with, or the quality of the hotdogs for sale or the length of the toilet queue? Let alone understand which contributes to longstanding well-being or momentary happiness? Distinguishing between important changes to well-being and spurious ones is difficult, and therefore well-being data do not always meet Dolan et al.'s (2011a, b) criteria. Evidence of the impacts of particular activities and interventions on well-being is often criticised, as we discovered in Chap. 3: generally, if you ask certain questions because you seek a causal relationship, you are most likely to find it. The same is therefore an issue for well-being research more gener-ally. The theory of confirmation bias is an account of how people tend to respond to causal messages which reinforce what they already believed or which suits their way of living and or thinking.

Thinking of the Facebook posts that have appeared on my feed in recent years, many different accounts, traditions and philosophies (that we have touched on briefly in this book) appear in the posts: we should try harder, we are trying too hard; we should visualise what we want and go for it, we spend too much time living in the future and not enough in the present and so on. All of these memes get shared because they appeal to things the person sharing already believes. Well-being wisdom repackaged is a large part of the wellness industry without any of the concerns with contradictions or evidence against the claims made. It appears that happi-ness economics may be similarly equipped to package simple ideas and positive psychology with long-held traditions, empirical evidence and call itself a new science.

There are several takeaways from this overview of the new sciences of happiness. First, that happiness economics seems to dominate the social sciences of well-being. Bearing in mind that all social sciences could be argued to be about understanding and improving well-being in some way, it is happiness economics that appears to be at the forefront—and that has certainly seen the largest increase as a discipline. This is because it has gained 'scientific authority' based on a couple of factors. First, is the com-bination of historical examples of moral philosophy, narratives of innova-tion and claims that the measures are growing increasingly robust. Second, these aspects are presented as simply as possible for media, policy and public audiences. Yet, the multidimensional nature of well-being means that it remains extremely difficult to remove confounders which include philosophical and empirical contradictions. It is, therefore, challenging to make and substantiate simple claims to *know* 'the causes of well-being', for example. Econometric models typically used to analyse subjective well-being data may lay claims to robustness, but are still not economically sound (see Cooper, in McKenzie 2015) and use data collected by questions that do not necessarily translate to the general public (as we shall discover later in the chapter).

These measures are, by the admission of prominent well-being experts, not neutral or objective measures of subjective well-being, but also involve subjective categorisation lists of people's strengths or moral character (such as that in positive psychology) or a country's development (as in the Human Development Index), as well as being the result of a process of decision-making when it comes to which data and how to model them. Having looked at the disciplines that have led to this new science of well-being, we will now turn to the data that inspired it and are generated by it. Specifically, we look at the ideas of subjective well-being and the methods that have shaped subjective well-being data and their prominence.

4.4   What Is Subjective Well-being?

Notions of subjective well-being or happiness have a long tradition as central elements of quality of life. (OECD 2013, 10)

How Is This Well-being Measure Subjective?

This portrayal of the 'new science[s]' of happiness is (as Seligman hints) not as new as implied, but also results from fundamental theories and indicators of well-being that date back centuries. One important—yet confusing—distinction is that there is the idea of experienced well-being (how we experience well-being or happiness) that gets called subjective well-being and then there are measures of well-being that form objective lists, like the OECD's, that are based on subjective data.

As we have seen, objective approaches to measuring well-being investigate the objective dimensions of a good life (using largely proxy indicators). However, the subjective approach examines people's subjective evaluations of aspects of their own lives by collecting numeric data. For example: 'on a scale of 1–10, how safe do you feel walking home at night?' This is not the same as how people feel about their well-being.

As we have also seen already, a number of well-being indices that were established around the same time have recognised the importance of taking people's perceived well-being into consideration alongside objective lists in order to measure overall well-being. Subjective well-being data are generally captured using questions about how people feel they are doing. We are going into more detail about this now, in order to understand how these data can differ, and how they are different from the objective well-being indicators and the qualitative data described at length in the previous chapter. Crucially, it is the subjective well-being data about how we think our own well-being is that are the driving force of happiness economics and the second wave of well-being (Bache and Reardon 2013). As we shall discover, this is largely down to the influence of key advocates, such as Layard, in the well-being agenda.

Let's consider the UK's ONS' subjective well-being data. As we have previously discovered, it uses four questions to understand what it calls 'personal well-being'. The questions are:

1. Overall, how happy did you feel yesterday?
2. Overall, how satisfied are you with your life nowadays?
3. Overall, to what extent do you feel the things you do in your life are worthwhile?
4. Overall, how anxious did you feel yesterday?

How are these data used? The answers to these questions are on a scale of 0–10 and could be traced over time to see how an individual is doing. This is not going to happen in an anonymous national-level survey; instead aggregated data are used to understand population-level well-being over a specific period or to compare population sub-groups by geography or ethnicity, for example.[15] Some of these questions with almost identical wording have been in surveys, and therefore generated data, for decades before 'the ONS4' were invented. Therefore, there are baselines to measure change against. The fact that these data have been collected over time can help establish how a major event such as COVID-19 has affected the well-being of the population, as well as more minor events. Chapter 7 runs through an example of how a policy change over ten years affects life satisfaction scores over a decade, for example.

These subjective well-being data can therefore be used to see how a particular event affected anxiety, alongside other social and structural issues, such as, say, poverty. Again, this does not mean that, for example, an individual's household income is looked at against their anxiety levels, but that average anxiety of everyone who was asked the question (or, as we might say, the population sampled) is measured against the average household income levels. There are two things to remember about samples, the first is that few surveys are completed by a whole population, so the data collected almost always come from a sample; the second is that sampling is cleverly worked out so that if you sample enough of the population, you can make generalisable claims. Therefore, while national-level surveys do not measure nations in their entirety, they can make good estimations using mathematical rules. The other thing to say is that poverty can be measured using whatever indicator has been decided to represent poverty. There are numerous poverty indicators, which could be household income, for example, or the IMD (index of multiple deprivation). As we discovered in Chap. 1, 'Introducing Well-being Data', poverty is not one absolute, objective thing when it is discussed in parliament. Politicians cherry-pick from absolute and relative poverty measures and across different timeframes to arrive at the most complimentary statistics for their argument. So, what subjective well-being is measured against can also be subjective, in that the data and their uses are not automatically neutral or without bias, but are indeed chosen.

What Well-being Means to People Is Subjective

While we have covered what subjective well-being means previously, it is important to note that what well-being means for people in their everyday lives is subjective. Recalling the free text field analysis discussed in Chap. 2, when people are asked what is important to their well-being, they present different kinds of answers, about different areas of their life.[16] Similarly, you might look at the aforementioned four questions from the ONS and think, 'well they don't capture my well-being!' You might also think about how your answer to a question about life satisfaction will have fluctuated across a year, or even a day: meanings may not be constant and bad days at work or a bad commute will make it fluctuate, affecting how you might answer the questions on how satisfied and happy you are overall. Alongside these smaller, more everyday interferences to our mood are the major events, such as grief, injury, sudden or long-term unemployment, divorce, or of course, the generalised anxiety caused by an international pandemic. Answers to these questions can reflect a fleeting positive experience, such as attending a concert, or reflect something you are missing out on, on a longer term: good relationships, a stable job, mobility or good mental health. When we come to the different measures, we shall see how these are accounted for—to a degree.

As we shall discover, subjective well-being is complex to capture in a way that can inform behaviour. There are often trade-offs to supposedly positive choices. People who enter into adult education as mature students, for example, gain the pleasure of learning and feeling purpose in their life (Duckworth and Cara 2012), and although the negative effects are less studied (Field 2009), people miss many hedonic aspects of subjective well-being that they were previously used to, because time and energy for social and leisure activities are further compromised (Aldridge and Lavender 2000). The same can be seen in data about parenthood (i.e. Pollmann-Schult 2014): it's rewarding, but you lose fun, time, money and autonomy; other relationships suffer and it can be unexpectedly lonely (Oman and Edwards 2020). A simpler binary, as found by White and Dolan (2009), is that time spent with children is relatively more rewarding than pleasurable, whereas time spent watching television is relatively more pleasurable than rewarding.

The measurement of well-being aims to capture how life is lived in society so that we can know how people are getting on. But this happens at a scale that means the subjective experience of well-being can be lost. Different people have different opinions on whether this is important to the overall measurements of well-being of populations. Experts who are great with numbers work on the basis that if your unit of analysis is a population (as in population level), and as long as those whose experiences don't fit the story are outliers, then, it will statistically even out. Therefore, crucially, these measures are not necessarily meant to capture how everyone feels about everything. Instead, they are meant to be able to compare whether particular groups are affected or how things might change over time. The aim of these measures is to do better at measuring how people are doing overall, so that better policy decisions can be made.

Others argue that measuring well-being can obscure ill-being,[17] particularly in already marginalised populations (Ahmed 2012; Tate 2016, 2017). There is concern that people who are already vulnerable are placed at further risk through the way that policy deals with data. For example, an issue which has gained prominence since the #MeToo movement is sexual harassment in universities. These cases can be obscured as they might be considered 'outliers', and so not get picked up by data which looks for overall well-being trends (Oman and Bull 2021, forthcoming). Similarly, marginalised experiences of ill-being are generally less visible

(Tate 2016; Oman and Bull 2021, forthcoming; Oman et al. 2015). In Chap. 3, we briefly touched on the capacity of the domains and indicators in the OECD index, and how unlikely they would be to find the impact of policy change, like Bogue's research on the 'bedroom tax'. Capturing well-being data at scale, therefore, does not always pick up the complexity or subjectivities of ill-being.

The second wave of well-being is distinguished from the first, because it sees the collection of data about how people feel, at scale. For this to be effective, people need to relate to the ideas of well-being they are being asked to think about in the survey questions used. However, people do not always relate to the task at hand, or, even understand the questions asked. In my primary research, people talked about how they felt about the idea of measuring well-being (Oman 2017a), as they did in the ONS' national consultations (as discussed in Oman 2015a, 2020). In both cases, some said it was a waste of time; that we have more important things to worry about. Others said that they didn't understand how what is measured reflects their experience, or they didn't understand the questions (Oman 2015a). As we will discover, the ONS also found this when they trialled the ONS4. So, although subjective well-being measures are thought more democratic (because they are about how people feel), they are—of course—by and large decided by experts and defined by experts, who preside on advisory boards and write influential working papers to the ONS and international agencies. What we see is a tension between 'robust approaches' and 'understandable to everybody'.

Definitions of Subjective Well-being

Subjective well-being encompasses different aspects (cognitive evaluations of one's life, happiness, satisfaction, positive emotions such as joy and pride, and negative emotions such as pain and worry): each of them should be measured separately to derive a more comprehensive appreciation of people's lives. (Stiglitz et al. 2009, 16)

Subjective well-being measures aim to capture a number of aspects of how well-being is experienced. This moves the focus from the idea that what matters in a good life is the presence of a specific set of life circumstances or material conditions. Nevertheless, using objective indicators with subjective well-being ones enables estimates of the impact that material conditions (measured with objective indicators) have on how people feel about their life (subjective well-being measures).

Measuring subjective well-being therefore lends itself to analyses of which circumstances and conditions are important for well-being (Kahneman and Krueger 2006). Looking at subjective well-being data also, then, helps to understand the gap between material living conditions and people's own evaluation of their circumstances (Helliwell 2003). These sorts of relationships are normally tested with a specific research question, for example: 'how does wealth improve subjective well-being?' You would pick what variable or data you would like to use to measure wealth: personal income, household income, property value, or identify where someone sits on a scale of poverty and wealth using a marker, such as their postcode. You would then pick how you wanted to measure subjective well-being. Using the ONS4 example, you might want to test the difference between how satisfied someone is with their life nowadays, or overall (life satisfaction) with how happy they say they were yesterday and the relationship between these two and wealth. One such example of this is a paper called 'High Income Improves Evaluation of Life but Not Emotional Well-Being' (Kahneman and Deaton 2010).

The OECD which 'exist[s] to promote policies that will improve the economic and social well-being of people around the world' (oecd.org) have also reported guidelines on measuring subjective well-being. The OECD propose a relatively broad definition:

> Good mental states, including all of the various evaluations, positive and negative, that people make of their lives and the affective reactions of people to their experiences. (OECD 2013, 16)

As this book is not aiming to provide a definition or statement of determinants of well-being, but offer the tools to understand how others use and understand well-being data, we are going to look at an overview of subjective well-being.

The diagram (Fig. 4.1) illustrates the key components of subjective well-being, contextualising them in the theories we have encountered before. You may remember from Chap. 2 that the eudaimonic is based on Aristotelian (c. 330 BC) teachings, and can most simply be understood as purpose or flourishing. The hedonic begins with Epicurious ([341–270 BC] 1994), but is more familiar with the well-being agenda as a utilitarian

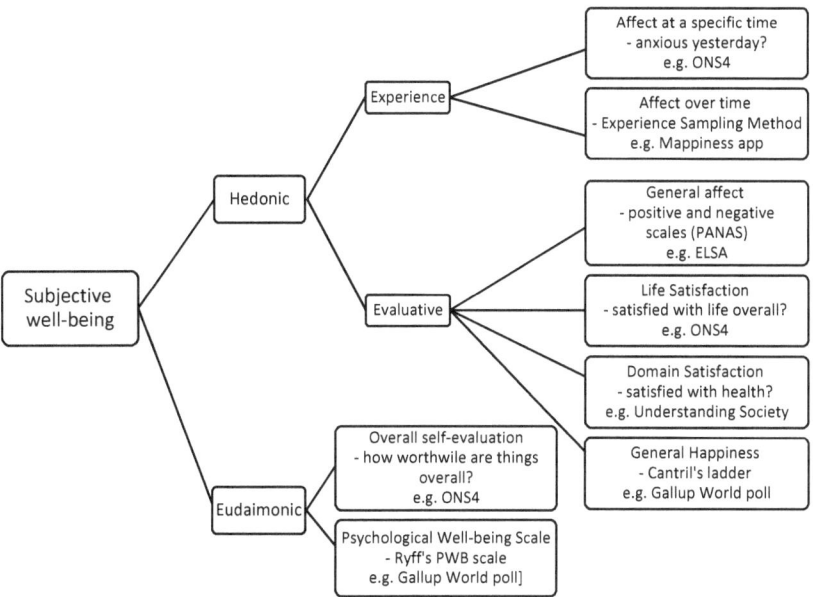

Fig. 4.1 Accounts and examples of subjective well-being measures. (Adapted from Oman 2017a)

principle (Bentham 1996 [1789]). It is most simply understood as pleasure, but more accurately means positive feeling.

You will see how the divide of pleasure versus purpose is then captured as measurable aspects of life, and how they relate to each other, whether that is in someone's experience and feeling, their satisfaction or a sense that their life is worthwhile in various ways.[18] Inside each bubble on the right-hand side is the name of the type of subjective well-being measure (i.e. Life Satisfaction), underneath that is an example of the question or method used, and underneath that, a survey in which these questions have been used (the anomaly being ESM, which is not really used in national-level surveys, as I will explain, but is suitable in mobile apps data collection). I found it took me a long time to acclimatise to the idea that all of these measures and approaches are called subjective well-being; that they are related, yet so varied in approach, and use similar language. The next section walks you through this diagram, with examples from each 'bubble', to hopefully give you a better idea of how they work together.

Table 4.1   Subjective well-being measures and their uses in policy

	Monitoring progress	*Informing policy design*	*Policy appraisal*
Evaluation measures	Life satisfaction	Life satisfaction Domain satisfaction, for example: Relationships; health; work; finances; area; time; children	Life satisfaction Domain satisfactions Detailed 'sub'-domains satisfaction with services
Experience measures	Happiness yesterday Worried yesterday	Subjective well-being measures	Happiness and worry Affect associated with particular activities 'Intrusive thoughts' relevant to context
Eudaimonic measures	Worthwhile things in life	Worthwhile things in life 'Reward' from activities	Worthwhile things in life 'Reward' from activities

Adapted from Dolan et al. (2011a)

4.5   Subjective Well-being Measures for Decision-Making

There have been many attempts to classify the different ways in which subjective well-being can be measured for policy purposes (Kahneman and Riis 2005; Dolan et al. 2011a, b; Waldron 2010). According to the recommendations on measuring well-being to the ONS, there are three uses for any well-being measure in policy: monitoring progress, informing policy design and policy appraisal (Dolan et al. 2011a). There are also three broad types of subjective well-being measure: evaluation (global assessments), experience (feelings over time or at specific times) and eudaimonic (reports of purpose and meaning, and worthwhile things in life). Table 4.1 shows how each of the three 'types' of subjective well-being can be used to measure well-being in a way which best informs policy. This section walks you through the array of subjective well-being measures and methods that feature in Fig. 4.1.

Evaluation Measures

Life satisfaction is the most commonly used evaluative measure of well-being (Fleche et al. 2012). Life satisfaction data are collected using questions similar to question 2 in the ONS4, 'Overall, how satisfied are you with your life nowadays?' The measure is popular with economists for policy-relevant research for numerous reasons. First, because of its longstanding prevalence in international and national-level surveys, such as Health Survey England, and more recently, the OECD's high-profile Better Life Index. Second, it is thought to be accessible to policy-makers (Donovan and Halpern 2002). Third, some believe it to be the idea of subjective well-being that overlaps most successfully with how people make decisions in their own lives (Kahneman et al. 1999). However, some evidence suggests that, as a concept, life satisfaction is not understood by all members of the general public, particularly those who are marginalised in some way (Oman 2017a; Ralph et al. 2011). We might also question how universal a measure it is in developing contexts, which calls into question its utility on a global scale.

General happiness has been used as an alternative to life satisfaction and features in many international-level surveys. Key happiness variables seem to impact on general happiness responses in a similar way as life satisfaction (Dolan et al. 2011a, b; Waldron 2010). The measure aims to assess a person's general happiness, and a popular example of trying to collect data on this concept is Cantril's (1965) 'ladder of life'[19] (see Fig. 4.2). The Gallup World Poll uses the principles of Cantril's ladder, where the questions are asked using a scale. This is a 'self-anchoring ladder', which asks respondents to evaluate their current life from 0 (*worst possible life*) to 10 (*best possible life*).

The term 'general happiness' can be used in reports (i.e. World Happiness Reports Helliwell et al. 2017, 2019) to mean the general happiness of a nation, or indeed, as John Stuart Mill[20] intended, 'the sum of individual *happinesses*' (Mill, cited in Crisp 1997, 78). This can be confusing and is something to be mindful of. It is not always clear if the term general happiness, when used to refer to population happiness, means taking individual-level data from something like Cantril's ladder and multiplying it to derive a population-level measure, or if it is another measure, such as life satisfaction, used at scale.

Domain satisfaction is an approach which is interested in how people evaluate different features of their life, such as 'work-life balance' or 'relationships'. These different features of our lives are grouped together into domains, which we have seen as a prominent feature in the objective lists approach. With the UK's national well-being domains, that would be: personal finance, the economy, what we do, health (Physical and mental),

Best Possible

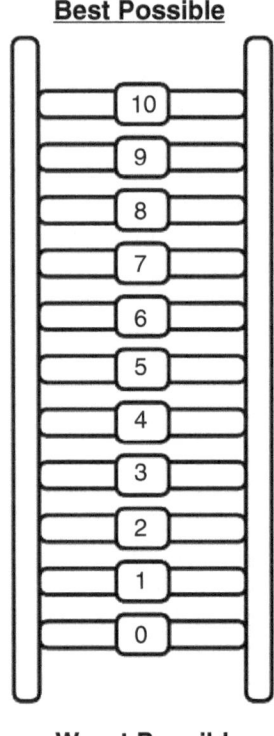

Worst Possible

Assume that this ladder is a way of picturing your life. The top of the ladder represents the best possible life for you. The bottom rung of the ladder represents the worst possible life for you.

Indicate where on the ladder you feel you personally stand right now by marking the circle.

Fig. 4.2 Cantril's ladder. (Adapted from Cantril 1965)

education and skills, our relationships, governance, where we live, the environment. In theory you could collect satisfaction data about each domain, and if a person were satisfied with all domains this could demonstrate overall 'life satisfaction'.

An example of a question to derive domain satisfaction data is from Understanding Society: UK Household Longitudinal Study (University of

Essex et al. 2020), in which respondents are asked to rate their satisfaction with their general health on a scale from 'completely dissatisfied' to 'completely satisfied'. Domain satisfaction data can be used to compare the reality of life with various standards of success (Veenhoven 1996, 30). Various domain satisfaction measures have been shown to correlate with numerous socio-demographic characteristics relative to income, health and gender, for example, and this has been replicated across studies (Dolan et al. 2008). Confusingly, sometimes the term 'domain satisfaction' is used to describe satisfaction across all domains (van Praag et al. 2003) but it more frequently refers to satisfaction within a specific domain, such as 'satisfaction with personal relationships', or 'satisfaction with health' which both appear in the UK's national well-being measures. As with the case in this index, domain satisfaction is most often used in an objective list approach with other administrative data. This means not all the domains are measured using satisfaction data, but with proxy data, such as crime rate or education level.

Affect is a term used to describe the experience of feeling or emotion and is prevalent in psychology. As an aside, the term has recently been taken up in the broader social sciences and humanities to describe emotion and experience in a less medicalised way (Sedgwick and Frank 2003; Thrift 2004; Massumi 2002; Ahmed 2010; Berlant 2011; Wetherell 2012, etc.). While the concept is linked, these theoretical uses of the concept of affect are not really captured by surveys, which is an important distinction that is rarely acknowledged.

General Affect means how people are doing overall and is a concept which is understood in evaluation questions. In psy-sciences,[21] it is the relative frequency of positive and negative affect that is thought to be key to how we experience well-being. The Affect Balance Scale (Bradburn 1969) and the Positive and Negative Affect Scale, or PANAS (Watson et al. 1988; see Fig. 4.3), involve questionnaires that are designed to gain numerical responses to general statements about different affects. These questions are also used in some large-scale surveys, such as the English Longitudinal Study of Ageing (ELSA n.d.).

Influential psychologists Huppert and Whittington have cautioned for some time that different versions of positive and negative scales are less similar than implied. Also, these scales are susceptible to change and adaptations in surveys. This must be accounted for when considering subjective well-being metrics which use them. Affect is also a key part of experience measures, which want to capture affect at a particular time or context.

This scale consists of a number of words that describe different feelings and emotions. Read each item and then list the number from the scale below next to each word. **Indicate to what extent you feel this way right now, that is, at the present moment OR indicate the extent you have felt this way over the past week (circle the instructions you followed when taking this measure)**

1 Very slightly or not at all	2 A little	3 Moderately	4 Quite a bit	5 Extremely

_____ Interested		_____ Irritable	
_____ Distressed		_____ Alert	
_____ Excited		_____ Ashamed	
_____ Upset		_____ Inspired	
_____ Strong		_____ Nervous	
_____ Guilty		_____ Determined	
_____ Scared		_____ Attentive	
_____ Hostile		_____ Jittery	
_____ Enthusiastic		_____ Active	
_____ Proud		_____ Afraid	

Scoring instructions:
Positive Affect Score: Add the score on items 1, 3, 5, 9, 10, 12, 14, 16, 17, and 19. Scores can range from 10 – 50, with higher scores representing higher levels of positive affect. Mean Scores: Momentary = 29.7 (SD = 7.9); Weekly = 33.3 (SD = 7.2)

Negative Affect Score: Add scores on items 2, 4, 6, 7, 8, 11, 13, 15, 18, and 20. Scores can range from 10 – 50, with lower scores representing lower levels of negative affect. Mean Score: Momentary = 14.8. (SD = 5.4); Weekly = 17.4 (SD = 6.2)

Fig. 4.3 PANAS questionnaire. (Adapted from Watson et al. 1988)

Experience Measures

Experience measures aim to capture a person's feelings at a given, specific time which can be thought of as 'the amount of affect felt in any moment' (Dolan et al. 2011a, 7). Measures are constructed with the *Benthamite* view that certain aspects of life are good or bad, based on their qualities of 'pleasurableness' or painfulness (Crisp 2006). How happy, sad or anxious any person is at a particular time is re-conceived as well-being by taking the average balance of pleasure (or enjoyment) over pain, measured over the relevant period. As already pointed out directly above, there is some evidence that positive and negative affect do not directly predict each other and should therefore be measured separately. Heeding Huppert and Whittington's concerns (2003), positive psychology has more recently begun to conceive of well-being as a continuum (ONS n.d., 3; Diener et al. 2009), rather than something which can be assessed by taking the average of positive and negative measures. The experience approach relied on in surveys will tend to specify a period of time for you to remember how you felt. In the ONS4, this is the only account with two questions, one for happy yesterday and one for anxious yesterday (see also Table 4.1). As well as specifying the exact moment you want someone to recall, other methods capture people's emotions at multiple points in a day or week, and for that reason, they are not really included in national-level surveys, which would be difficult to administer. However, they are suitable for mobile apps, as we shall discover.

The Day Reconstruction Method (DRM) (Kahneman et al. 2004) is perhaps the most renowned of numerous measures which attempt to capture experienced well-being over time which is called the *experience sampling method (ESM)*. The DRM is a diary-based technique, through which participants reflect on the main episodes that affected them on the previous day and recall the type and intensity of feelings. In other words, it literally takes a sample of feelings from specific days and weeks. Affect is an aspect of subjective well-being that is particularly sensitive to immediate surroundings and activities (Smith and Exton 2013, 230). This is why it is considered suitable for understanding the relationship between what we do and how we feel, as well as situational aspects of life that affect us.

For example, short-term affect data can be collected through DRM approaches to include information about both activities and locations, as well as the affective states accompanying them (Kahneman and Sugden 2005). Such an approach has the potential to capture data on how people spend their time and the 'experienced utility' (Kahneman and Sugden 2005) of such activities. For example, 132 teachers in the Netherlands completed a daily diary on three consecutive work days as well as a background questionnaire (Tadić et al. 2013). The researchers found that despite a lack of work-life balance, working hard was not necessarily detrimental to the teachers' happiness scores. If you take these scores at face value, then if the teachers were ambitious, then striving towards their goals was satisfying, but this motivation was not necessarily constant.

The Ecological Momentary Assessment (EMA) (Stone et al. 1999) is based on self-reports of well-being at specific, but often randomly chosen points in time. Reports explicitly include self-assessments of behaviours and physiological measures, but also the recording of events. In Chap. 5, we discuss how an app alerts its users to record how happy they feel at random moments, allowing the user (and whoever is capturing their data) to track their mood over time and establish what is good for their mood. The researcher who developed 'mappiness' has used these data to measure a number of aspects of happiness: that we are most miserable commuting, on the one hand, and that 'happiness is greater in natural environments', for example (MacKerron and Mourato 2013; Krekel and MacKerron 2020). These data have also been used (Fujiwara and MacKerron 2015) to compare how happy people feel doing different kinds of activities from birdwatching, to making love; and more specifically, between artforms, such as watching the performing arts or reading alone.

An exploration of the determinants of, and changes to, affect and time-use may offer understandings of how people's 'experiences of utility' vary. Returning to the example of the local, subsidised concert in Chap. 3, again, the questions we asked there can help us understand how people's responses to the cost, amount of time and effort vary, and how that changed their declaration of how they felt. This may be at odds with the 'utility' assumed by 'the provider', whether that is the local council, a theatre company or another funder.

However, it is important to remember that people who attended our hypothetical park concert, self-selected to do so. This is one of the key issues with valuing how people experience social and cultural activities: it makes it difficult to say how a particular experience might affect others in the future (Dolan et al. 2011b, 12). Also, people are liable to 'mind wanderings', which can mean they are not thinking of what you think they are when you ask them how they are feeling (ibid.: 8). Furthermore, what makes sense, or represents the experience of one person may not manifest in the average of a sample.

These approaches ostensibly measure at different points during the day and they relate to experiences associated with specific activities and time points. However, because in a national-level survey, large population samples are questioned at certain points during the year, it is not feasible to repeatedly survey respondents during a particular day. As an alternative, the rationale with the ONS4 experience measures is to 'replicate' or 'proxy' ESM approaches by asking respondents for their experiences and feelings relating to a whole day (yesterday).

While there is potential for the measurement of change in affect and time-use longitudinally, questions remain as to whether existing national-level survey data can capture the sensation and emotion of 'situated experience' (how it felt, to be there, in that moment) in a meaningful way, and to do so over time. In cultural policy studies, there is often a call for longitudinal measurement of the relationship between cultural participation and aspects of well-being. It is thought that this will solve some of the proclaimed issues with the evidence base (around data and causation, discussed in the latter chapters of the book). However, while longitudinal analysis can help address issues of causal direction in the evidence, they will not address issues related to capturing the duration of the impact of an experience, and this also is not always clearly understood (Oman 2017b).

'Eudaimonic' Measures

Some conceive of eudaimonia as part of subjective well-being (Dolan et al. 2011a, b), while others choose to conceive of subjective well-being as purely hedonic ('happiness', 'life satisfaction' and 'affect'). Eudaimonic or 'eudemonic' theories conceive of people needing purpose and as having various underlying psychological needs, such as control and connectedness (Ryff 1989). Likewise, that satisfying these needs contributes towards well-being independently of any pleasure they may bring (Hurka 1993). These accounts draw on Aristotle's 'eudaimonia' as what makes for a good life.

Psychological Well-being
In the 1960s, Harold Dupuy, psychologist at the National Center for Health Statistics, developed his Psychological General Well-being *(PGWB) Schedule*, a questionnaire of 68 items to measure the psychological distress of the American population. It was reduced and simplified to 18 items for introduction to a general health survey in the 1970s and then increased to

22 items to become the *PGWB Index*. One of the case studies in Chap. 7 uses the PGWBI, adapted again for an Italian survey.

Developed by psychologist Carol D. Ryff, the 42-item *Psychological Wellbeing (PWB) Scale* measures six aspects of well-being and happiness: autonomy, environmental mastery, personal growth, positive relations with others, purpose in life and self-acceptance (Ryff 1989). Again, different versions of the scale have been adapted to suit different contexts, including an 18-item version (Ryff and Keyes 1995). Ryff and Keyes (1995) compared their eudaimonic measures with evaluations of life satisfaction and happiness, finding that self-acceptance and environmental mastery were associated, but that positive relations with others, purpose in life, personal growth and autonomy were less well correlated.

Worthwhileness and Overall Evaluation

More simply, eudaimonia is related to ideas of worthwhileness that are connected to the diagnosed psychological needs listed above and, but can also be addressed with one question, as with the ONS in Fig. 4.1. White and Dolan (2009) measured the 'worthwhileness' associated with activities using the DRM method. They found some discrepancies between those activities that people find 'pleasurable' as compared to 'rewarding'. The example they used is that spending your time watching telly brings pleasure, but few rewards, while spending time with children is the opposite.

How These Measures Can Be Applied

There are important distinctions when considering how aspects of happiness economics can apply value to what we do. Recalling the photo album versus TV example from Chap. 2, it can be difficult to ascribe value to others' activities. Ateca-Amestoy has tried to explain the value of leisure as a psychological need for different kinds of experiences, and which impact on how we evaluate our quality of life.

> [L]eisure is a human need to be fulfilled by household production and consumption of what we may call 'leisure experiences'. Those experiences are commodities that fall directly within the individual's determination and assessment of his/her quality of life. This means that leisure is one of the arguments of the individual's utility function, one of the instances from which he/she will achieve well-being. (Ateca-Amestoy 2011, 53)

The importance of understanding the different kinds of well-being benefits offered by different types of leisure has been an aim of high-profile research over the isolated periods of COVID-19 lockdowns (https://www.covidsocialstudy.org/). That some activities offer hedonic utility, such as streaming and television watching, and some offer eudaimonic, such as reading (and some both, of course), is being studied (Bu et al. 2020; Mak et al. 2020; Nuffield 2021). However, what people do is often polarised as 'watching television excessively' (Bu et al. 2020, 7), with claims that 'these changes in behaviours and mental health are reflected in people's assessments of the differences in their lives between this lockdown and that of spring 2020' (Nuffield 2021). This is slightly misleading: from the evidence presented, we do not know that it is people's behaviour that has changed people's assessments of their lives, when policy-making and poor weather in a pandemic are arguably having a greater affect than watching the telly. As you may recall, this is one limit of applying the 'Greatest Happiness' principle and can also be the consequence of confirmation bias. For example, the Sarkozy Commission contrasted 'cultural events' with 'poor leisure'[22] (Stiglitz et al. 2009, 49) and Layard's analysis of television's negative effects was inevitably biased by an idea of good leisure.[23] However, as we have discovered, assumptions as to what qualifies as good leisure and poor leisure are problematic ethically, and will not present universal results.

That pleasure and reward do not map onto each other neatly aligns with Aristotelian thinking. The think tank, New Economics Foundation (NEF), has been highly influential in UK well-being research since the mid-2000s. Its definition of well-being is 'developing as a person, being fulfilled, and making a contribution to the community' (Shah and Marks 2004, 2). The report, 'A Well-Being Manifesto for a Flourishing Society' (Shah and Marks 2004), called for well-being to be foregrounded and for governments to work towards a 'flourishing society' with 'happy, healthy, capable and engaged' citizens (Shah and Marks 2004, 2). In 2008, NEF introduced a set of guidelines called the 'Five Ways to Wellbeing', based 'around the themes of social relationships, physical activity, awareness, learning, and giving' (Aked et al. 2008, 17), summarised as connect, be active, take notice, keep learning and give.

The 'Five Ways' have proven successful, and have been adopted in parts of the National Health Service and by organisations such as Mind, the mental health charity,[24] as well as many other social policy areas. Individual institutions have chosen to adapt it when offering well-being advice to staff and other members of the institution. The University of Manchester, for example (The University of Manchester n.d.), has adapted it into its 'six ways to well-being' which is used to frame its advice to students and staff. The cultural sector has embraced the guidelines, both in arts practices aimed at improving well-being (Dodd and Jones 2014) and as a means of evaluation of eudaimonic and broader well-being aspects of cultural engagement (Daykin and Joss 2016). According to a review of the evidence from international arts and health literature, '[t]he benefits from arts programmes resonate strongly with the evidence-based "five ways to wellbeing" model of mental health: connect, take notice, keep learning, be active, give' (Bidwell 2014, 3).

The success of the 'Five Ways' is down to legibility of its framework to many policy sectors, people in the general population and policy-makers. Let us briefly return to the takeaway conclusions from how the new sciences of happiness generate knowledge that is both policy-ready and accessible (popular, even 'pop') rests on clear and encouraging messaging (positive), innovation (new), authority (science) and morality (philosophy). The Five Ways to well-being meet all of these criteria, perhaps more than the idea of subjective well-being in and of itself. We will move towards closing, by looking at the ONS4 as a case study to understand the importance of legibility, transparency and understanding, when deciding on how to collect subjective well-being data.

4.6   Case Study: Subjective Well-being, by the Office for National Statistics' Design

The UK's national well-being measures are categorised into ten domains. These are as follows: Our Relationships; Health; What we do; Where we live; Personal Finance; Economy; Education and Skills; Governance; Environment; Personal Well-being.[25] Each of the ten domains is composed of multiple indicators, just like the OECD's index that is described in detail in Chap. 3. The subjective well-being domain was named personal well-being, because it was thought to make this domain more understandable to a general audience, which was considered particularly important to the MNW programme.[26] This domain comprises 'the ONS4'.[27] Table 4.2 presents the questions, together with their rationale.

'The ONS4' were designed to capture three types of subjective well-being: evaluative, eudaimonic and affective experience. The four

Table 4.2 The ONS4 capture different aspects of well-being

ONS' questions on personal well-being	Specific perspectives on personal well-being, from which the questions are drawn
'Overall, how satisfied are you with your life nowadays?'	This comes from the evaluative approach to measuring subjective well-being (i.e. a cognitive assessment of how life is going)
'Overall, to what extent do you feel the things you do in your life are worthwhile?'	From the eudaimonic approach
'Overall, how happy did you feel yesterday?'	This is about experience, specifically positive affect
'Overall, how anxious did you feel yesterday?'	Experience, negative affect

Source: Adapted from Allin and Hand (2017)

individual subjective well-being questions ask people to give their answers on a scale of 0 to 10, where 0 is 'not at all' and 10 is 'completely'. The ONS considered consolidating the figure of all four measures to provide a single measure of personal well-being. Just as with the HDI in Chap. 2's discussion of objective lists, this single number is easier to communicate and is most often discussed in national media and by politicians. It was, however, not considered conceptually robust to do so. Here, again, we see a tension between robust and easy to understand.

The first results from trialling the ONS4 were published in April 2011 (ONS 2011a). The aim was to gather responses from survey participants which are an 'assessment of their life overall, as well as providing an indication of their day-to-day emotions' (ONS 2015a, 5). 'The ONS4' gained National Statistics status in September 2014 and, since then, have continued to be introduced to surveys across government. They are, therefore, not necessarily intended to be used by themselves. Table 4.3 shows the variety of these surveys and the sorts of data they capture. The Government Statistical Service has more recently published advice on the harmonisation of the ONS4 (Nickson 2020). This aims to ensure subjective well-being statistics and data are 'comparable, consistent and coherent' across government departments and beyond.

While we know that the ONS4 capture the different aspects of subjective well-being, and there were many reports and working papers from the time, it was quite difficult to find methodological or administrative detail readily

Table 4.3 Surveys containing the ONS4

Organisation	Survey	Topics covered	First asked	Frequency of update
Office for National Statistics (ONS)	Annual population survey	Labour market data including employment and unemployment, as well as housing, ethnicity, religion, health and education.	April 2011 to March 2012	Annual
	Wealth and assets survey	Level of assets, savings and debt; saving for retirement; how wealth is distributed among households or individuals; and factors that affect financial planning.	July 2011 to June 2012 (Wave 3)	Bi-annual
	Living costs and foods survey	Household spending patterns for the consumer prices index and for GDP figures and detailed information on food consumption and nutrition.	April 2011 to March 2012	Annual
	Crime survey for England and Wales	Experience of crime and attitudes to crime-related issues such as the police, the criminal justice system, and perceptions of crime and anti-social behaviour.	April 2012	Annual with quarterly updates
	Opinions and lifestyle survey	Collects information on a variety of topics that are too small to have surveys of their own. Topics that have been previously commissioned include smoking habits, cancer awareness, charitable giving, climate change and disability.	April 2011	Monthly
University of Oxford and ONS	Time-use survey	Diary entry survey. The substantive domains are main activity (49 categories), secondary activity (10 categories), location and means of transport (11 categories) and with whom (8 categories). The temporal identifier holds information on the time when episodes start and end.	April 2014 to March 2015	Annual

(*continued*)

Table 4.3 (continued)

Organisation	Survey	Topics covered	First asked	Frequency of update
Cabinet Office	National Citizenship Services Evaluation	Social mixing; transition to adulthood; teamwork, communication and leadership; and community involvement.	2014	Not updated
	Youth social action survey	Social action (only satisfaction and worthwhile included).	2014	Annual
Department for Work and Pensions (DWP)	Life opportunities survey	Measures how disabled and non-disabled people participate in society in a number of areas which include: • work • education • social participation	2013 to 2014	Not updated
	The National Study of work search and well-being findings	Psychological health and well-being of jobseekers allowance (JSA) claimants.	2011	Not updated
	English longitudinal study of ageing (ELSA)	Information on the health, social, well-being and economic circumstances of the English population aged 50 years and older.	April 2012 to March 2013	Annual
Department of Health	What about YOUth? Survey	Young people's health, diet, what they do in their free time, bullying and whether they smoke, take drugs or drink alcohol.	2014	Not updated
Ministry of Defence (MoD)	Armed forces continuous attitude survey (AFCAS)	Information on the views and experiences of MoD personnel which helps shape policies for training, support, and the terms and conditions of service.	2012	Annual
Department for Business, Energy and Industrial Strategy (BEIS)	Families continuous attitude survey (FAMCAS)	Information on personals in the MoD spouses in a number of areas including accommodation, healthcare, education and childcare, and deployment.	2012	Annual
	Impact of FE learning survey	Attitudes towards further education, including funding, readiness of information, guidance and decision-making process.	2012	Not updated

(continued)

Table 4.3 (continued)

Organisation	Survey	Topics covered	First asked	Frequency of update
Department for Communities and Local Government (DCLG)	English housing survey	Age, type, condition and energy efficiency of housing stock and the characteristics of households.	2013 to 2014	Annual
The Department for Digital, Culture, Media & Sport (DCMS)	Taking part survey	Participation in and engagement with cultural and sporting activities at the individual level, and pathways in and out of participation and engagement.	2013 to 2014	Annual
	Community life survey	Volunteering, charitable giving, local action and networks, and well-being.	2013 to 2014	Annual
Food Standards Agency	Food and you	Reported behaviours, attitudes and knowledge relating to food issues such as reported food purchasing, storage, preparation and consumption. It also looks at eating habits, influences on where respondents choose to eat out and experiences of food poisoning.	2014	Bi-annual
Welsh Government	The National Survey for Wales	Opinions on a wide range of issues affecting people living in Wales and their local area.	April 2012 to March 2013	Annual
Central Statistics Office Ireland	Quarterly national households survey	Labour force estimates that include the official measure of employment and unemployment in the state (International Labour Organisation (ILO) basis).	2013	Well-being module not updated
Natural England	Monitor of engagement with the natural environment (MENE): The natural survey on people and the natural environment	How people use the natural environment, includes the: • type of destination • duration • mode of transport • distance travelled • expenditure • main activities • motivations • barriers to visiting	2012 to 2013	Annual

(continued)

Table 4.3 (continued)

Organisation	Survey	Topics covered	First asked	Frequency of update
UK Civil Service	Civil service people survey	Civil service staff attitudes and experiences of work.		
Sainsbury's, Oxford Economics and National Centre for Social Research	Living well index	What does it mean to live well? How well are we really living as a nation, and why? This study aims to provide the answers—by defining, measuring and tracking, over a number of years, what it means to live well in Britain.	2012	Annual
Higher Education Statistics Agency	Measuring graduate subjective well-being outcomes through destination of leavers from higher education (DLHE)	The survey which will gather insightful and comprehensive information about graduate outcomes. The four ONS personal well-being questions are optional.	2017	Annual
One Parent Families Scotland and Scottish Poverty and Inequality Research Unit at Glasgow Caledonian University	Single parents' community connections survey	Aims to be the largest ever survey of single parents in Scotland. The results will feed into OPFS and GCU's community connections project funded by the Scottish government innovation fund. The project aims to tackle isolation, loneliness and poor mental health among single parents.	2018	Not updated
The Land Trust	Perceptions survey and social value study	The Land Trust is dedicated to providing free public open space for the benefit of communities. Land Trust commissioned carney green to undertake a social value assessment of its sites.	2015	Not updated
Natural Resources Wales	People Survey 2015	Our people survey was carried out in order to gauge honest opinions from staff on how they feel about working for Natural Resources Wales.	2016	Not updated

(*continued*)

Table 4.3 (continued)

Organisation	Survey	Topics covered	First asked	Frequency of update
Active Lives survey	Sport England	Measuring the number of people aged 14 and over taking part in sport and physical activity.	2015	Annual
Centre for Regional Economic and Social Research	Active lives survey— children and young people survey	Includes 3 of the ONS4—does not include the anxiety question.	2017	Annual
(CRESR) and Institute for Employment Research (IER), University of Warwick	Big lottery talent match survey	An evaluation survey of the initial entrants onto the talent match programme. The overall objectives of the programme are to support 25,000 individuals with the goal of 5400 entering employment.	2014	Not updated
Isle of Man Government	Health and Lifestyle Survey 2017	The areas of interest for this survey were: • general health • diet and physical activity • smoking • alcohol and drug consumption • well-being	2016	Annual
Higher Education Policy Institute	Student academic experience survey	The survey investigates the learning and teaching experiences of students, including satisfaction with courses, reasons for dissatisfaction, experience of different-sized classes, total time spent working, perceptions of value for money, institutional spending priorities and a focus on student well-being.	2014	Annual

Source: ONS

available on how the questions themselves were decided on. In particular, the final wording chosen. In parallel to my PhD research, and after much searching, I found a detailed report to the Technical Advisory Group (Ralph et al. 2011) on the findings from 44 interviews.

This report is phase 2 of qualitative findings from testing the ONS4. Notably, not all the responses to the trials were positive in this report. Limitations were found in how able people were to answer the questions.

Interestingly, when it came to the life satisfaction question (thought to be the most robust, as you may remember), not everyone thought that being satisfied with life was positive; some believed it neutral and some thought it a negative commentary on their lives (Ralph et al. 2011, 5). With the 'worthwhile' question, answers were affected by what was seen as social desirability, leading to inflated scores. This is known as response bias, and meant that certain people (arguably with lower subjective well-being) did not want to appear as if they did not have worthwhile lives to the interviewer (Ralph et al. 2011, 5). A later phase in the cognitive testing also details how, when the questions are administered face to face, people felt uncomfortable giving negative scores in front of loved ones (ONS 2012, 7).

When it comes to understanding the meaning of the questions, the qualitative report also states that:

> Where the question was not understood this tended to be by those with lower educational attainment. This group simply did not understand the term 'worthwhile'. (Ralph et al. 2011, 5)

In some ways, what is more concerning is that:

> For the most vulnerable respondents, answering this question was distressing and in some cases respondents became visibly upset. It is recommended that ONS investigate the possibility of creating a flier that interviewers can leave with respondents, which tells them where they can seek help if it is required. (Ralph et al. 2011, 5)

Having a protocol at the end of research interview, should the interview have covered sensitive issues, is standard ethical practice in qualitative research, but less so in survey collection methods. It is not clear whether filers were trialled after asking participants these questions.

In summary, there were a number of issues that the qualitative research in 2011 uncovered with these four questions. These include: how accurately people were able to answer, based on their understanding of the questions; how honestly people felt capable of being when answering sensitive questions; and that arguably these questions could be detrimental for someone who was not experiencing good well-being. These issues revealed by the testing were brought to the attention of the programme's advisory groups.

The minutes from the Technical Advisory Group in 2011 outline the importance placed on these four questions. Lord Layard refers to these questions as 'the work of the ONS' and outlines that it is the status of this work that is the aim of the wider MNW programme, which reiterates the importance of this new subjective well-being data to the broader agenda. Layard also outlined his concerns that the 'UK is less likely to set international agenda if introducing unnecessary changes' (ONS 2011b). These minutes might suggest that what was learnt from the trials were unlikely to be able to change the new measures, which we have discovered were built from a synthesis of disciplines and authority.

The Technical Advisory Group (TAG) had disappeared from the ONS publications archive when I was originally undertaking this research to try and 'follow the data', and understand the methodological origins of the questions. However, I was able to find a record of the group by way of a fellow researcher. The National Statistician, Jill Matheson, refers to a National Statistician's Advisory Forum and a Technical Advisory Group. All traceable records of TAG meetings are headed by a list of those present. Only ONS, civil service and academic economists were present at the meetings in the minutes I was able to locate. However, another academic researcher confided to me during my ethnography fieldwork that there was a clear hierarchy in the programme and psychologists were rarely listened to, with the economics experts dominating proceedings. This appears to be substantiated by minutes regarding the development of the SWB measures (ONS 2011a). It also corroborates claims that economists dominate how evidence is presented, acknowledged and applied in these forums. However, it is important to note that these are not impartial accounts, either.

Psychologists reflecting on phase 2 of the testing of the questions advised that they could cause psychological distress in some participants, but this concern is absent from other outputs. Notably the report on phase 3 (ONS 2012) mentions it found no issue of difference in legibility for different people, unlike phase 2 (Ralph et al. 2011). More importantly, however, it does not acknowledge that one phase of research found the ONS4 questions to be detrimental to well-being. As you can see, looking under the bonnet of the data presents questions about how the measures work in practice, how they are decided on and by who, and what evidence of success becomes part of record and what disappears. It also reveals issues with regards to how data collection on well-being can be detrimental to well-being that are rarely considered.

4.7   Summarising What Measuring Subjective Well-being Does

So, as we have discovered, subjective well-being is often characterised as being concerned with happiness alone (OECD 2013, 10). Instead, subjective well-being is a more complex combination of various aspects of the lived experience; it involves several distinct ideas with disciplinary and theoretical histories. While these concepts can sometimes correlate when measured, the evidence for this remains inconclusive (Clark and Senik 2011 in Fleche et al. 2012, 9). Research using secondary subjective well-being data, therefore, should clearly establish the conceptual differences between different components of subjective well-being, to be sure that what is aimed to be measured is what is actually being measured. Furthermore, this could be better communicated.

While subjective well-being has been thought to predict behaviour in meaningful ways (Diener and Tov 2012), the subjective well-being measures we have encountered are thought valuable because they enable an empirical examination of the factors which cause improved or reduced well-being (Fleche et al. 2012, 10). Some economists (such as Layard) believe that these qualities make these approaches an improvement on traditional micro-economics approaches which rely on notions of utility. Utility, as we discovered in Chap. 2, is the idea that satisfaction is experienced by consuming a good or service and that 'rational choice' drives consumers to remove dissatisfaction (or discomfort) and to maximise on this satisfaction.

In general, subjective well-being data allow for an assessment of the positive or negative contribution of one factor (such as public libraries) over another, which may seem unrelated (such as being made redundant), to well-being. This therefore allows an appraisal of different factors which can be both monetary and non-monetary (Fleche et al. 2012). However, we must also remember that it can be difficult to separate spurious from essential well-being effects, and doing so often relies on human judgement.

The qualities of these newer measures of subjective well-being have led to influential figures, such as Lord O'Donnell[28] arguing for 'a well-being approach' to inform decisions that manage COVID-19 (O'Donnell 2020). O'Donnell and other advocates for this type of well-being approach argue that well-being measures should inform 'trade-offs' and 'the true costs of lockdowns', for example, by declines in mental health and access to healthcare (O'Donnell 2020). It could be a means of deciding the balance between how one policy move related to protecting the economy (which includes people's jobs) to another, such as healthcare (which includes its own financial considerations and multiple mortality rates). It is also this approach that helps unpick the assumed correlation between having money and attaining happiness that we opened this chapter with.

The different definitions of subjective well-being further complicate issues for those wanting to use well-being data in their research or to understand the research of others. The confusing naming conventions, overlapping definitions and disagreements as to what counts as subjective well-being, objective well-being, personal well-being or societal well-being also don't help those wanting to understand the ways in which well-being measurement more broadly furthers knowledge of the human experience. There is also work to be done on how the different ideas of subjective well-being overlap with longstanding cross-disciplinary beliefs and assertions regarding the value of different domains of life to well-being that we will encounter later in the book. In short, there is a transparency gap in the discussions of rigour, classifications and measures in the 'science' and the legibility of what that means to everyday people, despite the efforts made to do so.

4.8   CONCLUSION

Looking at the invention of subjective well-being measures in the UK offers context behind the ubiquity of well-being measurement practices. Understanding the recent history behind a specific way of measuring a particular idea of well-being, that is considered robust and universal, is vital to appreciate the limitations of such projects. This chapter's comprehensive survey and critical lens aims to offer tools to promote better understanding of the power of these well-being data, their capacity to change culture and society, and the limits of their application in areas of social and cultural policy and practice.

In short, 'the new science of happiness' has much to offer understandings of well-being and the human experience more generally. The techniques, whether originating as national-level social survey questions or personal psychological tests, can be adapted and applied to other environments and have been used widely to understand the impacts of COVID-19. Yet, politics, disciplinary and international competition compromise their neutrality. These contexts are vital to understanding the subjective well-being data generated through survey questions and their uses to inform important decisions in policy development, monitoring and evaluation, and the way these, then, promote behaviour change in people.

We have seen evidence that the national well-being *measurers* want to be top of the class, with possibilities that complexities of the questions in certain contexts were disregarded. This leaves us with questions. Could it be that in the keenness to compete in the new science and the international game of devising the best measures, considering the subjective experience of people answering questions on subjective well-being may have been side-lined? It transpires that less attention is paid to the qualitative trials of questions that end up as 'robust measures' than you may imagine, as I also found with some questions long-used to measure class (discussed in Chap. 9). Yet, should it be a great surprise that quantitative researchers and national statistics offices tend to overlook the qualitative aspects of their methodologies? It is hard to say because such evidence is hard to find.[29]

We have used data on the contexts behind subjective well-being data to understand them better: who collected them, interpreted them, looks after them and uses them. We have seen some trends emerge across people and policy, but found these contextual data have limits to what can be understood, too. It can be hard to find all the archival information we need, and it can be easy to interpret the absence of evidence as some sort of cover-up, when actually in policy-making and public services, institutional memory is often lost through the 'churn' of staff and these issues of paper trails. There is, sadly, 'no culture of a repository of knowledge' (Hallsworth et al. 2011, 8). Thus, the data we have on how data are made can be as compromised or limiting as the quantitative or qualitative data we have been discussing in these last two chapters.

This chapter has looked at the new sciences of happiness as people, publications, projects, politicians, agencies and disciplines. Easterlin is presented as the turning point in this tale, because he offers a useful narrative device. However, the limitations of how economics was used to understand human flourishing have been known longer—as presented in Chap. 2—and indeed in the introduction to Easterlin's paper. Discovering the stories behind data in this way, we are able to see how all these different components work together to make the well-being agenda. We can also see that it is the subjective measures, rather than the compiling of objective lists, that are the greater driver of the agenda, and that this is—in part—owing to claims to innovation.

Essentially, however, the new sciences of happiness: the new measures and uses of data from old questions (Allin and Hand 2017), are the driving force behind the well-being agenda. At least what we have referred to as 'the second wave' in this book. Without the technological advances and the advocacy for the new measures, we might ask, would we have seen calls for the change in policy? Thus, the terms data-driven decision-making and evidence-based policy-making take on new meaning—where the promise of the possibilities of well-being data changes the policy rhetoric and call for more data to be collected. Data do not only capture social change, but ensure it, and as the next chapter demonstrates, it feels as if Big Data increase this pace of change, but how do they impact on well-being?

NOTES

1. It is difficult to pinpoint exactly when Layard's nickname became so prevalent. One of the earliest references is in Jeffries (2008). UK Prime Minister Tony Blair began appointing special policy advisors in 1998, which led to the media nickname of 'tsars' (see Levitt and Solesbury 2012 on policy tsars).
2. Crucially, causes of well-being and objective lists of well-being indicators are similar, but not the same. With the OECD example from Chap. 3, perception of safety of the local neighbourhood is a proxy indicator of well-being, but is not necessarily a primary cause. There is a conceptual difference between a condition indicating well-being and a cause of well-being.
3. It may be helpful to know that index is a rare word that has two plurals, indices and indexes.
4. Both Layard (2006) and Davies (2015) offer engaging commentaries on Bentham and his relationship to the Greatest Happiness principle that are worth referring to if this history interests you.
5. While equality, diversity and inclusion are ostensibly the same agenda, and the words are used interchangeably, there are differences in the separate agendas.
6. Further descriptions of the hedonic treadmill can be found in Layard (2006), 48–49.
7. For a comprehensive engagement with how the logic of competition has bled into all aspects of everyday life, see Davies, W. 2014. *The Limits of Neoliberalism: authority, sovereignty and the logic of competition.* London: Sage.
8. See particularly Chapter 1.2 'Assessing the sustainable competitiveness of nations'.
9. Will Davies describes the cherry picking in the weell-being agenda succinctly in this 2015 interview, see Oman (2015b) https://theconversation.com/why-government-issued-well-being-may-not-make-us-happier-42153.

10. These classifications include hope; wisdom; purpose; creativity; future mindedness; courage; emotional intelligence; spirituality or purpose; perseverance; and being an active citizen, socially responsible, loyal, and a team member (Peterson and Seligman 2004).

11. Cloninger's review stated that 'the major accomplishment of this book is in showing that empirically minded humanists can measure character strengths and virtues in a rigorous scientific manner'.

12. There is a tension in this mode of measuring happiness at individual level, aggregating data, and analysing patterns at population level. Many of the world's societies act as collectives, with this idea of the individual and the nation being specific to a particular way that western societies work, which some consider to be bad for well-being (as described at the end of the previous section). This is also interlinked with the concerns of Chap. 2: that measurement and management of populations have developed in tandem and structured the ways societies work. In Chap. 6, we discuss the Bhutanese context of well-being measures which retain culture, community, values and understanding in their approach.

13. I encountered this in my observations, discussions and informal interviews with well-being experts in my PhD fieldwork (2012–2015).

14. Much of the commercial side of happiness economics, as with Paul Dolan's book *Happiness By Design* (2014) is about finding our own 'route to happiness' through exercises to locate pleasure and purpose in relation to what we do, and to be more strategic. In a broader sense, a crucial critique of positive thinking (which is different from positive economics, but linked) is Barbara Ehrenreich's *Smile or Die: How Positive Thinking Fooled America and the world* (2009). She states in a presentation to the Royal Society of Arts, 'Encouraging patients to "be positive" only may add to the burden of having cancer while providing little benefit' (Ehrenreich 2010).

15. See the ONS n.d. Well-being. Office for National Statistics: https://www.ons.gov.uk/peoplepopulationandcommunity/wellbeing.

16. In Oman 2015a , where I discuss my reanalysis of the UK's Measuring National Well-being debate, I present the complex, heart-breaking and rich narrative of a specialist nurse, who had become unemployed owing to her own ill-health (pp. 81–82). This might be compared with more expedient free text answers of only a few words.

17. Ill-being, as you might expect, describes poor well-being, or to be more exact a deficiency in well-being.

18. I began mapping how the accounts and measures of subjective well-being fitted together in my PhD, initially drawing from Dolan et al. (2011a, b), primarily because it informed the ONS measures. Figure 4.1 and the subsequent section use this briefing paper as a starting point, with many elaborations I found useful along the way.

19. Despite the popularity of the ladder of life, concerns have been raised about the integrity of the research behind it from an ethical and methodological perspective. An interesting history can be found in Zubaida 1967.

20. John Stuart Mill was the son of one of Jeremy Bentham's proteges. Mill's own depression at 20 caused him to question Bentham's assumptions about happiness. He decided there were better versions of happiness that are linked to noble pursuits.

21. The psy-sciences are generally considered to be: psychology, psychiatry, psychotherapy and psychoanalysis

22. Stiglitz et al. (2009, 176) specify this as a measure, 'such as the proportion of individuals, families or children that cannot afford a week of holidays away from home at least once a year'. 'Among EU countries, close to 10% of households in the Netherlands and in most Nordic countries report that they could not afford a week away from home, as compared to levels above 50% in some countries in Southern and Eastern Europe'.

23. For more on good and bad leisure, see Chap. 6.

24. Mind's use of the Five Ways can be found online (Mind n.d.).

25. See ONS 2019, 'Measures of National Well-being Dashboard'.

26. The MNW debate was more than simply a data collection exercise; it was also a way of engaging the public in the new measures of well-being (Oman 2015a).

27. The personal well-being domain also includes a measure of 'population mental well-being', using data from Understanding Society: UK Household Longitudinal Study. I found it difficult to establish why his additional measure was in the domain, as it gets overshadowed by 'the ONS4', with numerous ONS pages on personal well-being, only showing 'the ONS4'. However, the population mental well-being (SWEMWBs) question was developed to capture a broad concept of positive mental well-being, including psychological functioning and affective emotional aspects of well-being. Respondents to Understanding Society complete the seven-question SWEMWBs survey questions. Eachresponse is given a score of between 1 and 5, resulting in a total score of between 7 and 35.

28. Gus O'Donnell served as the Cabinet Secretary between 2005 and 2011, the highest official in the British Civil Service.

29. As my research has found, records of the qualitative aspects of largely quantitative evidence projects for policy-making can be an afterthought or overlooked (Oman 2017a). That the minutes of civil service meetings from a decade ago have been re-archived a number of times, and are no longer easily findable is fairly common. In the writing of this book, I discovered my own reports on policy that I had published less than 12 months earlier had been re-archived, with changed links, and the document titles changed. This is one of the trials of a policy researcher—or of trying to understand the origins of the data presented to us as facts.

References

Adler, M. 2013. Happiness Surveys and Public Policy: What's the Use? *Duke Law Journal* 62: 1509–1601.

Ahmed, S. 2010. *The Promise of Happiness*. Durham: Duke University Press.

———. 2012. *On Being Included: Racism and Diversity in Institutional Life*. Durham: Duke University Press.

Aked, J., et al. 2008. *Five Ways to Wellbeing*. Accessed 31 March 2021. https://neweconomics.org/2008/10/five-ways-to-wellbeing.

Aldridge, F., and P. Lavender. 2000. *The Impact of Learning on Health*. Leicester: National Institute of Adult Continuing Education.

Alexandrova, A. 2017. *A Philosophy for the Science of Well-being*. Oxford: Oxford University Press.

Allin, P. 2007. Measuring Societal Wellbeing. *Economic & Labour Market Review* 1 (10): 46–52. https://doi.org/10.1057/palgrave.elmr.1410157.

Allin, P., and D.J. Hand. 2017. New Statistics for Old?—Measuring the Wellbeing of the UK. *Journal of the Royal Statistical Society: Series A (Statistics in Society)* 180 (1): 3–43. https://doi.org/10.1111/rssa.12188.

Ateca-Amestoy, V. 2011. Leisure and Subjective Well-Being. In *Handbook on the Economics of Leisure*, ed. S. Cameron. Edward Elgar Publishing.

Bache, I., and L. Reardon. 2013. An Idea Whose Time has Come? Explaining the Rise of Well-Being in British Politics. *Political Studies* 61 (4): 898–914. https://doi.org/10.1111/1467-9248.12001.

Beckett, A. 2017. PPE: The Oxford Degree that Runs Britain. *The Guardian*. http://www.theguardian.com/education/2017/feb/23/ppe-oxford-university-degree-that-rules-britain.

Benjamin, D.J., et al. 2012. What Do You Think Would Make You Happier? What Do You Think You Would Choose? *American Economic Review* 102 (5): 2083–2110. https://doi.org/10.1257/aer.102.5.2083.

Bentham, J. 1996 [1789]. *An Introduction to the Principles of Morals and Legislation*. Oxford: Clarendon Press.

Berlant, L. 2011. *Cruel Optimism*. Duke University Press.

Bidwell, S. 2014. *The Arts in Health: Evidence from the International Literature*. Pegasus Health.

Blanchflower, D.G. 2008. *International Evidence on Well-Being*. 3354. Bonn: Institute for the Study of Labor.

Bradburn, N. 1969. *The Structure of Psychological Well-Being*. Chicago: Aldine.

Bu, F., et al. 2020. Time-Use and Mental Health during the COVID-19 Pandemic: A Panel Analysis of 55,204 Adults Followed across 11 Weeks of Lockdown in the UK. *medRxiv*, p. 2020.08.18.20177345. https://doi.org/10.1101/2020.08.18.20177345.

Cantril, H. 1965. *The Patterns of Human Concern.* New Brunswick, NJ: Rutgers University Press.

Clark, A., and C. Senik. 2011. *Is Happiness Different from Flourishing? Cross-Country Evidence from the ESS.* HAL Archives-Ouvertes.fr. School of Economics (Working Paper). https://halshs.archives-ouvertes.fr/halshs-00561867.

Cloninger, C.R. 2005. Character Strengths and Virtues: A Handbook and Classification. *American Journal of Psychiatry* 162 (4): 820-a. https://doi.org/10.1176/appi.ajp.162.4.820-a.

Cresswell, J. 2010. *Oxford Dictionary of Word Origins.* Oxford: Oxford University Press.

Crisp, R. 1997. *Routledge Philosophy Guidebook to Mill on Utilitarianism.* Psychology Press.

———. 2006. Hedonism Reconsidered. *Philosophy and Phenomenological Research* 73 (3): 619–645. https://doi.org/10.1111/j.1933-1592.2006.tb00551.x.

Davies, W. 2015. *The Happiness Industry: How the Government and Big Business Sold Us Well-being.* Verso.

———. 2018. *Nervous States: How Feeling Took Over the World.* Jonathan Cape.

Daykin, N. and Joss, T. 2016. Arts for health and Wellbeing: An Evaluation Framework. 2015595. Public Health England. https://www.gov.uk/government/publications/arts-for-health-and-wellbeing-an-evaluation-framework.

Diener, E., Scollon, C. N., and Lucas, R. E. 2009. The evolving concept of subjective well-being: The multifaceted nature of happiness. In *Assessing well-being: The collected works of Ed Diener* (pp. 67–100). Springer Science + Business Media. https://doi.org/10.1007/978-90-481-2354-4_4

Diener, E., and W. Tov. 2012. National Accounts of Well-Being. In *Handbook of Social Indicators and Quality of Life Research,* ed. K.C. Land, A.C. Michalos, and M.J. Sirgy, 137–157. Dordrecht: Springer Netherlands. https://doi.org/10.1007/978-94-007-2421-1_7.

Dodd, J., and C. Jones. 2014. *Mind, Body, Spirit: How Museums Impact Health and Wellbeing.* Report. University of Leicester. Accessed 31 March 2021. Available at: https://leicester.figshare.com/articles/report/Mind_Body_Spirit_How_museums_impact_health_and_wellbeing/10137716/files/18270350.pdf

Dolan, P., and Metcalfe, R. 2012. Measuring Subjective Wellbeing: Recommendations on Measures for use by National Governments. *Journal of SocialPolicy,*41(2),409–427.https://doi.org/10.1017/S0047279411000833

Dolan, P., T. Peasgood, and M. White. 2008. Do We Really Know What Makes Us Happy? A Review of the Economic Literature on the Factors Associated with Subjective Well-Being. *Journal of Economic Psychology* 29 (1): 94–122. https://doi.org/10.1016/j.joep.2007.09.001.

Dolan, P., R. Layard, and R. Metcalfe. 2011a. *Measuring Subjective Well-Being for Public Policy.* Office for National Statistics.

———. 2011b. *Measuring Subjective Well-Being for Public Policy: Recommendations on Measures.* London School of Economics: Centre for Economic Performance.

Donovan, N., and D. Halpern. 2002. *Life Satisfaction: The State of Knowledge and Implications for Government*. London: Prime Minister's Strategy Unit.

Duckworth, K., and O. Cara. 2012. *The Relationship between Adult Learning and Wellbeing: Evidence from the 1958 National Child Development Study*. London: Department for Business, Innovation & Skills (BIS Research Paper). http://hdl.voced.edu.au/10707/236318.

Easterlin, R. 1973. Does Money Buy Happiness? *The Public Interest* 30 (3): 3–10.

Easterlin, R.A. 1974. Does Economic Growth Improve the Human Lot? Some Empirical Evidence. In *Nations and Households in Economic Growth*, ed. P.A. David and M.W. Reder, 89–125. New York: Academic Press. https://doi.org/10.1016/B978-0-12-205050-3.50008-7.

———. 2001. Income and Happiness: Towards a Unified Theory. *The Economic Journal*. https://doi.org/10.1111/1468-0297.00646.

Easterlin, R., et al. 2010. The Happiness–Income Paradox Revisited. *Proceeding of the National Academy of Sciences* 107 (52): 22361–22362.

EconLit. n.d. *EconLit, American Economic Association*. Available at: https://www.aeaweb.org/econlit/. Accessed: 28 April 2021.

Ehrenreich, B. 2010. Barbara Ehrenreich—Smile or Die. *RSA*. Accessed 28 April 2021. https://www.youtube.com/watch?v=PJGMFu74a70.

———. 2021. *Smile or Die: How Positive Thinking Fooled America and the World*. S.l.: Granta Publications Ltd.

ELSA. n.d. *The English Longitudinal Study of Ageing (ELSA), ELSA*. Accessed 28 April 2021. https://www.elsa-project.ac.uk

Field, J. 2009. Good for Your Soul? Adult Learning and Mental Well-Being. *International Journal of Lifelong Education* 28 (2): 175–191. https://doi.org/10.1080/02601370902757034.

Fleche, S., C. Smith, and P. Sorsa. 2012. *Exploring Determinants of Subjective Wellbeing in OECD Countries: Evidence from the World Value Survey*. 921. Pari: Organisation for Economic Cooperation and Development.

Fujiwara, D., and G. MacKerron. 2015. *Cultural Activities, Artforms and Wellbeing*. London: Arts Council England.

Gray, C. 2004. Joining-Up or Tagging On? The Arts, Cultural Planning and the View From Below. *Public Policy and Administration* 19 (2): 38–49. https://doi.org/10.1177/095207670401900206.

Grimes, A., and M. Reinhardt. 2019. Relative Income, Subjective Wellbeing and the Easterlin Paradox: Intra- and Inter-national Comparisons. In *The Economics of Happiness: How the Easterlin Paradox Transformed Our Understanding of Well-Being and Progress*, ed. M. Rojas, 85–105. Cham: Springer International Publishing. https://doi.org/10.1007/978-3-030-15835-4_4.

Hallsworth, M., S. Parker, and J. Rutter. 2011. *Policy Making in the Real World: Evidence and Analysis*. London: Institute for Government.

Helliwell, J.F. 2003. How's Life? Combining Individual and National Variables to Explain Subjective Well-Being. *Economic Modelling* 20 (2): 331–360. https://doi.org/10.1016/S0264-9993(02)00057-3.

Helliwell, J., L. Richard, and J. Sachs. 2015. *World Happiness Report 2015*. New York: UN Sustainable Development Solutions Network.

Helliwell, J., R. Layard, and J. Sachs. 2017. *World Happiness Report 2017*. New York: Sustainable Development Solutions Network. Accessed 28 April 2021. https://worldhappiness.report/ed/2017/.

———. 2019. *World Happiness Report 2019*. New York: Sustainable Development Solutions Network. Accessed 28 April 2021. https://worldhappiness.report/ed/2017/.

Holden, J. 2012. New Year, New Approach to Wellbeing?, *The Guardian*. https://www.theguardian.com/culture-professionals-network/culture-professionals-blog/2012/jan/03/arts-heritage-wellbeing-cultural-policy.

Huppert, F.A., and J.E. Whittington. 2003. Evidence for the Independence of Positive and Negative Well-Being: Implications for Quality of Life Assessment. *British Journal of Health Psychology* 8 (1): 107–122. https://doi.org/10.1348/135910703762879246.

Hurka, T. 1993. *Perfectionism*. New York: Oxford University Press.

Jeffries, S 2008. Will This Man Make You Happy?, *The Guardian*. http://www.theguardian.com/lifeandstyle/2008/jun/24/healthandwellbeing.schools.

Kahneman, D., and A. Deaton. 2010. High Income Improves Evaluation of Life But Not Emotional Well-Being. *Proceedings of the National Academy of Sciences* 107 (38): 16489–16493. https://doi.org/10.1073/pnas.1011492107.

Kahneman, D., and A.B. Krueger. 2006. Developments in the Measurement of Subjective Well-Being. *Journal of Economic Perspectives* 20 (1): 3–24. https://doi.org/10.1257/089533006776526030.

Kahneman, D., and J. Riis. 2005. Living and Thinking About It: Two Perspectives on Life. In *The Science of Wellbeing: Integrating Neurobiology, Psychology, and Social Science*, ed. F. Huppert, N. Baylis, and B. Kaverne. Oxford: Oxford University Press.

Kahneman, D., and R. Sugden. 2005. Experienced Utility as a Standard of Policy Evaluation. *Environmental and Resource Economics* 32 (1): 161–181. https://doi.org/10.1007/s10640-005-6032-4.

Kahneman, D., E. Diener, and N. Schwarz, eds. 1999. *Well-being: The Foundations of Hedonic Psychology*. New York: Russell-Sage.

Kahneman, D., et al. 2004. A Survey Method for Characterizing Daily Life Experience: The Day Reconstruction Method. *Science* 306 (5702): 1776–1780. https://doi.org/10.1126/science.1103572.

Krekel, C., & MacKerron, G. 2020. How Environmental Quality Affects Our Happiness. In J. F. Helliwell, R. Layard, J. Sachs, & J.-E. De Neve (Eds.), *World Happiness Report 2020*, 95–112. Sustainable Development Solutions Network. https://happiness-report.s3.amazonaws.com/2020/WHR20.pdf.

Layard, R. 2003. Happiness: Has Social Science a Clue? In *Lionel Robbins Memorial Lecture*. London: London School of Economics. https://digital. library.lse.ac.uk/objects/lse:vuk454feq.

———. 2006. *Happiness: Lessons from a New Science*. London: Penguin.

Le Guin, U.K. 2017. *The Unreal and the Real: The Selected Short Stories of Ursula K. Le Guin*. London: Gallery/Saga Press.

Levitt, R., and W. Solesbury. 2012. Debate: Tsars—Are They the 'Experts' Now? *Public Money & Management* 32 (1): 47–48. https://doi.org/10.108 0/09540962.2012.643057.

LSE Centre for Economic Performance. n.d. *CEP | Topics | Wellbeing, Centre for Economic Performance*. Accessed 31 March 2021. https://cep.lse.ac.uk/ wellbeing/.

MacKerron, G., and S. Mourato. 2013. Happiness Is Greater in Natural Environments. *Global Environmental Change* 23 (5): 992–1000. https://doi. org/10.1016/j.gloenvcha.2013.03.010.

Mak, H.W., M. Fluharty, and D. Fancourt. 2020. Predictors and Impact of Arts Engagement during the COVID-19 Pandemic: Analyses of Data from 19,384 Adults in the COVID-19 Social Study. *PsyArXiv*. https://doi.org/10.31234/ osf.io/rckp5.

Massumi, B. 2002. *Parables for the Virtual: Movement, Affect, Sensation*. Duke University Press.

McKenzie, L. 2015. Policymakers Don't Know How to Value Culture, Says AHRC Report. *Research Professional*. Accessed 1 October 2016. https://www. researchprofessional.com/0/rr/news/uk/researchcouncils/2015/10/ PolicymakersdontknowhowtovaluecuituresaysAHRCreport.html.

Nickson, S. 2020. *Personal Wellbeing Harmonised Standard*. Government Statistical Service. Accessed 31 March 2021. https://gss.civilservice.gov.uk/ policy-store/personal-well-being/.

Nuffield. 2021. People Exercising Less and Watching More TV Than in First Lockdown. *Nuffield Foundation*. Accessed 31 March 2021. https://www. nuffieldfoundation.org/news/people-exercising-less-and-watching-more-tv-than-in-first-lockdown.

Oakley, K., O'Brien, D. and Lee, D. 2013. Happy Now? Well-being and Cultural Policy, *Philosophy and Public Policy Quarterly*, 31(2), pp. 18–26. doi: 10.13021/ G8pppq.312013.131.

O'Donnell, G. 2020. *Handling Covid Crisis Required Stronger Leadership and a Better Use of a Wider Range of Evidence Says Gus O' Donnell*. Institute for Fiscal Studies. The IFS. Accessed 31 March 2021. https://www.ifs.org.uk/ publications/15042.

O'Donnell, G., et al. 2014. *Wellbeing and Policy*. London: Legatum Institute.

OECD. 2013. *How's Life? 2013 Measuring Well-Being*. OECD (OECD Better Life Initiative). http://www.oecd.org/sdd/3013071e.pdf.

———. 2014. *Competition.* http://www.oecd.org/daf/competition/.

Oman, S. 2015a. Measuring National Well-Being: What Matters to You? What Matters to Whom? In *Cultures of Wellbeing: Method, Place, Policy*, ed. S. White and C. Blackmore. London: Palgrave Macmillan.

Oman, S. 2015b. Why government issued well-being may not make us happier. *The Conversation.* Available at: http://theconversation.com/why-government-issued-well-being-may-not-make-us-happier-42153. Accessed 11 August 2021.

———. 2017a. *All Being Well: Cultures of Participation and the Cult of Measurement.* PhD. The University of Manchester.

———. 2017b. *Mainstream Cultural Activities and Subjective Well-Being. A Review of the Literature.* A Report to the Wellcome Trust.

———. 2020. Leisure Pursuits: Uncovering the 'Selective Tradition' in Culture and Well-Being Evidence for Policy. *Leisure Studies* 39 (1): 11–25. https://doi.org/10.1080/02614367.2019.1607536.

Oman, S. and Edwards, D. 2020. Temporalities and Typologies of Loneliness: A Methodology to Understand New Parents, Self-predicted Loneliness & the Role of NCT', In *Loneliness & Social Isolation in Mental Health Research Network Symposium*, London. Available at: https://www.ucl.ac.uk/psychiatry/events/2020/jan/loneliness-social-isolation-mental-health-research-network-symposium.

Oman, S., J. Rainford, and H. Stewart. 2015. Stories of Access in Higher Education: A Triumph (or Failure) of Hope over Experience? *Discover Society*, 1 December. Accessed 28 April 2021. https://archive.discoversociety.org/2015/12/01/stories-of-access-in-higher-education-a-triumph-or-failure-of-hope-over-experience/.

Oman, S., and A. Bull. 2021, forthcoming. Joining up well-being and sexual misconduct data and policy in HE: 'to stand in the gap' as a feminist approach. *The Sociological Review.*

ONS. n.d. *Measuring National Well-being: Conceptual Framework.* Resource Pack.

ONS. 2011a. *Initial Investigation into Subjective Well-Being from the Opinions Survey.* Office for National Statistics. http://www.ons.gov.uk/ons/rel/well-being/measuring-subjective-wellbeing-in-the-uk/investigation-of-subjective-well-being-data-from-the-ons-opinions-survey/index.html.

———. 2011b. *Measuring National Well-Being Technical Advisory Group.* Office for National Statistics. Accessed 5 April 2014. http://www.ons.gov.uk/ons/guide-method/user-guidance/well-being/measuring-national-well-being-technical-advisory-group/Notes-from-the-meeting-on-4-february-2011.pdf.

———. 2012. *Overview of ONS Phase Three Cognitive Testing of Subjective Well-Being Questions.* Office for National Statistics. http://www.ons.gov.uk/ons/guide-method/user-guidance/well-being/about-the-programme/advisory-groups/well-being-technical-advisory-group/overview-of-latest-ons-cognitive-testing-march-13-version.pdf.

———. 2015a. *Measuring National Well-Being: Life in the UK, 2015*. Office for National Statistics. https://webarchive.nationalarchives.gov.uk/20160106 094809/http://www.ons.gov.uk/ons/dcp171766_398059.pdf.

———. 2015b. *Measuring National Wellbeing: Personal Well-Being in the UK, 2014 to 2015*. Newport: Office for National Statistics.

———. *Measures of National Well-being Dashboard. Office for National Statistics*. https://www.ons.gov.uk/peoplepopulationandcommunity/wellbeing/articles/measuresofnationalwellbeingdashboard/2018-04-25. Accessed 30 March 2021.

Peterson, C. and Seligman, M. E. P. 2004. *Character Strengths and Virtues: A Handbook and Classification*. New York: Oxford: American Psychological Association.

Pollmann-Schult, M. 2014. Parenthood and Life Satisfaction: Why Don't Children Make People Happy? *Journal of Marriage and Family* 76 (2): 319–336. https://doi.org/10.1111/jomf.12095.

van Praag, B.M.S., P. Frijters, and A. Ferrer-i-Carbonell. 2003. The Anatomy of Subjective Well-Being. *Journal of Economic Behavior & Organization* 51 (1): 29–49. https://doi.org/10.1016/S0167-2681(02)00140-3.

Ralph, K., K. Palmer, and J. Olney. 2011. *Subjective Well-Being: A Qualitative Investigation of Subjective Well-Being Questions*. Working Paper for the Technical Advisory Group on 29 March 2012.

Rustin, S. 2012. The Conversation: Can Happiness be Measured?, *The Guardian*. Accessed 28 April 2021. https://www.theguardian.com/commentisfree/2012/jul/20/wellbeing-index-happiness-julian-baggin.

Ryan, F. 2021. Cake and Inner Calm: 10 Ways to Improve Your Mood—Without Exercising. *The Guardian*. Accessed 29 March 2021. http://www.theguardian.com/lifeandstyle/2021/feb/23/cake-and-inner-calm-10-ways-to-improve-your-mood-without-exercising.

Ryff, C.D. 1989. Happiness Is Everything, or Is It? Explorations on the Meaning of Psychological Well-Being. *Journal of Personality and Social Psychology* 57 (6): 1069–1081. https://doi.org/10.1037/0022-3514.57.6.1069.

Ryff, C.D., and C.L. Keyes. 1995. The Structure of Psychological Well-Being Revisited. *Journal of Personality and Social Psychology* 69 (4): 719–727. https://doi.org/10.1037/0022-3514.69.4.719.

Sedgwick, E.K., and A. Frank. 2003. *Touching Feeling: Affect, Pedagogy, Performativity*. Duke University Press.

Seligman, M.E.P. 1998. *APA President's Address 1998*. Positive Psychology Center. https://ppc.sas.upenn.edu/sites/default/files/APA%20President%20 Address%201998.docx.

Seligman, M. 2002. *Authentic Happiness*. Random House Australia.

Seligman, M.E.P., and M. Csikszentmihalyi. 2000. Positive psychology: An introduction. *American Psychologist* 55 (1): 5–14. https://doi.org/10.1037/0003-066X.55.1.5.

Seligman, M.E.P., et al. 2005. Positive Psychology Progress: Empirical Validation of Interventions. *American Psychologist* 60 (5): 410–421. https://doi.org/10.1037/0003-066X.60.5.410.

Shah, H., and N. Marks. 2004. *A Well-Being Manifesto for a Flourishing Society.* London: New Economics Foundation.

Smith, C., and C. Exton. 2013. *OECD Guidelines on Measuring Subjective Well-Being.* Paris: OECD Publishing. https://read.oecd-ilibrary.org/economics/oecd-guidelines-on-measuring-subjective-well-being_9789264191655-en#page258.

Stevenson, B., and J. Wolfers. 2008. Economic Growth and Subjective Well-Being: Reassessing the Easterlin Paradox. *Brookings Papers on Economic Activity* 2008 (1): 1–87. https://doi.org/10.1353/eca.0.0001.

———. 2012. Subjective and Objective Indicators of Racial Progress. *The Journal of Legal Studies.* The University of Chicago Press. https://doi.org/10.1086/669963.

Stevenson, D., K. McKay, and D. Rowe. 2010. Tracing British Cultural Policy Domains: Contexts, Collaborations and Constituencies. *International Journal of Cultural Policy* 16 (2): 159–172. https://doi.org/10.1080/10286630902862646.

Stiglitz, J.E., A. Sen, and J.-P. Fitoussi. 2009. *Report by the Commission on the Measurement of Economic Performance and Social Progress.* OECD. https://ec.europa.eu/environment/beyond_gdp/download/CMEPSP-final-report.pdf.

Stone, A., S. Shiffman, and M. DeVries. 1999. Ecological Momentary Assessment. In *Well-being: The Foundations of Hedonic Psychology*, ed. D. Kahneman, E. Diener, and N. Schwarz, 26–39. New York: Russell-Sage.

Tadić, M., A.B. Bakker, and W.G.M. Oerlemans. 2013. Work Happiness Among Teachers: A Day Reconstruction Study on the Role of Self-Concordance. *Journal of School Psychology* 51 (6): 735–750. https://doi.org/10.1016/j.jsp.2013.07.002.

Tate, S.A. 2016. 'I Can't Quite Put My Finger on It': Racism's Touch. *Ethnicities* 16 (1): 68–85. https://doi.org/10.1177/1468796814564626.

———. 2017. *Putting Feelings into Words: Racism and Wellbeing in Universities.* Leeds Beckett University. https://www.youtube.com/watch?v=bbLXxRSKi5s.

The University of Manchester. n.d. *Student Support | Taking Care of Your Wellbeing | Wellbeing | Six Ways to Wellbeing | The University of Manchester, Student Support.* Accessed 28 April 2021. https://www.studentsupport.manchester.ac.uk/taking-care/wellbeing/six-ways-to-wellbeing/.

Thrift, N. 2004. Intensities of Feeling: Towards a Spatial Politics of Affect. *Geografiska Annaler: Series B, Human Geography* 86 (1): 57–78. https://doi.org/10.1111/j.0435-3684.2004.00154.x.

University of Essex, Institute for Social and Economic Research, NatCen Social Research, Kantar Public. 2020. *Understanding Society: Waves 1-10, 2009-2019 and Harmonised BHPS: Waves 1-18, 1991-2009.* [data collection]. 13th Edition. UK Data Service. SN: 6614, http://doi.org/10.5255/UKDA-SN-6614-14.

Veenhoven, R. 1996. The Study of Life Satisfaction. In *A Comparative Study of Satisfaction with Life in Europe*, ed. W. Saris et al., 11–48. Budapest: Eötvös University. https://repub.eur.nl/pub/16311/.

———. 2010. Greater Happiness for a Greater Number. *Journal of Happiness Studies* 11 (5): 605–629. https://doi.org/10.1007/s10902-010-9204-z.

Waldron, S. 2010. *Measuring Subjective Wellbeing in the UK: Working Paper.* Newport: Office for National Statistics. http://www.mas.org.uk/uploads/artlib/measuring-subjective-wellbeing-in-the-uk.pdf.

Watson, D., L. Clark, and A. Tellegen. 1988. Development and Validation of Brief Measures of Positive and Negative Affect: The PANAS Scales. *Journal of Personality and Social Psychology* 54 (6): 1063–1070. https://doi.org/10.1037/0022-3514.54.6.1063.

Wetherell, M. 2012. *Affect and Emotion: A New Social Science Understanding.* SAGE Publications.

White, M.P., and P. Dolan. 2009. Accounting for the Richness of Daily Activities. *Psychological Science* 20 (8): 1000–1008. https://doi.org/10.1111/j.1467-9280.2009.02392.x.

World Economic Forum. 2013. *The Global Competitiveness Report 2013–2014.* Geneva: World Economic Forum. http://www3.weforum.org/docs/WEF_GlobalCompetitivenessReport_2013-14.pdf.

Zubaida, S.D. 1967. Review of the Pattern of Human Concerns. *The British Journal of Sociology* 18: 212–212. https://doi.org/10.2307/588624.

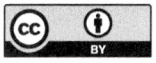

CHAPTER 5

Getting a Sense of Big Data and Well-being

5.1 WHAT *EVEN IS* 'BIG DATA'?

Big data generally capture what is easy to ensnare—data that are openly expressed (what is typed, swiped, scanned, sensed, etc.; people's actions and behaviours; the movement of things)—as well as data that are the 'exhaust', a by-product … It takes these data at face value, despite the fact that they may not have been designed to answer specific questions and the data produced might be messy and dirty. (Kitchin 2014, Chap. 2, p. 3 of individual chapter version)

Rob Kitchin is possibly one of the most cited definers of 'Big Data', opening books and dissertations up and down the land. Yet, as we are about to discover, Kitchin himself tells us that while the term 'Big Data' is repeatedly defined (Kitchin 2014, Chap. 2, p. 3), big data themselves defy categorical labelling. So, it is not clear-cut, because differentiating what 'it' is and what *they are not* is often side-stepped, or comes with caveats.[1] We encountered something similar before, if you remember, in Chap. 2. When it comes to understanding what well-being is, those *inclined* to measure are sometimes keen to measure well-being to understand it, rather than define what it is that is being measured. In a similar way, those describing Big Data are often more concerned with what Big Data *does* (or do), rather than what Big Data *is*, or are.

© The Author(s) 2021   175
S. Oman, *Understanding Well-being Data,*
New Directions in Cultural Policy Research,
https://doi.org/10.1007/978-3-030-72937-0_5

In this chapter on Big Data, we will discover that how they are used can defy some of the old definitions of *how* to use data or what data are *for*. So, let us start with some definitions and what is different. For Kitchin, the lack of 'ontological clarity' of Big Data (as the individual concepts and categories of Big Data and the relations between them) means the term acts as a vague, catch-all label for a wide selection of data (Kitchin 2014, Chap. 2, p. 3). Despite this, he has reviewed how other people define it and proposes the key traits of Big Data. These qualities are outlined in Table 5.1. Given the word 'big', it is probably no surprise that volume is one of 'the 3Vs' identified by Doug Laney back in 2001. The other two being velocity and variety. Other qualities include exhaustivity, resolution, indexicality, relationality, extensionality and

Table 5.1 Ways that Big Data are different

Label/definition	Origin	Meaning	Pre Big Data	Big Data
Volume	Laney (2001)	Consisting of enormous quantities of data	Limited to large	Very large
Velocity	Laney (2001)	Created in real-time	Slow, freeze-framed/bundled	Fast, continuous
Variety	Laney (2001)	Being structured, semi-structured and unstructured	Narrow²	Wide
Exhaustivity	Mayer-Schönberger and Cukier (2013)	An entire system is captured, Rather than being sampled	Samples	Entire populations
Resolution and identification	Dodge and Kitchin (2005)	Fine-grained (in resolution) and uniquely indexical (in identification)	Coarse and weak to tight and strong	Tight and strong
Relationality	Boyd and Crawford (2012)	Containing common fields that enable the conjoining of different datasets	Weak to strong	Strong
Flexible and scalable	Marz and Warren (2012)	Can add/change new fields easily and can expand in size rapidly	Low to middling	High

Adapted from tables in Kitchin (2014) and Kitchin and McArdle (2016)

scalability (Kitchin and McArdle 2016; Kitchin 2014). But what does this mean? How do these characteristics help us understand the data?

Having established a series of classifications for Big Data, Kitchin tested his taxonomy of traits with co-author McArdle a few years later (Kitchin and McArdle 2016). They applied the categories to 26 datasets which are widely considered Big Data and drawn from across seven sources: mobile communication, websites, social media/crowdsourcing, sensors, cameras/lasers, transaction process generated data and administrative data (2016). The authors find all seven traits in Table 5.1 are only applicable to 'a handful' of these datasets (Kitchin and McArdle 2016, 9). This shows how difficult it is to diagnose what Big Data actually are. Rather than the qualities of the data themselves, it might be more useful to instead turn to thinking about the contexts of data again: where they come from, and what they do (Oman n.d.).

The key differences in the characteristics of Big Data are context, which is often missing when presented. Table 5.2 represents how difficult it is to diagnose what Big Data actually are, without considering the qualities that affect their use. It shows there are additional Vs: veracity, value and variability—these are concerned with how the data suit their re-purposing. Given the multiple insights and applications of data outside of their original setting, it can be difficult—even more difficult—to find certainty from them. This is because the data were collected, generated and produced for a specific reason, or as a by-product, that differs from how they are re-used.

The *value* of Big Data is the *variety* of insights that are possible and that can be used for other purposes. However, there are many things in the data that may not be useful. This also means using Big Data can increase the risk of confounding more traditional causal explanations. Instead, the mess of Big Data lends them to correlation with many insights, which can

Table 5.2 Some qualities of Big Data

Label / definition	Origin	Qualities of data that affect their use
Veracity	Marr (2014)	The data can be messy, noisy and contain uncertainty and error.
Value	Marr (2014)	Many insights can be extracted and the data repurposed.
Variability	McNulty (2014)	Data whose meaning can be constantly shifting in relation to the context in which they are generated.

Synthesised from Kitchin and McArdle (2016)

be used to enable prediction of well-being for individuals and society. We shall return to correlations and well-being in our case studies later in this chapter.

Table 5.3 looks at sources of different kinds of data typically used to predict well-being along with their pros and cons. These sources were drawn from an article in a journal for Data Science Analytics (Voukelatou et al. 2020), and I have synthesised these with Kitchin's seven sources (mobile communication, websites, social media/crowdsourcing, sensors, cameras/lasers, transaction process generated data and administrative data) retaining commentary from Voukelatou et al. on the pros and cons for their use to understand well-being. You may look at these and feel like these data sources seem like strange ways to understand people's well-being: the difference in origins and what they may be used for. You may also note that the authors' presentation of the pros and cons, based on these sources, does not really prompt consideration for the people whose data they are, more their ease of use for the Data Scientist.

Returning to contexts of use: mobile phone data, for example, have a primary purpose which is for billing, or because apps need location data to work (such as maps or for local restaurant recommendations). This is very different from these data being used to understand trends about people and society. Our previous examples of data re-use (or secondary analysis) have largely involved data that were collected in national surveys, or through more qualitative methods with smaller samples to understand a specific aspect of people and society more deeply in some way. Notably, even if the research question is different when data are re-used in Chap. 3's examples, the purpose of the data's collection is not *as* different, or *as* removed, as this 'exhaust', 'by-product' nature of the data Kitchin refers to.

The process which has come to be known as 'datafication' (as coined by Mayer-Schönberger and Cukier 2013) describes the increased demand for and uses of data. As we have seen in previous centuries, appetite for numbers (pandemics being one accelerator of data desire) has coincided with technological evolutions with numbers. In turn, and as we have seen over the last four chapters, different disciplines have increased and expanded their capacities for data and knowing the human experience in their own, particular way, and 'new sciences' have been declared. 'Big Data', as data with the qualities presented above, result from mounting capacity and faster instruments that increase the possibilities for the origins and volumes of data that can be stored in expanding databases, or in different databases which can be readily linked for a variety of purposes. As we have

Table 5.3 Sources of Big Data and their pros and cons for well-being measurement

Data Source	Pros	Cons
Mobile communications data (including GPS)	Captures temporal, spatial and social dimensions, Worldwide diffusion, Repeatability Unbiased and classified, real-time monitoring	Not publicly available, sparsity, geographically Imprecise Limited coverage in rural areas Indoor/altitude spatial inaccuracy
Social media	Measuring social dynamics, publicly available	Privacy issues, overrepresentation, Social desirability bias Disturbance of normal activities to post
Health and fitness (including mental health and well-being apps)	Cost-effective, Prediction of near-term risk of events Reduced respondent burden	Not publicly available, not necessarily representative of the population Requests for data input can disrupt daily activities Data can neglect moment-to-moment variations in mood.
News	Variety of subject domains, Variety of data Range of targets, 24/h updated, Archived historical news	Gatekeeping bias, Coverage bias, Statement bias
Transaction process generated data	Modelling of dynamic household behaviour, Temporal accuracy, Long-term coverage, Quality	Dependency on retailer's permission, Legal constraints
Websites and searches	Publicly available. Speed, convenience, flexibility, ease of analysis Timeliness, observation of people's behaviour through searches	Population size varies across domains. Relevant queries difficult to identify Bias of content and terms Comparability of different search terms on different days

(*continued*)

Table 5.3   (continued)

Data Source	Pros	Cons
Crowdsourcing	Large number of data Speed, relative low-cost measurement of daily behaviour and activity	Risk of low-quality results, trade-off between quality and cost Use of self-reports Paid participation of users
Administration data	Accurate, temporal stability, valid for community-level understanding and cross-cultural comparisons	Limited understanding of human experience in administration data

NOTES: Made from synthesising across Rob Kitchin's 7: mobile communication; websites; social media/crowdsourcing; sensors; cameras/lasers; transaction process generated data; and administrative data & Voukelatou et al. (2020)—with the data examples in this chapter

also seen before, it can be difficult to decide which came first: appetite for data, or capacity to expand on data possibilities.

In the age of Big Data, these newer data sources hold a wide variety of easy-to-capture data points, including observations of how we feel, where we are (or were), who we know, what we spend—and on what. These provide information on what products we have clicked on, and those we have not bought (Turow 2011). They can show how and where we spend our spare time and our money, both off and online. They are, therefore, incredibly valuable for research and commerce.

It is not these individual data points that are important, per se, but the links between them, that make them valuable. Through linking, assumptions can be made about how our behaviour, such as online spending, or improved mood, can be replicated in another place or time. These insights are also linked with other more familiar data points from administrative records, for example: where we were born, how much we earn, whether we own our own house. Other data are produced by loyalty cards, smartphones and in-house devices, such as Alexa, expanding such linking opportunities. Those who may try to avoid 'being known' by these other data will try to bypass the systems that gather these data. However, this resistance also becomes data in and of themselves; avoidance still produces digital traces that can be used to gather insights. Corporations may still create an automated profile of sorts, and assumptions will be made about the kind of products 'the resistors' buy. The persistence of data practices and their seeming inescapability are the reason we are starting to think about the experience of Big Data as something we 'live with' (Kennedy et al. 2020) and as something we 'feel'.

This chapter covers some of the pervasiveness of Big Data, alongside the possibilities that come with that. Crucially, we look at what that means for well-being. We start by looking at the ways that data about mundane aspects of our lives is increasing, alongside how normalised increasing data collection, analysis and re-use are. These 'data practices' present new possibilities and realities of data-driven systems and decision-making that affect culture and society.

In this chapter, we touch on some of the uncomfortable aspects of these new realities, before historicising Big Data as well-being data to contextualise contemporary concerns regarding data practices that can be harmful. The second half of the chapter uses case studies to explore these concerns about well-being and data. Firstly, we consider a high-profile case that was billed as the promise of Big Data: Google Flu Trends (GFT), looking back from the age of COVID-19. Three further, short examples show the possibilities of social media data, place-based data, and health and fitness data to understand well-being for social and cultural policy and culture and society more generally.

5.2   BIG DATA: A NEW WAY TO UNDERSTAND WELL-BEING?

"Big Data", was cited 40,000 times in 2017 in Google Scholar, about as often as "happiness"! (Bellet and Frijters 2019)

The datafication of social life has led to a profound transformation in how society is ordered, decisions are made, and citizens are governed. (Hintz and Brand n.d., 2)

Digital devices and data are becoming an ever more pervasive and part of social, commercial, governmental and academic practices. (Ruppert et al. 2013, 2)

The majority of Big Data are collected in a different way to the national surveys and interviews we encountered in Chaps. 3 and 4, and consequently has numerous different qualities. One is that surveys and questionnaires are, by and large, overt methods, in that it is obvious you are asking questions to generate data. The new technologies use data which are collected covertly and so often gathered on individuals without their 'considered consent', and are often processed without transparency. Figure 5.1 shows just a small selection of the types of personal data that are useful and valuable for social analytics and that are covered in this chapter.

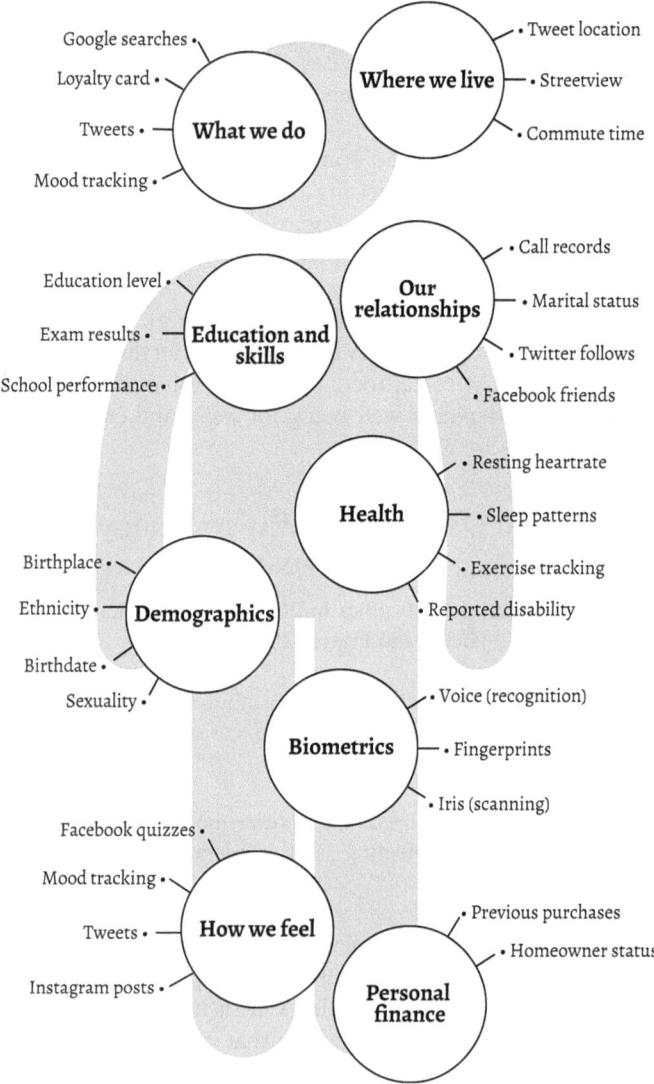

Fig. 5.1 Some examples of personal data used for social analytics in the era of Big Data

Social analytics involve the: monitoring, analysing, measuring and interpreting of data about people's movements, characteristics, interactions, relationships, feelings, ideas and other content. Figure 5.1 shows only a few of many more examples. Here, they are categorised into domains that share the same names as the UK's well-being measures, to enable you to cross reference the different kinds of insights available under each domain from these data (although biometrics is a new addition). The data are from 'observations' of how we move around the on and offline world. They can include behaviours collected by sensors (think of how your mobile phone uses data via GPS to tell you when the next bus is, or that you are about to encounter traffic on the motorway). They include our feelings, shared by social media data, or in apps. While demographic data have long been collected, as we know, these newer forms of data can say much more about us, our well-being and quality of life. As we shall discover, this is both for good and bad and any insights gained need to be put into context.

As we have also discovered, data are not only numbers or text, but can be sound and pictures. Analysing these kinds of qualitative data as Big Data holds new possibilities. In some ways it is these new possibilities that feel the most uncomfortably non-human. Whether it is concern that your phone is always listening to you, or, rather, that Alexa or Siri are (to humanise these technologies). Even the Street View option of Google Maps allows us to look at other people's homes. I remember keenly finding the image of the flat I rented in London for years, only to see my washing-up through the kitchen window. I couldn't help but think, I wish I had known they were coming.

More notable than my neglected washing-up being on public view for judgement are other visual data used for training datasets, particularly for facial recognition. There are the moments when you know that facial recognition technology is being used: to log in to your phone, or at passport control at the airport, perhaps. However, they are also being developed for schools, public transport systems, workplaces and healthcare facilities (Ada Lovelace Institute 2019). Revelations about its use in shopping centres prompted media and public outrage, regulatory investigation and political criticism (Denham 2019; BBC 2019). These reactions are in part about the further encroachment on the way we live (like the call centre example from the 1990s that opens the book) and in part the lack of consent and knowledge about these data being collected about us.

Some people who uploaded photos to Flickr, some 10–15 years ago, more recently discovered they (as in the people's faces and their photos) appeared in a huge facial-recognition database called MegaFace (Hill and Krolik 2019). They found the database held facial data on around 700,000 individuals, including their children, and was being downloaded by various companies to train face-identification algorithms. These algorithms were then being used to track protesters, surveil terrorists, spot problem gamblers and spy on the public at large (Hill and Krolik 2019). Notably, a colleague who read this chapter before publication—a digital sociologist,[3] no less—confessed to me their shock at reading this anecdote, as they had used Flickr and were not aware of this story. Therefore, not only are our personal data collected and used without our knowledge, but the controversies surrounding their re-use are not even shared with users. This poses questions for accountability and transparency.

The questions of who is collecting these data, and who is using them, and for what, present a more complex issue than before. Public support for the police to use facial recognition technology is conditional upon limitations and subject to appropriate safeguards, but there is no trust in private company use (Ada Lovelace Institute 2019). As we have been discovering—it is the contexts of data collection and uses that we need to understand: it is the who, what, where, why and what for? that are important.

Why We Need to Ask Critical Questions of Data in the Context of Well-being

Many issues related to Big Data don't have clear-cut answers, especially where well-being is concerned. While data reveal details of the vulnerable, often involving risk for these people and their communities, the State uses data systems that people increasingly need to be a part of to access healthcare and welfare support (Dencik 2020). This is why the growing amount of research which problematises the utility and ethics of Big Data, and how they are used, is vital. In this area of critical data science (see Bates 2016), some researchers use Big Data to reveal the limits and social issues connected to everyday datasets that we all use, such as a search engine's image database (e.g. Otterbacher et al. 2017). These critical studies of data and their effects on society reveal how data are capable of not only new problems, but persistent racism and misogyny, as we discovered in Chap. 1 with Virginia Noble's example of what happens when you search for the phrase 'black girls' (Noble 2018). These projects reveal data's negative social effects, and how they are already embedded in society, exacerbating issues.

Other research aims to investigate what people know and think is going on. Also looking at the possibilities of Big Data (and their associated technologies) to understanding aspects of well-being. One such example (Living With Data n.d.) presents real-life cases of public sector data practices to members of the public. It wants to understand how much people appreciate the possible benefits and how much they doubt or distrust the possible implications of data systems and sharing in their everyday lives. One option being, of course, that many people may not really care as much as we think they do, or should.

We touch on these issues in this chapter. Most notable is the increase in concerns regarding the harms that Big Data and new technologies are capable of, and which are happening unchecked (i.e. the UK's Data Justice Lab n.d.; Eubanks 2018; O'Neil 2016; Noble 2018; Benjamin 2019). There are two main problems here. One is that we are compromising well-being in the so-called aim of better understanding the human condition. The second is that we are not only using these data and technologies to understand people but also sorting and managing them in different ways that suit those who are already more powerful.

It is vital to note that key to concerns about datafication are how these practices disproportionately affect the well-being of those already most vulnerable. Facial recognition, for example, negatively impacts people already disadvantaged, owing to its own gendered, heteronormative classed and racialised biases (Ada Lovelace Institute 2019). These technologies are also being trialled in policing in the UK and have reported more than 90% of incorrect matches (Fussey and Murray 2019; Davies et al. 2018). In a more general way, all public services are adopting new data practices and possibilities.

Data-driven decision-making is growing as an everyday feature of public services. Who receives welfare (Eubanks 2018, 37) housing (Eubanks 2018, 93) and other interventions, such as child protection (Eubanks 2018, 135) or education (O'Neil 2016, 5-9; 52–60) are decisions increasingly made by algorithms, rather than people. Even when automated decisions are questioned by people (Eubanks 2018, 141), it is unclear whether 'experienced workers' (Eubanks 2018, 77) or the data system has the greater influence in key decisions.

Beyond welfare, algorithms intervene in other social policy areas. They monitor the 'quality' of education, using dubious proxies (O'Neil 2016), with various bad outcomes, including teachers undeservedly losing their jobs.[4] In COVID-19 UK in 2020, an algorithm also decided the grades awarded to school-leavers in the absence of exams, owing to social distancing measures. One national media headline (Pidd 2020) called this 'punishment by statistics'.

The UK's A Level algorithm example was extremely high profile, causing outrage that data-driven decision-making would have such an enormous effect on the futures of these young people. It was seen as morally outrageous for a number of reasons. First, because our society dictates that these young people's well-being should be protected. Second, this algorithm used data that no one had consented to: no one knew at the time that their prior grades could be used as a final grade. Third, the data model also included proxies for expected performance which were nothing to do with each student's own academic record. Instead, they used their school's overall performance in previous years, which were scores based on previous students' grades, not theirs. While the governing body, Ofqual, insisted its standardisation arrangements 'are the fairest possible to facilitate students progressing on to further study or employment as planned' (Pidd 2020), there were further controversies over transparency around how they had arrived at 'fair'. After which, Ofqual published a 319-page document explaining its methodology (Pidd 2020) which was criticised for not being accessible to the general public. Therefore, not only did the whole thing seem far from fair, but Ofqual didn't make explicit how the approach was fair to those affected.

Here we see public services failing to look after well-being through the use of data in ways which go against the moral code of fairness, accountability and transparency[5]—and without the young people's consent. Beyond their high-profile nature, what is different about these data uses? While Chap. 2 discussed the greater role of data in public services from the 1980s onwards, this ostensibly had a different rationale. It aimed to evaluate qualities of these services, such as efficiency or cost-effectiveness. While these approaches led to flawed decisions and evaluations, assessments were made at a societal level. Contemporary data-driven decision-making, whether the allocation of resources to people or the labelling of individuals at risk, is a different approach and uses data on a different level. Or, to use the language of Chap. 3, there is a different unit of analysis, and that unit could be a vulnerable person.

In sum, why do we need to ask critical questions about how people and their well-being are being understood or about how data and data systems used to understand people can compromise well-being? Going back to those definitions, people are often concerned with the speed and size, and so on, of Big Data. Actually, as Kitchin indicates, it is the contexts of these data that are the most important ways that they are different. Not only are the contexts of origin of Big Data more different, and further from the contexts of use, than before, but the practices of analysing data feel less human. By this I mean that less human attention is now required in data analysis and in important processes that require data. What does that mean for decisions made about people and well-being?

As we will discover in a few sections, the response to COVID-19 required older data and data systems—and more human judgement—than you would have imagined if you were looking at media reports of the promise of artificial intelligence (AI) in the first half of 2020. However, as the financial value of data increases, the more expediently they can be analysed, and here we must ask other questions. Who stands to gain and who stands to lose? Who has chosen to participate? But then did people ever get to choose to participate in systems of well-being data? Or were we even thinking about data as 'a thing' about us, that affects our lives and was valuable? The next two sections deconstruct the financial value of Big Data and whether this reality is even new.

Value

Another major reason why we need to ask critical questions about Big Data and well-being concerns the financial value of knowing more about people and the financial value of the systems that sort people for public services and welfare distribution (Eubanks 2018). Beyond public services, the value of the new ways that Big Data can work is not just in *knowing* more about people, but because of the potential this knowledge has to orient people's thinking through suggestion and in some high-profile cases to manipulate what they do. They enable marketers to sell you products you might be most tempted by, knowing when you might be most susceptible too, based on your previous sales or what else you've looked at (Turow 2011). They also enable political campaigns to target their messages in the same way and change voting behaviour (Avila 2019; Bates et al. 2016; Murgia 2017). The recent Cambridge Analytica scandal saw Facebook implicated in not only the unethical use of people's data, and knowledge it had on their behaviour, but in misinformation that is thought to have changed the results of the US presidential election 2016 and Brexit in the UK the same year.

The first and second waves of well-being (Bache and Reardon 2013) from Chap. 2, and to which we keep returning, evolved as historical moments in which data capabilities married policy-makers' aims: improving the way we think about measuring human progress. Similarly, well-being metrics became more viable because well-being methodologies were evolving in a way that politicians saw as favourable. Political will and academic developments work with evolving infrastructure and technological development to enable datasets to be created with more detailed and nuanced information about quality of life. These factors work together for new methodologies to generate new kinds of data and analytical approaches which then, by extension, affect research and policy-making, which in turn impact upon our quality of life.

The increasing emphasis on Big Data as 'the new oil'[6] (a misnomer, of course) is not because datasets are 'better' (which would need some qualification) or because the technologies are new (though admittedly this is partly why it has become such a fixation). Instead, 'Big Data' datasets offer data with different *qualities* than more traditional data acquired by surveys. This means big datasets offer capacity to answer different research questions—or answer the same research questions differently. Most importantly, they have been called the new oil because: (1) 'data powers today's most profitable corporations, just like fossil fuels energized those of the past' (Matsakis 2019) and (2) this means these qualities can be financialised.

The amount of data on individuals that are now collected is almost impossible to visualise in our minds. The growing number of devices and sensors means we are generating more and more data than can be collected: the International Data Corporation predicts that by 2025, the total amount of digital data created worldwide will rise to 163 zettabytes (Coughlin 2018). That is 10^{21} (1,000,000,000,000,000,000,000 bytes) or one trillion Gigabytes. The European Commission forecasted the European 'data market' to be worth as much as €106.8 billion by 2020 (Ram and Murgia 2019). These kinds of numbers reinforce the importance of looking at Big Data as social phenomena—with social effects, but how new are large datasets about people and populations?

5.3   Are Big Data *Even* Actually New?

While data are 'sold' to us as 'the new oil' (The Economist 2017), large datasets, and their use to understand human behaviour, are not new; neither is the relationship between governments, commerce and value, when it comes to data. Mary Poovey's *A History of the Modern Fact: Problems of Knowledge in the Sciences of Wealth and Society* (1998) describes the rise of merchants and their influence over the State, including campaigns to promote the balance of trade as the index of national well-being from the early seventeenth century onwards (Poovey 1998, 93–94). The new 'enthusiasm for numbers' in the early to mid-nineteenth century (Hacking 1991, 186; Porter 1986, 1996) coincided with a growing infrastructure to collect and analyse data. This desire for numbers, and the data processes that were required to provide them, led to the 'great explosion of numbers that made the term statistics' (Porter 1986, 11). If truth be told, the term 'statistics' originated for governments to understand 'the quantum of happiness' (Sinclair 1798, vol. 20, p. xiii). In this 'avalanche of numbers', 'nation-states classified, counted and tabulated their subjects anew' (Hacking 1990, 2; 1991, 186). However, while 'statistics' may be hundreds of years old, large datasets go back further.

Managing land, agricultural hierarchies and the desire to control populations have long required systems of recording. One of the oldest-known writing systems is Sumerian script, which is approximately 6000 years old (Bellet and Frijters 2019). This script is called cuneiform, and its uses are said to include the tracking of trade and taxes: you need records on who has paid, how much; who has not paid, and what they owe (Harford 2017). While the clay tablets these records were written on may not seem like a database, or feel like the Big Data futures outlined in the previous and subsequent sections, they were a dataset of sorts. Crucially, these data were used to monitor and control resources, including the management of people.

Most countries now undertake a census of sorts. The UK Census takes place every ten years and has done since 1801.[7] The first four were only headcounts, with the 1841 Census being the first to intentionally record names of all individuals in a household or institution. The UK's ONS website offers an interesting history of censuses in the UK, back to the Domesday book ordered by the Norman (French) King, William the Conqueror in 1086 (ONS 2016). Again, censuses precede these European data moments by some 4000 years in both Egypt and China, whose governments (as they would have been formed and named in those days) recorded who lived where and how wealthy they were. The Romans held regular censuses to keep track of their expanding—and then contracting—empire. Evidence of other institutionalised data practices exists in the Bible: the book of Genesis talks of kinship and marriage records and

Exodus mentions a population census to support the tabernacle. The Church collected information on births, christenings, marriages, wills and deaths; this tracked the business of a church and its parish, but was also a means of counting the faithful and tracking their wealth.

You will note that the recording of trade and births, marriages and deaths is not so different from the administrative data that appear in all our examples of well-being data, from Table 3.1 to 5.3. So, what is new about Big Data? We've long had large datasets that hold multiple data points on people and nations, but these are thought to be 'state simplifications' for officials (Scott 1998). Rationalisation and standardisation mean these representations 'did not successfully represent the actual activity of the society depicted, nor were they intended to; they represented only the slice of it that interested the official observer' (Scott 1998, 3). What the historian James Scott tells us here is that the sorts of information that were collected on scale lacked detail that could be used to improve quality of life. He implies, of course, that those in charge did not *actually care* about quality of life, only quantity of resource, whether this was people to work the land, make armies, or pay taxes. More recently, as we have seen, governments were charged with responsibility for people's well-being, and therefore, more complex data were required.[8] One such development was the social survey.

The social survey has been used to collect data which capture various qualities of lives in richer ways, and for longer, than it is often credited for. For example, surveys in the UK in the mid-1940s (in World War II) discovered almost one in ten households did not have the number of cups deemed necessary for essential use, and 'the shortage of scrubbing brushes seems to have been extensively felt' (Oman 2015, 88; ONS 2001, 9). Whilst still administrative records of resource and scarcity, the survey began to be used to articulate more qualitative aspects of quality of life as proxies for well-being. This presents richer detail than many of the contemporary surveys that generate the well-being data we have seen as either objective or subjective data so far.

These more qualitative data were not only collected using government social scientists that we might imagine with clipboards. A project called Mass Observation was established in 1937 by anthropologist Tom Harrisson, poet Charles Madge and filmmaker Humphrey Jennings.[9] Mass Observation aimed to record everyday life in Britain. There were paid investigators who anonymously recorded people's conversations and their behaviour: at work, on the street and at memorable occasions, including public meetings or sporting and religious events.

This project was reminiscent of the current idea of 'Big Data', not only in the scope of the data gathered, but also in *how* they were gathered. Mass Observation had numerous phases and at one point also used a panel of around 500 voluntary 'observers'. The initial aims of Mass Observation were to research everyday life, making use of 'the untrained observer, the man in the street'[10] as much as those who were thought to be skilled and qualified in gathering data of this sort (Madge and Harrisson 1937, 10). The observers used various data collection methods to generate large datasets on different topics: some maintained diaries, while others replied to open-ended questionnaires. In 1938, there was 'a competition' for the residents of Bolton, Lancashire (see Fig 5.2), asking people what happiness meant for them. This was one of many themes, and people would reply to what were called directives with often very long texts describing what they thought and how they felt. The data from these and from the 1938 project can still be accessed via a vast archive at the University of Sussex.[11]

Mass Observation began with a positive vision of democratising the processes behind how data were gathered to better understand people's lives. However, over time, much qualitative social research shifted towards the narrower analysis of consumer choice, and Mass Observation became a market-research firm in 1949 (Albert 2019). Mass Observation re-launched in 1981, returning to its original egalitarian ideals and the archives are testament to the ways that Mass Observation aims to engage the public in the documenting of their own lives.

These historical examples of large datasets are, therefore, not so different from the qualities found in previously crowdsourced, location-based, time-based data on how people feel about things, as seen in Table 5.3. The purchasing of scrubbing brushes was used as proxy data for other qualities of life in the same way our purchasing data are analysed to better understand us. Similarly, a lack of cups was indicative of a particular kind of poverty and lack of resources at a point in time, and this was analysed across the population. However, the democratic promise of Mass Observation and other projects of the time were superseded by the potential of understanding what makes people happy for commercial gain.

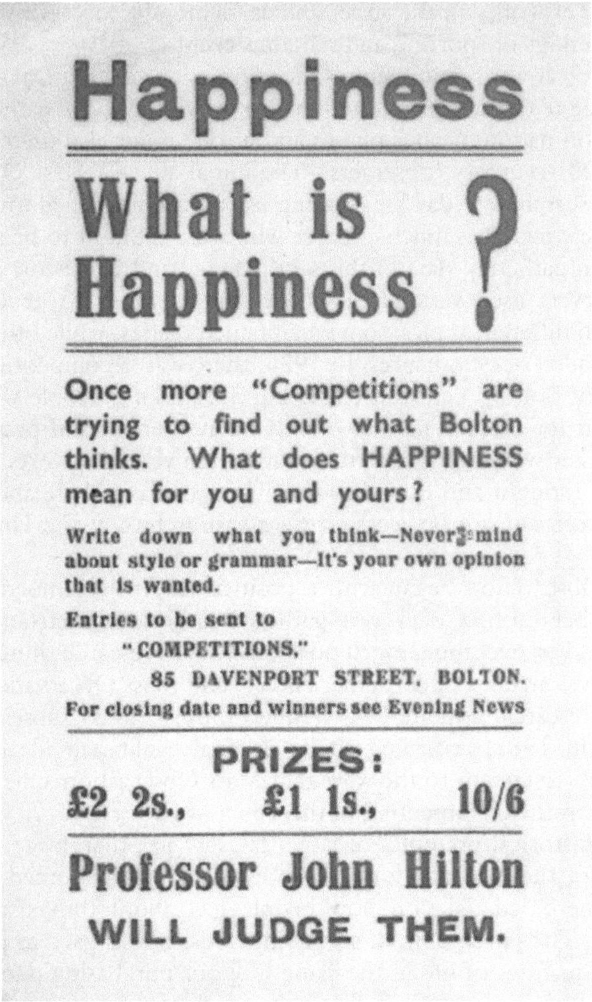
Happiness

What is Happiness ?

Once more "Competitions" are trying to find out what Bolton thinks. What does HAPPINESS mean for you and yours?

Write down what you think—Never mind about style or grammar—It's your own opinion that is wanted.

Entries to be sent to
"COMPETITIONS,"
85 DAVENPORT STREET, BOLTON.
For closing date and winners see Evening News

PRIZES:
£2 2s., £1 1s., 10/6

Professor John Hilton
WILL JUDGE THEM.

Fig. 5.2 What is happiness? Mass Observation competition flyer, 1938

The Darker Side of Historical Well-being Data and Commercial Gain

With the rise of market research came increased interest in people's preferences, and in what made them happy or gave them pleasure (Davies 2015; Savage 2010). This involved capturing subjective well-being data, as well as cultivating communications to imply that owning or consuming certain things would increase someone's well-being in some way. The aim here in this context, of course, was to change people's purchasing choices. With this shift, people as citizens became consumers. Over the years, 'consumer sentiment' indices have been assessed to see if these data can predict people's behaviours on a macro level, from economic cycles (Carroll et al. 1994) to presidential popularity (Suzuki 1992). This marriage of mood and economics is not new to us, of course. In Chap. 4, we encountered the development of subjective well-being data, a newer shinier well-being data, as a marriage of economics and psychology, known as happiness economics that was able to measure subjective well-being at population level.

Mood and sentiment analysis are not new, then. Neither are big datasets. Even Fitbits and Apple watches are not new; not really, as attaching technologies to people's bodies has been used to study and improve productivity and surveillance of workers and citizens for around a hundred years (Davies 2015; Cryle and Stephens 2017). So, what is new? The amount and variety of data on the well-being of individuals and populations are increasing as technologies develop to manage greater amounts of different kinds of data, not only faster, but faster together.[12] Therefore, it is not necessarily how one thing (not that Big Data are one thing, really) is new. Instead, it is a far more complex picture of how different aspects of, and different people across fields of, politics, science, research and technology work together—and work with commerce. These all combine as developments in *what* we know, and *ways of knowing*, about society.

The question is, what does that mean for well-being? How can we learn from previous mistakes regarding the context of who is using what data—and to what end? COVID-19 will offer us many data insights and many insights into how data can help us understand and look after well-being better. The next section looks at the role of data and learning in a pandemic, of old and new infrastructures and commercial and governmental data practices in the management of a pandemic.

5.4   A CASE STUDY ON THE PROMISE OF COMMERCIAL BIG DATA

One of the most high-profile cases of the possibilities of Big Data involves a tale that begins in 2009 when a new virus was discovered. This new illness spread quickly and combined elements of bird flu and swine flu. This story opens Mayer-Schönberger and Cukier's book, *Big Data: A Revolution That Will Transform How We Will Live, Work and Think*, which you may remember is mentioned earlier in the chapter as a much-cited originator of the term 'datafication' (2013). The authors explain that the only way authorities could curb the spread of this new virus was through knowing where it was already.

In the US, the Centres for Disease Control and Prevention (CDC) requested that doctors inform them of cases. However, the information on the pandemic that the CDC had to work with was out of date. This was by nature of the data collected, and its 'data journey' (Bates et al. 2016). There were multiple data journeys to consider: data were collected at the point someone went to the doctor, which could be days after initial symptoms, let alone contraction; sharing data with the CDC was a time-consuming procedure; the CDC only processed the data once a week. Thus, the picture was probably weeks out of date, making intervention or behavioural analysis difficult. In other words, while the datasets were large, even potentially fairly detailed, these Big Data were too slow.

Coincidentally, so Mayer-Schönberger and Cukier tell us, a few weeks before the new disease made the headlines, Google engineers published a paper in a high-profile journal, *Nature*, which explained how Google could 'predict' the spread of the winter flu in the US. This was possible just through analysing what people had typed into their search engine (and, of course, knowing where those people typing were). It compared the CDC data on the spread of seasonal flu from 2003 to 2008 with the 50 million most common search terms in America.

The Google engineers looked for correlations between what people typed into the Google search engine and the spread of the disease. Mayer-Schönberger and Cukier point out that.

Google's method doesn't require traditional infrastructures to distribute mouth swabs or for people to go to doctors' surgeries.

'Instead, it is built on 'big data'—the ability of society to harness information in novel ways to produce useful insights or goods and services of significant value. With it, by the time the next pandemic comes around, the world will have a better tool at its disposal to predict and thus prevent the spread. (Mayer-Schönberger and Cukier 2013, 2–3)

Sadly, a pandemic with wider societal and well-being effects arrived after I started writing this book, and despite the promise of Big Data, it did not prevent the spread. Data hold a very important place in the story of COVID-19 and its management, but all data have limitations in how it can inform human action to change reality, as do the different ways of analysing data. Indeed, data are not just *there* but are managed and *used* by people with their own interests. Data do not speak for themselves but are interpreted. All data realities also involve selective processes in what data are important and what data are not. These limits are not always made as clear as they should be.

Mayer-Schönberger and Cukier's promise of Big Data as revolutionary and transformational in the US was clearly jumping the gun. Not only was the pandemic not prevented by way of predictive analytics, but actually, part of COVID-19 data management has very much involved doctors' surgeries and mouth swabs—in the UK at least. To clarify, I was randomly selected from data held on people registered with a GP to participate in a survey in August 2020.[13] I was contacted by the Real-time Assessment of Community Transmission (REACT) Study,[14] which is in fact a series of studies, using home testing to understand more about COVID-19, and its transmission in communities in England. The logic behind the study was that not all people with the virus were being tested at this point, either because they were asymptomatic or for some other reason. This was one of a few projects to collect data from a sample of the population, over time, in order to understand how it was spreading.

This process relied on old infrastructures: I received a letter by Royal Mail, I signed up online, and then I was sent a mouth swab—also by post. That all worked fine for me, but there was a series of steps registering different barcodes and I found myself wondering how accessible this was for everyone (when I say everyone, I often think of my once tech-savvy Dad, who'd have been bewildered at this whole process). After completing these steps, a courier was ordered to collect the test. I sat in patiently waiting for my test to be collected, slightly anxious about what felt like a huge responsibility, and acutely aware that I might need to be ready to run out and meet a courier with my test.

I live in a high-rise with no working bell or intercom (and a bunch of other things that don't work). For three separate days, I watched for details of the courier on the app, and out of my window, waiting for them to appear on the road, or call to say I should come down. But there was no sighting of the courier in real life and no phone call. When the app showed they were coming, they disappeared without attempting to deliver. After three attempts. I was told that this particular courier company was infamous for not bothering to try and collect from my flats, because it was too inconvenient. So, in my case, while some aspects of the traditional data infrastructure (the post) worked fine, they didn't necessarily all work together as they might. This meant that my test remained uncollected, expired and had to be securely disposed of. This meant my data became 'missing data'.

What I was surprised by was how the information system assumed you would live somewhere that was easy to access. As we know, many people from our poorest communities live in high-rises where the lift doesn't work, or the people in the flats themselves are difficult for a courier to access. Thinking about the contexts in which data are collected (or not) can be both extraordinary, and mundane, and we often don't hear of these stories—when they work, and the odd occasion when they don't, and what that might mean for the data. Yet, these contexts have huge impact on who is readable in data and how we understand well-being and inequality.

So why did COVID-19 data collection end up using more traditional infrastructures in the UK? On a larger scale, why did the world not use Google data as Mayer-Schönberger and Cukier predicted? As it turns out, Google Flu Trends (GFT) missed the peak of the 2013 flu season by 140%, and Google subsequently closed the project (REF). In 2014 a paper called 'The Parable of Google Flu: Traps in Big Data Analysis' was published in another high-profile academic journal, *Science* (Lazer et al. 2014). The authors concluded that while there was potential in these sorts of methodologies, and while Google's efforts in projecting the flu may have been well meaning (which could be called into question), the method and data were opaque. This made it potentially 'dangerous' (Lazer and Kennedy 2015) to rely on GFT for any decision-making, as the context of the data and the analyses were not made explicit to public decision-makers. Of course, it is also perhaps unlikely that Google had designed the tool for public decision-making contexts,[15] considering what government officials need to understand for this kind of decision-making.

There are other limits to the data: its sample. Google assumes this ubiquitous reputation, yet, it is not the only search engine available: people choose other search engines for various reasons. Crucially, Google also does not have global reach. Most services offered by Google China, for example, were blocked by the Great Firewall in the People's Republic of China. This was not even the first time it was banned in China. So, even if GFT were still in action, would it have pre-empted the COVID-19 outbreak in Wuhan, China, before more official announcements?

If we are to think about how Big Data have transformed how we live, as Mayer-Schönberger and Cukier want us to, then we must also consider how 'datafication' has changed people's practices. More and more of us scour the internet, hoping to reassure ourselves that recently developed symptoms are minor ailments. This is—as we discovered in Chap. 2—part of the anxiety introduced with audit culture: we consult technologies as a default because we can, rather than should. We search for confirmation that nothing is wrong, rather than only searching when something is wrong. In countries where access to healthcare is diminished, people are actively encouraged to search the internet before interacting with health services. Consequently, this limits the predictability of search data, as their contexts have changed.

In the case of COVID-19, people searched for symptoms they didn't necessarily have, especially in the second quarter of 2020, when most nations were in lockdown and the severity and ramifications of the disease were becoming clearer. The implications of this are that searches would not necessarily have reflected the infected state of an individual that could be aggregated to reveal community or population infections, or more importantly, predict transmission so that it might be controlled in some way. Instead, searches for COVID-19 symptoms may well be a predictor of concern or anxiety. Ironically, then, Google searches are arguably a better indicator of negative subjective well-being than of COVID-19.

The very idea of data being reliable has led to our need to feel sure—to have objective confirmation that all was OK, is OK or will be OK, and has led to an increased reliance on data. In the case of Google searches, this reliance has triggered people to search for verification of risk or safety. So how might we have cut through the 'noise' that the definitions at the beginning of this chapter point to, in order to *know* how it was spreading? We are back at the chicken and the egg dilemma: do people search about

COVID-19 because they have symptoms? Or do people search about COVID-19 because they are worried about it and feel compelled to search for confirmation—or search on behalf of friends or loved ones? I watched someone use their internet searches to check our colleague's proclaimed symptoms against the common signs of swine flu—a very collegiate individual, but one whose search history told a story of their friend's (potential) disease state, rather than their own. In this latter case, then, Google searches were more indicative of personality than health or even subjective well-being, although, perhaps well-being data all the same.

Bigger datasets make correlation more powerful than causation, explain Mayer-Schönberger and Cukier, devoting a whole chapter to it in their book (2013). Google queries went from 14 billion per year in 2000 to 1.2 trillion a decade later. There are even websites that show a live running tally of how many searches have been achieved in a day.[16] If Big Data were all about scale, then GFT would have been more, not less likely to work on the premise of correlation as search numbers increased. The scale at which we have correlations using 'Big Data' may be an *indicator* of causation, but not proof. Is this the end of the promise of Big Data, though? If we return to a case of COVID-19 and Big Data, what might we find?

Linking Big Datasets: For Well-being?

On New Year's Day, 2020, a Canadian health monitoring company alerted its customers to the COVID-19 outbreak, some days before the US' CDC or the World Health Organization (WHO) alerted anyone (Niiler 2020). Of course, the disease was not yet called COVID-19, and it was not known that it was to be a global pandemic. At this point, a cluster of unusual pneumonia cases had been detected. One of the companies said to have beaten the WHO to this discovery is called BlueDot, which uses AI-driven algorithm searches to look at datasets, much like GFT.

Unlike Google Flu Trends, BlueDot's algorithms consolidate and analyse data from numerous sources. BlueDot's owner, Dr. Kamran Khan explains:

> We can pick up news of possible outbreaks, little murmurs or forums or blogs of indications of some kind of unusual events going on. (Khan, in Niiler 2020)

Other data sources are more official, such as statements from health organisations, livestock and news reports in 65 languages. BlueDot also uses 'anonymous mobile phone data' (Whitaker 2020), flight sales and other records. These various data points enable a prediction of a possible new serious disease. Importantly, the logic is that this approach also offers insight into how that disease becomes mobile by the people who carry it and the planes who carry the people carrying the disease.

> What we have done is use natural language processing and machine learning to train this engine to recognize whether this is an outbreak of anthrax in Mongolia versus a reunion of the heavy metal band Anthrax. (Niiler 2020)

Also, crucially, 'epidemiologists check that the conclusions make sense from a scientific standpoint' (Niiler 2020). The company website states that 'BlueDot protects people around the world from infectious diseases with human and artificial intelligence' (BlueDot n.d.). Therefore, despite claims to its sophistication, the automated data-sifting still requires human analysis to make *sense* of what has been found.

Khan's company utilised technological developments at its disposal to synthesise many different types of data from multiple datasets to construct evidence. Only when the data were pieced together was the information useful, and only after human experts had checked it, were these insights deemed useful enough to share and use. BlueDot is a commercial company. The human and artificial intelligence are synthesised as an enterprise, and Khan is often presented as both an entrepreneur, as well as a professor of medicine and public health at the University of Toronto. Khan has also worked in hospitals, so understands how they work. Khan explains in one interview,

> Disease doesn't wait for the reviewers, so we need a more agile system. My motivation for creating a company—here to start supporting an entrepreneurial spirit—using business as the vehicle to do that. (Khan, on Charrington 20 February 2020)

There are two things to note here. Khan suggests that the old structures of peer review and scientific expertise are too slow in their use of data and evidence to tackle a global pandemic. He also suggests that his business successfully links together 'human and artificial intelligence' to provide what traditional science cannot: the analysis of data with veracity and variability, speed, resolution, relationality and so on. The *value* of BlueDot is in its claims to harnessing the qualities of Big Data.

To return to Mayer-Schönberger and Cukier, 'Google's method' may not have involved distributing mouth swabs, or been built on old infrastructures, but instead, they explain:

> [I]t is built on "big data"—the ability of society to harness information in novel ways to produce useful insights or goods and services of significant value. (Mayer-Schönberger and Cukier, 2)

So, there we have those familiar terms of insights (a marketing term) and valuation (that we discovered from economics in Chap. 2), alongside clear communications and the presentation of novelty (Chap. 4), goods and services. Mayer-Schönberger and Cukier hint at the complex politics at play on the value of data—and the values of data more broadly than we have already encountered.

Crucially, in a book about well-being and data, we have to note that BlueDot's business is entrepreneurial because it is profitable. In other words, the insights have to be sold to clients and customers. They were also not the only innovator (as acknowledged by the Lancet and MIT Review [McCall 2020; Heaven 2020]). Here, we must return to the economic value of data because of the possibilities of well-being insights and the ideological project of the well-being agenda.

If the well-being agenda is about improving redistribution of resources as an issue of social justice, we might want to think about what position we are coming from: rather than asking, 'what are the data limits of these well-being projects?', we might ask, 'what are the well-being limits of data projects like these?' Although, despite the clear sophistication of BlueDot's project, it also did not prevent COVID-19's spread. This criticism has been noted in the MIT Review:

> The hype outstrips the reality. In fact, the narrative that has appeared in many news reports and breathless press releases—that AI is a powerful new weapon against diseases—is only partly true and risks becoming counterproductive. (Heaven 2020)

The point this MIT article was making here is that the over-reaching claims of AI could be damaging to its future progression, in the same way that GFT overstretched its claims.

Data and the distribution of resources are very much part of the COVID-19 story, and not just of private companies profiteering, either.

Such competition is also reiterated by national politicians misleading the public about 'world-beating' systems of data (BBC 2020). In the same way that the social indicators movement was halted because it was not quite measuring what it thought it was measuring (Chap. 2), the 'promise' of Big Data has adjusted. The limits of Google's approach are in a lack of context: the nature of what people actually search for is different than was predicted. The limits on data are social, cultural, political and economic, and by extension, these limit the possibilities for a good society. We will explore social media and mobile communications data in the final few sections to better appreciate this relationship.

5.5   Social Media Data: A Game Changer?

I am sure that social media plays a role in unhappiness, but it has as many benefits as it does negatives. (Sir Simon Wessely, president of the UK's Royal College of Psychiatrists in Campbell 2017)

Social media platforms have an interesting relationship to well-being. They are often demonised as bad for well-being, especially for the younger generation who are thought to dwell on images of idealised bodies and lifestyles on Instagram (Campbell 2017). All ages feel a pang looking at the picture-perfect presentations on Facebook, and even the NHS warns people to take breaks from social media (NHS 2016). Credible, successful women leave themselves vulnerable to criticism from strangers in the sharing of thoughts, opinions and aspects of their identity on platforms like Twitter (Lewis et al. 2016). Similarly, hate speech against people of colour (Gayle 2018) or for their gender identity (Pearce et al. 2020) are realities of social media platforms. However, social media and online platforms also offer places for human connections, and have had beneficial effects for the social isolation brought about by measures to curb the spread of COVID-19. The jury is still out on many of the pros and cons of social media, including their propensity to spread disinformation, versus credible analysis of data and guidelines. Social media therefore hold an ambivalent place in the management of well-being.

These controversial aspects of social media are not their only connections to well-being. The data we share can make them useful for well-being analysis. The most mundane aspects of our feeds, the venting of minor irritations, celebrations of small wins or just feelings shared with friends and family mean our social media accounts are full of well-being data. Think about those ONS4 questions again (Table 4.2) that aim to gauge 'personal well-being'. For example, they all ask you to think about how you felt yesterday overall—in terms of happiness or anxiety, as well as whether you think what you do is worthwhile, and whether you are satisfied with your life. When you think about Facebook's most prolific posters in your timelines, for example, much of their content will indicate how they felt in similar ways at specific moments. The recent addition of emojis to Facebook means it is easier to proclaim whether you were happy, celebrating or anxious. The reminders of what you were doing this time last year or ten years ago means we are telling everyone on Facebook how we feel now, about how we were feeling in previous years. Crucially, this means it is even easier for Facebook to know this too, as you have essentially coded your own data for them.

This compulsion to share how we feel means we are also sharing our data with Facebook and other platforms. These platforms are able to analyse us alongside millions of others at scale. Companies like Brandwatch monitor social media and analyse several billion emoticons each year to inform brands whether they are provoking hatred or happiness with their products. It is also possible for a broad range of actors to mine social media data, whether commercial companies, government agencies, academic researchers or amateurs with the inclination to do so. The platforms are set up with open Application Programming Interfaces (APIs). APIs are what allow other (data mining) software to interact with social media platforms. Once access to social media data has been gained, it can be 'scraped' with comparative speed with the right skills and software. Scraping is a process which essentially involves gathering and copying data that meets specific search terms. It is then put into a database (that can be as crude as a spreadsheet), for later retrieval or analysis. This can be done by a person, although the term more typically refers to automated processes involving a bot or web crawler. The fact that APIs are generally open as a standard indicates that these data—your data—are made available by social media platforms to be used by various different actors. Not many people think about the fact that their public post on a social media platform is public in the sense that it is no longer their private property and can be used by others in research.[17]

There are practical limits to what can be known through analysing people's social media posts, of course. First, people are not neutrally representing themselves on social media. As we know, people feel compelled to publish reflections on an idealised version of their lives (Kruzan and Won 2019). Of course, our social media posts don't always represent our lives as happier than they actually are: people often exaggerate the impact of minor negative events that are as mundane as missing the bus or being rained on. Some people collectively engage in dissatisfaction with their lot in life, leading to Twitter bubbles and what has become known as 'the culture wars',[18] as the contemporary cultural conflict between social groups. This term describes a gap between those who side with a traditional, conservative approach, and those with a liberal, progressive approach to society and social issues, such as immigration, abortion, LGBTQIA+ rights, and so on. The contemporary culture wars, as a struggle for dominance of values and beliefs, now takes place on Twitter, and we might question the extent to which such rage and passion are indicative of someone's personal well-being, or some form of tribal rage on a larger scale. Essentially, we are seeing how important social media can be in both distorting and shaping our well-being for better or for worse. The key to appreciating the relationship of social media, data and well-being is understanding limits and context—of collection and use.

Social Media Data Mining in Social and Cultural Sectors

Social media data mining is not always a large-scale affair requiring APIs and special software. As found in a six-month research project with city councils and a city-based museums group in the north of England (Kennedy 2016), many small organisations use quite basic techniques to do this work. Social and cultural policy sectors are reliant on understanding well-being data, as improving well-being is at the core of what many of them do. Yet, as Chap. 1 of this book acknowledges, the sectors do not always have the skills or confidence to use data. We will look at these sectors as a whole in greater depth in the next three chapters.

The project exploring how these smaller social and cultural organisations were already using data mining, wanted to understand how they might use it more effectively. The researchers discovered that although software packages were adopted to analyse institutional impact and engagement on Twitter, this was largely unsystematic (Kennedy 2016, 71 & 72). Keen to improve their social media data mining capacity, these organisations signed up for training in new tools that would improve their capability. However, it became clear that less data mining was happening than expected and the capacity of workshop participants to engage with training in the new tools also fell away (Kennedy 2016, 74). Doing better with data seems a good idea, but is not always as easily resourced or incorporated into working practices as initially hoped.

Local councils, social and cultural sector organisations all have limited resources. Despite enthusiasm for being, or becoming, data-driven, capacity to invest time and money in new tools at the organisational level is often lacking (Kennedy 2016; Oman 2019a, b). In the case of the cultural sector, there is a tendency to invest in grand schemes, new metrics and reports at policy level that claim to investigate the value of new and/or Big Data and the associated technologies required to generate or analyse them (Gilmore et al. 2018; Oman 2013a). However, when considering the (already ill-defined) cultural sector[19] as a whole, differences are obscured in requirements and capacity for data technologies, which are multiplied by huge variability in organisation size, type, purpose, mission and cultural offering across and within sectors (Oman 2013a). These top-down resources and contributions are not always actually used or found useful at an organisational level or across the wider sector (Oman 2013a). Some organisations recognise that their audiences are full of people whose opinions are less easily captured by Big Data. Some people, for example, still prefer booking telephone lines to web pages and are certainly not tweeting or Instagramming their experience of a show. As such, some who attend a show are less likely to be generating data on their opinions that might then be mined. Advocates for using Big Data in small organisations acknowledge that Big Data can be 'debilitating' in their complexity and challenges. This is not always explored in a way that offers resolution (Oman 2013a), and as we have seen (Kennedy 2016) when recommendations, even training, are offered, there is not necessarily the capacity to take them up.

Yet, it can be very easy and fast to interact with Big Data as social media data, as long as you consider the limitations of the data and their origins, as well as how you might analyse them yourself. Organisations and individuals do not need Big Data analytics know-how or software, although there are excellent resources freely available to help them understand how,[20] as I found when I wanted to explore Twitter discussions about happiness. In 2013, Mass Observation recreated the Bolton happiness study on Twitter (see Fig. 5.3). This was still fairly experimental for them as much as me when I requested access to the tweets. There were 25 responses that they captured at the time.

The sample of 25 meant that—of course—I did not require data mining or sentiment analysis software—or any knowledge of APIs. In fact, I did not even need to request these tweets from Mass Observation directly, as

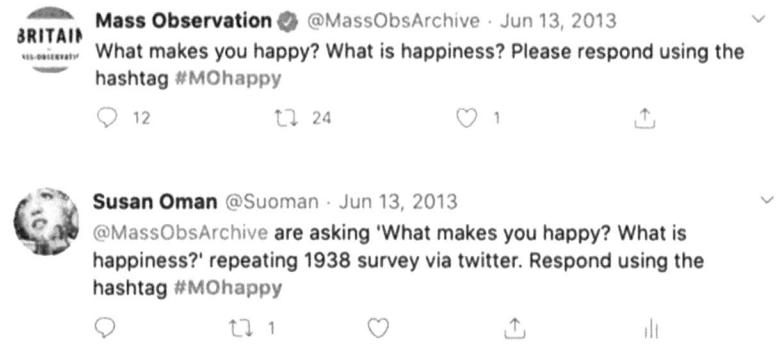

Fig. 5.3 Mass Observation happiness tweets

they are still available on Twitter by searching the hashtag (or were in August 2020 when I last checked). A cursory analysis in this case simply meant reading, and noting similarities and themes, which I could have done on a piece of paper.

So, what did this cursory analysis tell me? Whilst 20% mentioned pets, all of which were cats (it is the internet after all), one person replied with a single word: bacon. Mainly, however, people described informal, everyday participation,[21] including reading, going to gigs, watching films. There were lots of glasses of wine and some chocolate in there too. The textual content of these tweets is reproduced in Box 5.1, without Twitter handles. You might note the surprising varieties of theories of well-being we have encountered so far in the book can be present in 25 tweets. Some map onto clear areas of social policy, others are definitely in the private domain. Some people used negative language to imply life isn't currently great for them: 'Day off. Smoke in peace.' And 'Ability for women to walk down the street & not be catcalled or threatened. Few happy women here'. Some people were philosophical, others wistful. Some focussed on activities, others on the 'bliss' of doing nothing. The variety of tone and content makes for fascinating reading, but leaves these data wide open to interpretation—whether that is via human or artificial intelligence.

Box 5.1   Tweets Answering the Question: 'What Is Happiness?'

- Beer, maps, chocolate, quizzes, the unending pursuit of knowledge
- Ability for women to walk down the street & not be catcalled or threatened. Few happy women here
- Short term happiness is different for everyone. Long term happiness is about fulfilling your potential.
- Bacon
- 5 minutes to myself and a good book, with peppermint tea and the cats curled up around me. Absolute bliss!
- Volunteering, yoga, baking, being with loved ones, reading, warm days paddling in the sea, colourful things, exploring, my cat: D
- Doing what I love (#history), a safe home by the sea, someone to love & share things with
- Good company, fireworks, being smiled at, a job well done, 'sweet pea' by Manfred Mann, making someone else happy, good health.
- I am happiest when discovering/learning new things, such as reading books and finding new music.
- Happiness is cooking for those I love, with a glass of wine and giggles on the side.
- Day off. Smoke in peace.
- "What is happiness?" something to do with dopamine levels
- Making things that muself [sic], and hopefully other people will enjoy
- Loving and being loved and valued for who I actually am.
- More precisely: Time, a book, a view, a friend.
- Choices and control in life not just in shopping.
- Connecting with other people, being able to make a difference to someone else, a good book and a purring cat on my lap!
- My kids
- What is happiness?'—"A warm spot on the bed in the sunshine"
- Knowing that enough is plenty
- The scent of roses on a damp morning […] being where you are without wishing to be somewhere else
- Happiness is seeing my children flourish, Swansea City FC progress & succeed & cooking for husband. Ln that order!;)
- Love, health and a sense of purpose. Oh, and cake.
- What makes me happy? Cuddling up on the sofa with my partner & animals, a glass of wine, chocolate, a film & crochet- bliss
- Happiness is good relationships, a little more than enough money, satisfaction and contentment

I used these tweets as a light-hearted example, with my ever so light-touch analysis, in my first ever conference presentation in 2013. In Chap. 3, I explained that my research question at the beginning of my PhD was loosely: 'When people describe well-being, how often do they talk about participating in different kinds of activities—and what might that tell us about aspects of social and cultural policy?' or 'how can qualitative data collected to understand well-being tell us how people feel about what they do?'. I noted in this presentation that state-funded cultural practices (like art galleries and museums) were less frequently mentioned by people as making them happy than what is called everyday participation (Oman 2013b). This same finding emerged from my reanalysis of the ONS free text data I used in my PhD (Oman 2017, 2020). By extension, these data (with their caveats) were another dataset to suggest we should question whether cultural funding was supporting activities that made people happier or increased their well-being.

This was not the only way of analysing these tweets to make an argument about the relationship between culture and well-being. Someone else may have counted how many of these responses included something creative and used their analysis to argue they have found the value of culture to people, thereby justifying more funding. These are debates about data and their use in politics and policy that we return to in the next chapter. What is important here is that even with (arguably, especially with) such a small dataset we can see how human bias can interact with data and lead to different arguments.

If it is difficult for humans to make categorical claims from a form of sentiment analysis that is not much more systematic or technical than reading 25 tweets, we must remember these limits when these analyses are made through machine learning. This is especially vital as time-sensitive analyses of large-scale samples of emotional expressions are being used in research on COVID-19, particularly given they are seen to have the potential to inform mental health support and help tailor risk communication to change behaviours (i.e. Pellert et al. 2020). As with all data uses mentioned in this book, it is not that using social media data, or automated sentiment analyses are necessarily bad, but rather, that their limits should be recognised. As ever, it is an issue of methodology, transparency context and legibility.

Understanding Where People Are and How They Feel Using Twitter Data

Of course, it is not only what people say that can be mined, but also where they are. One research project attempted to gauge community well-being using Twitter data from between 27 September and 10 December 2010 (Quercia et al. 2012). Interestingly, as an aside, this coincided with the UK's Measuring National Well-being debate which launched in November of that year. The researchers were interested in a few things. They wanted to understand more than individuals, to measure the well-being of communities. They state their intention as moving the recent developments in subjective well-being measures that we discovered in the last chapter forward. Rather than administering questionnaires on an individual basis, or in a national-level survey, they wanted to explore the recent possibilities of sentiment analysis to understand community well-being,

Social media data can significantly reduce the time-consuming processes that make large-scale surveys and qualitative work resource-heavy. Once these data have been 'scraped' and saved into a database, they can be analysed in many ways. In the case of Querica and their co-authors, they were interested in the idea of using sentiment analysis to see if it could interpret community well-being. They created a sentiment metric, which was originally derived from studying Facebook status updates (Kramer 2010). This metric standardised the difference between the percentage of positive and negative words in a Facebook user's posts in one day. Kramer used the metric to make arguments at a national level, aiming to develop, as he suggests in the title of his paper, 'An Unobtrusive Behavioral Model of "Gross National Happiness"'.

His new standardised metric was found to correlate with self-reported life satisfaction. Looking at the US specifically, peaks were found in life satisfaction that correlated with national and cultural holidays. This is fine in and of itself, but what does that tell us about well-being? Christmas is good for well-being? Other research indicates otherwise (Holmes and Rahe 1967; Mutz 2016), suggesting it can cause feelings of stress for various reasons: financial, family, and so on. What about the days either side when people are travelling huge distances (with everyone else) using transport infrastructure which is not fit for purpose? Or the excesses of consumption that holidays like Christmas involve, as well as their impact on the planet? What about all those who do not celebrate Christmas, as they are not of a Christian denomination? In his limitations, the author acknowledges that there is a possibility that the likelihood to wish people 'Happy Christmas' could have affected these results. However, he decided not to control for this, as wishing someone happy holidays is a positive sentiment. We might wonder, then, whether this study was really interested in the possibilities for understanding the human experience using the details of the Facebook posts, or whether it was interested in deriving a metric that was comparable with more established methods.

Returning to the study on community well-being, the authors state, 'it is not clear whether the correspondence between sentiment of self-reported text and well-being would hold at *community level*, that is, whether sentiment expressed by community residents on social media reflects community socio-economic well-being' (Quercia et al. 2012, 965). Therefore, they do note some of the limitations of using this approach to answer their research question. However, notably, they do not acknowledge some of the limitations of the metric itself.

London was chosen for the study to understand about communities, socio-economics and well-being. Let's break down what they did and how. The study used four types of data gathering, it:

1. 'Crawled' Twitter accounts whose user-specified locations report London neighbourhoods.
2. Geo-referenced the Twitter accounts by converting their locations into longitude—latitude.
3. Measured socio-economic prosperity, using the UK's IMD.[22]
4. Conducted sentiment analysis on tweets between particular dates from their sample.

How did these processes work?

1. How the crawl worked: the researchers chose three popular London-based profiles of news outlets: the free newspaper *The Metro*, which was available in London on the Tube at the time (it has since expanded), a right-wing tabloid *The Sun* and the centre-left newspaper *The Independent*. These media were chosen because they are thought to capture different demographics of class and politics. Using these three accounts as 'seeds', they used 'a crawler' to trace linked accounts. Crawlers are software that allows you to gather various kinds of available data based on who interacts with a particular website or Twitter account. In this instance, every user following these accounts was 'crawled'.

2. Some Twitter users stated where they live in their profiles. Accounts were crawled to find 157k of 250k profiles had listed locations, with 1323 accounts specified London neighbourhoods. They then filtered out likely bots by also 'crawling' using another metric[23] for each profile. This brought the sample down to 573 profiles. Once these were established, locations were converted into longitude-latitude pairs, translating these data into geographical co-ordinates which are easier to work with.

3. The IMD is broken into 32,482 areas, 78 of these are within the boundaries of London used by the authors (these are not necessarily fixed). The IMD offered a score for each of London's 78 census areas. The authors use a census area to represent 'a community'. We shall return to this key point in a bit, but hold that thought. The data comes from the ONS' Census and is an objective list of sorts: income, employment, education, health, crime, housing, and the environmental quality. It is worth noting that in the IMD, the ONS talk about 'Lower Layer Super Output Areas' (LSOAs), rather than communities.

4. Sentiment analysis was undertaken on the tweets using two algorithms. (1) Kramer's metric described and (2) something called a 'Maximum Entropy classifier', which uses machine learning. The algorithm in Kramer's metric has a limited dictionary, so this second machine learning package was used to improve on the first, by using a training dataset of tweets with smiley and frown-y faces. The authors argue that the results across the two algorithms correlate and are accurate. They then measured the sentiment expressed by a profile's tweets and then compute, for each region, an aggregate sentiment measure of all the profiles in the region.

Findings: So what did they find? Through studying the relationship between sentiment and socio-economic well-being they found that 'the higher the normalised sentiment score of a community's tweets, the higher the community's socio-economic well-being'. In other words, the sentiment metric accounted for positive and negative sentiments, enabling each area's aggregated data to show an average score. This tended to correlate with the scale that they used that indicates poverty and prosperity in that locale (the IMD).

Limitations—What did the authors identify as limitations?

Demographic bias—Twitter users are certain types of people; therefore, these findings will over-represent the happiness of Twitter users—missing out on non-users.

Causality—our old friend. Though the causal direction is difficult to determine from observational data, one could repeatedly crawl Twitter over multiple time intervals, and use a cross-lag analysis to observe potentially causal relationships.

Sentiment—They tracked sentiment but not '*what* actually makes communities happy' (Quercia et al. 2012, 968). The intention was to compare topics across communities. Their example:

> given two communities, one talking about yoga and organic food, and the other talking about gangs and junk food, what can be said about their levels of social deprivation? The hope is that topical analysis will answer this kind of question and, in so doing, assist policy makers in making informed choices regarding, for example, urban planning. (Quercia et al. 2012, 968)

As evidenced with the possibilities for making an argument using the crude analysis of the Mass Observation tweets, and as suggested by the citation directly above, there is bias in the ways that Big Data can be used to inform social and cultural policy. However, this is not necessarily any more the case in these examples than in those using more traditional data sources explored earlier in the book. The ways our social worlds are ordered do not reside in the algorithms, but in the preconceptions, laziness and judgements which become reproduced through researchers and their research and through policy-makers and their decisions. While the Quercia et al. examples were presented as a binary of opposites for narrative effect, the ridiculousness of the proposition may not stop it coming into effect as a deductive study in future. The fact that gangs are unlikely to tweet about gangs is one thing. Furthermore, the idea that these gangs remain within their ONS-allocated geographical boundaries called LSOAs is also a nonsense.

This brings me to another point, LSOAs are not communities: not in the way that we think of community well-being as built on social relations and inter-related lives. People are not only active citizens where they live, and in a city like London especially, may actually be more likely to be active citizens where they work. Without the context of understanding London, what it is to *live in* London, and the complex, overlaid communities and social groups that comprise a postcode, this idea of community well-being is a misnomer. Instead, it matches one index that uses census data, which, while valuable, can be out of date, and is well-known for its various limitations as a metric of socio-economic deprivation or advantage.

Perhaps another way to look at a question of community well-being might be to look at people interacting in public space. Plunz et al. (2019) also used sentiment analysis with geo-located Twitter data. They were interested in finding well-being indicators associated with urban park space. Their goal was to assess if tweets generated in parks may express a more positive sentiment than tweets generated in other places in New York City. Their results suggest that tweets in Manhattan are different from other NYC boroughs. In Manhattan, people's tweets were more positive outside of parks than inside, whereas the opposite was true outside of Manhattan. They concluded that Twitter data could still be useful for aspects of social policy, including urban design and planning. They also note that one of the limitations of geo-located Twitter data is that GPS is less accurate than sometimes accounted for. It also does not account for elevation, so you could be on the metro underneath Central Park, or indeed, stuck in traffic alongside it. It is hard to establish whether people may have gone for a walk to let off steam, or commute to work, for example.

The relationships between where we are standing or where we live and our well-being are not new, but a feature of much philosophy on the nature of subjective experience, especially since the Enlightenment (which we shall come to in the next chapter). Big Data offer new ways to test what we know about place. However, these data and devices also make assumptions about place and experience (Wilmott 2016). The expectations and suppositions of what happens where, for whom and how drive these analyses with the same bias as other Big Data technologies, and we must be aware of the limitations of these data, technologies and the ideas of well-being they claim to measure. We also need to be vigilant about who holds the data and why they are analysing.

5.6   Fit for Purpose? Health and Well-being Tracking and Apps

Recent technological developments have seen a rise in people using wearable technologies and their mobile phones to track their movements and behaviour. These include: periods of activity, menstruation, what they have eaten, how they have slept, how far they have walked and their heart rate, in order to gain an overall picture of their health and general well-being. These practices are frequently called the Quantified Self movement (Ruckenstein and Pantzar 2017), which refers both to the cultural phenomenon of self-tracking using one's own data, as well as the community of people who use and share data in this way.

The technologies are increasingly popular and are being discussed as cost-savers for the NHS, but there are barriers to their use (Jee 2016). Around five years ago, 85% of the general population did not own wearable devices (Lee et al. 2016). Therefore, measures which use datasets from these technologies will only account for a proportion of the population, who are most likely to be younger and more affluent (Strain et al. 2019) and already demonstrating an investment in their current and future well-being by owning such a device in the first place. We also do not yet fully understand the impact of COVID-19 on wearable devices and app use, as at the beginning of the crisis there were stories about governments using these data to monitor compliance with lockdown measures (Digital Initiatives 2020). YouGov polling data[24] indicate that even in July 2020, 65% of the UK had still never owned a wearable device, with 22% currently using one (with everyone else having tried one, or owned one but not currently using one). However, the same YouGov data indicate that usage has increased from 22% to 27% in January 2021, and those who have never owned a device has decreased at a similar rate. Therefore COVID-19 has seen an increase in wearable technology, as people take an interest in their well-being data in new ways.

Self-tracking, or the practice of generating or capturing data about everyday activities like eating, exercise for purposes of self-improvement, puts data and control in the hands of people, as well as the corporations which produce self-tracking devices and the third parties with which these data are shared (Kennedy et al. 2020). The research is ambivalent as to whether the experience of self-tracking has positive benefits, such as perception of control, agency or, in the case of professional or amateur sporting, opportunities for new communities (Ajana 2017; Lupton 2019; Pink and Fors 2017). It is also thought that these practices in and of themselves, and in their relationship to control, may decrease well-being more generally (Kennedy et al. 2020).

Data collected via mobile phone apps present similar possibilities for community and compromise. Smartphone access and usage only account for certain sections of a national demographic, much like wearable devices. Similarly, people who download an app to better understand their well-being are already self-selecting as wanting to improve their well-being, and therefore may not be considered a representative sample. A number of apps in the early 2010s wanted to further develop the insights gained from better understanding subjective well-being measurement.

In 2012, experts in geography and the lived environment based at the London School of Economics created a mobile phone app to understand happiness (MacKerron and Mourato 2013). What they branded a 'hedonimeter' (after the nineteenth-century invention we discovered in Chap. 2), the 'Mappiness' app asked people to allow the app to collect objective data about where they were (automatically, using GPS data), what activity they were doing, and who they were with (as manual entries). It also asked them to provide hedonic responses (subjective well-being data) as to how awake, happy and relaxed they were. These data were collected using sliders instead of the more traditional scales we have previously encountered. The data collected by the app were used in a number of different ways to appreciate subjective well-being and we will touch on a couple here.

In 2015, a report which drew on this data was published. 'Cultural Activities, Artforms and Wellbeing' reported on research commissioned by Arts Council England (ACE). The authors evaluated the hedonic readings of various activities found in the data collected by the app (Fujiwara and MacKerron 2015). Table 5.4 shows what the authors describe as 'happiness activities rankings', with theatre, dance and concert appearing to have the highest effect, and reading the lowest, unless you incorporate

Table 5.4 'Happiness activities[a] rankings'

Activities	Coefficient
Theatre, dance, concert	8.735***
Singing, performing	7.731***
Exhibition, museum, library	7.457***
Hobbies, arts, crafts	5.737***
Talking, chatting, socialising	3.789***
Drinking alcohol	3.646***
Listening to music	3.518***
Childcare, playing with children	2.888***
Reading	2.331***
Watching TV, film	2.084***
Housework, chores, DIY	-0.651***

Source: Fujiwara and MacKerron (2015)

[a]The table shows coefficients, rather than rankings. Compared with the baselines, these coefficients report how much happier participants reported being when participating in these activities on a scale, when relevant variables have been controlled for. The coefficient shows the size of the impact on happiness from doing the activity (where happiness is measured on a scale of 0-100). All variables were statistically significant.

other 'everyday participation' activities, such as TV watching. As you can see housework, chores and DIY is negatively associated with happiness.

Other studies cited in this report indicate that theatre has less of an effect on life satisfaction, whereas reading fares much better (Leadbetter et al. 2013). As we encountered in Chap. 4, there are conceptual differences between life satisfaction and happiness, and common sense might tell us that reading and attending a theatre performance present different kinds of well-being experiences. Yet, seeing that reading looks quite *bad* for well-being is surprising at first glance. Elsewhere in the report are regression tables[25] for other activities, including birdwatching, gardening and hunting and fishing which are significantly better than watching a film—or indeed—poor old reading that doesn't win on these happiness scales. Interestingly, when you go back to the Twitter data answering the question: 'what is happiness?' (Box 5.1) there were many responses that answered reading, curling up on the sofa and watching a film, and so on. While the limited sample of the Twitter data makes it impossible to generalise, it certainly still poses questions as to what is going on with confounding results in various happiness data. One thing that struck me returning to these cases in 2020, a world changed by COVID-19, is the difference between activities in the home and outside the home.

Interestingly, the app's inventors co-authored an academic article for the journal *Global Environmental Change*. Using the same data, they found that outdoor activities were better for well-being. They state:

> [T]he predicted happiness of a person who is outdoors (+2.32), birdwatching (+4.32) with friends (+4.38), in heathland (+2.71), on a hot (+5.13) and sunny (+0.46) Sunday early afternoon (+4.30) is approximately 26 scale points (or 1.2 standard deviations) higher than that of someone who is commuting (-2.03), on his or her own, in a city, in a vehicle, on a cold, grey, early weekday morning. Equivalently, this is a difference of about the same size as between being ill in bed (-19.65) vs doing physical exercise (+6.51), keeping all other factors the same. (MacKerron and Mourato 2013, 997)

The numbers in the brackets refer to 'the scale points', showing the increase in probable happiness by where people are, what day of the week it is, what time of day it is. Interestingly, the greener the space you are in and the hotter the day (if sunniness seems less important than you might expect), the better. While this may appear to be common sense in one way, when you think back to how policy relies on evidence to improve well-being, what are the policy messages here from an investment point of view?

I had this app for a while and my results always told me that I was happiest in a pub beer garden with my best friends. Did I know that the data I was ploughing in when the app beeped me to do so was going to potentially be used to inform policy-making? Well, yes, of course, *I* guessed that, because I was researching well-being data and policy, which was why I downloaded the app in the first place. But did most people who were interested in how they felt doing certain things imagine the contexts of their data's potential future use?

What policy decisions should be made about beer gardens off the back of my interactions with some sliders on a mobile phone app after a few ciders on a summer's day? While these data were collected at a scale that means my personal data and my interactions are no longer visible on an individual level, it does pose questions for some of the correlations we make with these data. Are people happier on a weekend because they are not working or because they can go to the pub?

5.7   Conclusion

Despite the conflicting evidence from different approaches to 'Big Data', people are keen to find new ways to harness them to answer the age-old policy and philosophy questions around people's well-being. The increase in well-being research coincides with an increase in research with and on Big Data. Both have possibilities and challenges, but could they be exacerbated by combining well-being research with these data practices? Do Big Data have a capacity for good when making decisions about young people's exam grades or whether someone is eligible for social housing? We reflected on some important examples of where this went awry in this chapter.

New methods and metrics using Big Data, and indeed the research going into developing new tools to harness them, are not necessarily being checked for rigour before the approach is used elsewhere, as was the case with the Twitter community study, and its use of the sentiment metrics. Generalising people's happiness based on mobile phone data has its limitations. We cannot necessarily be entirely sure of whether it is the aesthetic grandeur of an old Victorian bandstand in the park, whether there is a classical concert inside, if you had enough sleep, whether you are picnicking with your favourite friends, with your kids, or having time away from your kids; indeed, whether you are stuck on a delayed tube underneath the park, or are walking in a hailstorm, that truly adds to (or detracts from) your momentary happiness.

The ethics of studying Big Data more broadly should be considered, and the behaviours of those who are outside the sample of users of wearable tech or smartphones, especially as these people may be older or poorer, for example, which we know intersects with well-being in very significant ways. Despite this, claims are still made that findings from these studies could be used to inform policy and investment. While they can offer some insights, we must be mindful of their limits—and crucially of their implications, especially in different contexts.

All in all, Big Data and new technologies, whilst not always revolutionary in kind, *can* offer insights into well-being that are useful for policymakers on a national scale, in international pandemics and for people who simply want to see what people think. But they are not without their limits, nor are they a magic bullet to the issues we have with existing data. If anything, they are also shown to have the potential to exacerbate existing problems as much as investigate solutions.

The capacity for Big Data to embrace complexity, and at greater speed, means they present new opportunities to analyse health data—and crucially how health intersects with social concerns. Reflecting back from today on how crude the Google Flu Trends analysis in 2013 now seems, it is clear that Big Data technologies and techniques are improving at pace. The COVID-19 example, BlueDot, shows that the value of Big Data analyses is in their capacity to now cope with more of Big Data's qualities at the same time, and in fact, to harness them: their messiness, variability, size and the capacity to link previously unconnected data sources from farming information to flight sales. The value was in the variety of data and sources used. Yet harnessing the power of Big Data was not powerful enough to prevent a worldwide crisis, despite the grand claims.

What we think of as 'Big Data' offer a peculiar perspective on 'well-being'. Consider the different things they capture, from sleep patterns to elite cycle trails to facial recognition and how many steps your walk to the post office takes. These devices exist to capture and produce data *because* data can be useful and commercialised. We are not even clear on whether more knowledge of the self is good for well-being or bad (yet?), let alone whether it is good at scale: that governments (and who else) know more about us. What is clear is that data are producing and changing culture and society, as much as they are capturing it.

We need to ask questions around the commercial value of these data practices alongside social justice issues. How would these data have had a greater chance of improving well-being were the contexts in which they were analysed different? Who should be included in these discussions, and who is excluded? Ultimately, how will decisions and trade-offs be made between the commercial and social justice dimensions?

NOTES

1. In fact, what a lot of people refer to as Big Data are not 'Big' at all by the initial standards of definition. They are just large datasets or newer types of data in not even large datasets, and so arguably not *Big* at all.
2. Kitchin and McArdle's (2016) original table says, 'Limited to wide' here (p2), but I think this makes more sense, as: 'Limited in width' or narrow.
3. A digital sociologist is interested in understanding the use of digital media (often data) as part of everyday life, and how these various technologies contribute to patterns of human behaviour, identity, relationships and social change.
4. O'Neil describes how the bottom scoring 2–5% of teachers were fired. Yet, the modelled target student scores and small classrooms made the scoring of teachers little better than random, and there was almost no correlation in a teacher's scores from one year to the next and qualitative data called one of the sacked teachers 'one of the best teachers I've ever come into contact with' (O'Neil 2016, 4).
5. Critical Data Studies are moving for more fairness accountability and transparency in data practices. Please see the FAccT conference for more on this: https://facctconference.org/.
6. This is largely credited to the 2017 article in the Economist, 'The world's most valuable resource is no longer oil, but data' (The Economist 2017).
7. With the exceptions of 1941 (during World War II) and Ireland in 1921.
8. Although, of course, given what we have seen elsewhere in the book, we might question whether the changing possibilities for what data could describe, changed policy, rather than the other way around.
9. There were a number of iterations of Mass Observation, with different people initiating them, but these were the original founding members.
10. There were no women observing anything in those days, of course.
11. See Mass Observation (n.d.) website for more on the data available and how to access them.
12. Several new methodologies are emerging that propose new possibilities for well-being measurement through combining new data sources with the survey data we have explored in previous chapters (Bellet and Frijters 2019; Daas et al. 2013; Jahani et al. 2017). These are not only hoping to understand well-being as personal or subjective experience, but to change the way that social justice issues such as poverty are approached (Blumenstock 2016). International organisations such as the United

Nations are supporting this kind of work, although primarily focussing on patterns of 'health and well-being' (United Nations 2014, 2015).

13. More information is available on the REACT's data collection and management here: https://www.ipsos.com/ipsos-mori/en-uk/covid-19-swab-test-faqs#nameaddress.

14. REACT was commissioned by the Department of Health and Social Care (DHSC) and is being carried out by Imperial College London in partnership with Ipsos MORI and Imperial College Healthcare NHS Trust. https://www.imperial.ac.uk/medicine/research-and-impact/groups/react-study/.

15. A review of literature on data and data practices, Kennedy et al. (2020), found that tech and policy were considered different worlds when it comes to data practices, and with different aims, although that is evolving.

16. See Internet Live Stats, 'Google search statistics' (Internet Live Stats n.d.). Internet Live Stats offer plenty more up-to-date data *on* data, if you are interested.

17. For the ethical concerns regarding social media research, see Townsend and Wallace (2016).

18. See Davies 2018 for a discussion on the greater implications of 'the culture wars' for politics and community.

19. If you are reading this chapter a while after reading the previous ones, then the cultural sector is a broad description of cultural institutions like libraries, heritage sites, museums, theatres and so on. Crucially, it is not only about the buildings themselves, but all the ways people make and consume culture and can include Netflix and outdoor festivals. In the UK, the cultural sector includes organisations funded by public subsidy as well as commercial organisations.

20. This post from Wasim Ahmed (2019) offers a clearly presented overview of the kinds of analyses available using different software https://blogs.lse.ac.uk/impactofsocialsciences/2019/06/18/using-twitter-as-a-data-source-an-overview-of-social-media-research-tools-2019/

21. 'everyday participation' (Miles and Sullivan 2010) has come to mean the everyday activities we participate in, which tend to fall outside of formal subsidy, which tendentially funds 'the arts'.

22. IMD is the UK government's Index of Multiple Deprivation.

23. This is called the PeerIndex realness score. This score is generated using information such as whether the profile has been self-certified on the PeerIndex site and/or has been linked to Facebook or LinkedIn. 'PeerIndex realness score is a metric that indicates the likelihood that the profile is of a real person, rather than a spambot or twitter feed. A score above 50 means this account is of a real person, a score below 50 means it is less likely to be a real person' (http://www.peerindex.net/help/scores).

24. See YouGov (n.d.) 'Brits use of wearable device'.

25. A regression table like the one reproduced in Table 5.4 will mainly be concerned with communicating the degree of association between variables. Chapters 7 and 8 go into this in far greater detail. The values will always lie between 0 and 1, and the way this table has been presented shows simplified detail. Ordinarily there is additional information to show not only the degree of association, but how sure we can be that this is a correct estimate. There will always be a degree of error that has to be accounted for. Typically in a regression table, you will find asterixes, as in Table 5.4. Asterisks in a regression table indicate the level of the statistical significance of a regression coefficient.

REFERENCES

Ada Lovelace Institute. 2019. *Beyond Face Value: Public Attitudes to Facial Recognition Technology.* Accessed 28 April 2021. https://www.adalovelaceinstitute.org/report/beyond-face-value-public-attitudes-to-facial-recognition-technology/.

Ahmed, W. 2019. *Using Twitter as a Data Source: An Overview of Social Media Research Tools (2019). Impact of Social Sciences.* Accessed 28 April 2021. https://blogs.lse.ac.uk/impactofsocialsciences/2019/06/18/using-twitter-as-a-data-source-an-overview-of-social-media-research-tools-2019/.

Ajana, B. 2017. *Self-Tracking: Empirical and Philosophical Investigations.* Springer International Publishing. https://doi.org/10.1007/978-3-319-65379-2.

Albert, A. 2019. *Citizen Social Science: A Critical Investigation.* PhD thesis. University of Manchester. https://www.escholar.manchester.ac.uk/api/datastream?publicationPid=uk-ac-man-scw:319481&datastreamId=FULL-TEXT.PDF.

Avila, R. 2019. Fixing Digital Democracy? The Future of Data-Driven Political Campaigning. *openDemocracy.* Accessed 28 April 2021. https://www.opendemocracy.net/en/fixing-digital-democracy-future-of-data-driven-political-campaigning/.

Bache, I., and Reardon, L. 2013. An Idea Whose Time has Come? Explaining the Rise of Well-Being in British Politics. *Political Studies,* 61(4), 898–914. https://doi.org/10.1111/1467-9248.12001.

Bates, J. 2016. Towards a Critical Data Science—The Complicated Relationship Between Data and the Democratic Project. *Impact of Social Sciences.* https://blogs.lse.ac.uk/impactofsocialsciences/2016/01/12/towards-a-critical-data-science-data-and-the-democratic-project/.

Bates, J., Lin, Y.-W., and Goodale, P. 2016. Data Journeys: Capturing the Socio-material Constitution of Data Objects and Flows. *Big Data & Society* 3 (2): p. 2053951716654502. https://doi.org/10.1177/2053951716654502.

BBC. 2019. London Mayor Quizzes King's Cross Developer on Facial Recognition. *BBC News*, 14 August. Accessed 29 April 2021. https://www.bbc.com/news/technology-49343822.

———. 2020. Coronavirus: UK to Have Test, Track and Trace System by June. *BBC News*. Accessed 28 April 2021. https://www.bbc.co.uk/news/av/uk-politics-52745202.

Bellet, C. and Frijters, P. 2019. *Big Data and Well-being*, p. 26. Accessed 28 April 2021. https://worldhappiness.report/ed/2019/big-data-and-well-being/.

Benjamin, R. 2019. *Race After Technology: Abolitionist Tools for the New Jim Code*. Medford, MA: Polity.

Boyd, D., and Crawford, K. 2012. Critical Questions for Big Data. *Information, Communication & Society*, 15(5), 662–679. https://doi.org/10.1080/1369118X.2012.678878.

BlueDot. n.d. *BlueDot | Who We Are, BlueDot*. Accessed 2 May 2021. https://bluedot.global/team/.

Blumenstock, J.E. 2016. Fighting Poverty with Data. *Science* 353 (6301): 753–754. https://doi.org/10.1126/science.aah5217.

Campbell, D. 2017. Facebook and Twitter 'Harm Young People's Mental Health'. *The Guardian*. Accessed 28 April 2021. http://www.theguardian.com/society/2017/may/19/popular-social-media-sites-harm-young-peoples-mental-health.

Carroll, C., J.C. Fuhrer, and D.W. Wilcox. 1994. Does Consumer Sentiment Forecast Household Spending? If So, Why? *The American Economic Review* 84 (5): 1397–1408.

Charrington, S. 2020. *How AI Predicted the Coronavirus Outbreak with Kamran Khan—#350*. Accessed 28 April 2021. https://www.youtube.com/watch?v=V6BpKSGquRw.

Coughlin, T. 2018. 175 Zettabytes By 2025. *Forbes*. Accessed 29 March 2021. https://www.forbes.com/sites/tomcoughlin/2018/11/27/175-zettabytes-by-2025/.

Cryle, P.M., and E. Stephens. 2017. *Normality: A Critical Genealogy*. Chicago: The University of Chicago Press.

Daas, P. J. et al. 2013. Big Data and Official Statistics. In *Proceedings of the NTTS. New Techniques and Technologies for Statistics*, pp. 5–7.

Davies, B., Innes, M. and Dawson, A. 2018. An Evaluation of South Wales Police's Use of Automated Facial Recognition. Cardiff: Crime and Security Research Institute, p. 46. https://www.statewatch.org/media/documents/news/2018/nov/uk-south-wales-police-facial-recognition-cardiff-uni-eval-11-18.pdf.

Davies, W. 2015. *The Happiness Industry: How The Government and Big Business Sold Us Well-Being*. London: Verso.

———. 2018. *Nervous States: How Feeling Took Over the World*. Jonathan Cape.

Dencik, L. 2020. *The Datafied Welfare State: A Perspective from the UK*, 24. Cardiff: Cardiff University. https://datajusticeproject.net/wp-content/uploads/sites/30/2020/09/The-Datafied-Welfare-State_draft.pdf.

Denham, E. 2019. Statement: Live facial recognition technology in King's Cross. ICO. Accessed: 19 August 2019. https://ico.org.uk/about-the-ico/news-and-events/news-and-blogs/2019/08/statement-live-facial-recognition-technology-in-kings-cross/.

Digital Initiatives. 2020. Strava: Striving in the Time of Corona? *Digital Innovation and Transformation*. Accessed 28 April 2021. https://digital.hbs.edu/platform-digit/submission/strava-striving-in-the-time-of-corona/.

Dodge, M., and Kitchin, R. 2005. Codes of Life: Identification Codes and the Machine-Readable World. *Environment and Planning D: Society and Space*, 23(6), 851–881. https://doi.org/10.1068/d378t.

Eubanks, V. 2018. *Automating Inequality: How High-Tech Tools Profile, Police, and Punish the Poor*. St. Martin's Publishing Group.

Fujiwara, D., and G. MacKerron. 2015. *Cultural Activities, Artforms and Wellbeing*. London: Arts Council England.

Fussey, P., and D. Murray. 2019. *London-Met-Police-Trial-of-Facial-Recognition-Tech-Report.pdf*. Essex: University of Essex, p. 128. Accessed 28 April 2021. https://48ba3m4eh2bf2sksp43rq8kk-wpengine.netdna-ssl.com/wp-content/uploads/2019/07/London-Met-Police-Trial-of-Facial-Recognition-Tech-Report.pdf.

Gayle, D. 2018. Diane Abbott: Twitter Has 'Put Racists into Overdrive. *The Guardian*. Accessed 28 April 2021. https://www.theguardian.com/politics/2018/dec/18/diane-abbott-calls-for-twitter-to-clamp-down-on-hate-speech.

Gilmore, A., Kostas, A., and Albert, A. 2018. 'Never Mind the Quality, Feel the Width': Big Data for Quality and Performance Evaluation in the Arts and Cultural Sector and the Case of 'Culture Metrics'. In G. Schiuma and D. Carlucci (Eds.), *Big Data in the Arts and Humanities: Theory and Practice*. Boca Raton: Taylor and Francis.

Hacking, I. 1990. *The Taming of Chance*. Cambridge: Cambridge University Press.

———. 1991. How Should We Do the History of Statistics? In *The Foucault Effect: Studies in Governmentality*, ed. G. Burchell, C. Gordon, and P. Miller. Chicago: The University of Chicago Press.

Harford, T. 2017. How the World's First Accountants Counted on Cuneiform. *BBC News*. Accessed 28 April 2021. https://www.bbc.co.uk/news/business-39870485.

Heaven, W.D. 2020. AI Could Help with the Next Pandemic—But Not with This One, MIT Technology Review. Accessed 2 May 2021. https://www.technologyreview.com/2020/03/12/905352/ai-could-help-with-the-next-pandemicbut-not-with-this-one/.

Hill, K., and A. Krolik 2019. How Photos of Your Kids are Powering Surveillance Technology. *The New York Times.* Accessed 28 April 2021. https://www.nytimes.com/interactive/2019/10/11/technology/flickr-facial-recognition.html.

Hintz, A., and J. Brand. n.d. *Data Policies: Approaches for Data-Driven Platforms in the UK and EU.* Cardiff: Data Justice Lab, p. 30. https://datajustice.files.wordpress.com/2020/01/data-policies-research-report-revised.pdf.

Holmes, T.H., and R.H. Rahe. 1967. The Social Readjustment Rating Scale. *Journal of Psychosomatic Research* 11 (2): 213–218. https://doi.org/10.1016/0022-3999(67)90010-4.

Internet Live Stats. n.d. *Google Search Statistics—Internet Live Stats.* Accessed 28 April 2021. https://www.internetlivestats.com/google-search-statistics/.

Jahani, E., et al. 2017. Improving Official Statistics in Emerging Markets Using Machine Learning and Mobile Phone Data. *EPJ Data Science* 6 (1): 1–21. https://doi.org/10.1140/epjds/s13688-017-0099-3.

Jee, C. 2016. Wearable Tech: Could It Save the NHS?, Techworld. Accessed 15 September 2016. http://www.techworld.com/wearables/could-wearables-save-nhs-3621960/.

Kennedy, H. 2016. *Post, Mine, Repeat: Social Media Data Mining Becomes Ordinary.* New York; Secaucus: Palgrave Macmillan UK. https://doi.org/10.1057/978-1-137-35398-6.

Kennedy, H., Oman, S., Taylor, M., Bates, J., and Steedman, R. 2020. *Public Understanding and Perceptions of Data Practices: A Review of Existing Research.* Sheffield: The University of Sheffield. https://livingwithdata.org/project/wp-content/uploads/2020/05/living-with-data-2020-review-of-existing-research.pdf.

Kitchin, R. 2014. *The Data Revolution: Big Data, Open Data, Data Infrastructures and Their Consequences.* SAGE.

Kitchin, R., and G. McArdle. 2016. What Makes Big Data, Big Data? Exploring the Ontological Characteristics of 26 Datasets. *Big Data & Society* 3 (1): p. 2053951716631130. https://doi.org/10.1177/2053951716631130.

Kramer, A.D.I. 2010. An Unobtrusive Behavioral Model Of 'Gross National Happiness'. In *Proceedings of the SIGCHI Conference on Human Factors in Computing Systems. CHI 10*, 287–290. Atlanta: Association for Computing Machinery.

Kruzan, K.P., and A.S. Won. 2019. Embodied Well-Being Through Two Media Technologies: Virtual Reality and Social Media. *New Media & Society* 21 (8): 1734–1749. https://doi.org/10.1177/1461444819829873.

Laney, D. 2001. 3D data management: Controlling data volume, velocity and variety. *Meta Group.* Accessed: 16 January 2013. http://blogs.gartner.com/doug-laney/files/2012/01/ad949-3D-Data-Management-Controlling-Data-Volume-Velocity-and-Variety.pdf.

Lazer, D., et al. 2014. The Parable of Google Flu: Traps in Big Data Analysis. *Science* 343 (6176): 1203–1205. https://doi.org/10.1126/science.1248506.

Lazer, D., and R. Kennedy. 2015. What We Can Learn from the Epic Failure of Google Flu Trends. *Wired*. Accessed 28 April 2021. https://www.wired.com/2015/10/can-learn-epic-failure-google-flu-trends/

Leadbetter, C., O'Connor, N., and Commonwealth Games, Culture & Sport Analysis Scottish Government. 2013. *Healthy Attendance? The Impact of Cultural Engagement and Sports Participation on Health and Satisfaction with Life in Scotland*. Scotland: The Scottish Government. Accessed 17 May 2021. https://www.gov.scot/publications/healthy-attendance-impact-cultural-engagement-sports-participation-health-satisfaction-life-scotland/.

Lee, L. et al. 2016.Information Disclosure Concerns in The Age of Wearable Computing. In *Proceedings 2016 Workshop on Usable Security*. *Workshop on Usable Security*, San Diego, CA: Internet Society. https://doi.org/10.14722/usec.2016.23006.

Lewis, R., M. Rowe, and C. Wiper. 2016. Online Abuse of Feminists as An Emerging form of Violence Against Women and Girls. *The British Journal of Criminology* 57 (6): 1462–1481. https://doi.org/10.1093/bjc/azw073.

Living with data. n.d. *Living with Data*. https://livingwithdata.org/.

Lupton, D. 2019. Data Mattering and Self-Tracking: What Can Personal Data Do? *Continuum* 34 (1): 1–13. https://doi.org/10.1080/10304312.2019.1691149.

MacKerron, G., and S. Mourato. 2013. Happiness is Greater in Natural Environments. *Global Environmental Change* 23 (5): 992–1000. https://doi.org/10.1016/j.gloenvcha.2013.03.010.

Madge, C., and T.H. Harrisson. 1937. *Mass Observation*. London: Frederick Muller Ltd.

Marr, B. 2014. Big Data: The 5 vs everyone must know. Accessed: 4 September 2015. https://www.linkedin.com/pulse/20140306073407-64875646-big-data-the-5-vs-everyone-must-know.

Mass Observation. n.d. *Mass Observation*. http://www.massobs.org.uk.

Matsakis, L. 2019 The WIRED Guide to Your Personal Data (and Who Is Using It). *Wired*. Accessed: 28 April 2021. https://www.wired.com/story/wired-guide-personal-data-collection/.

Mayer-Schönberger, V., and K. Cukier. 2013. *Big Data: A Revolution that Will Transform how We Live, Work, and Think*. London: John Murray.

Marz, N. and Warren, J. 2012. *Big Data: Principles and Best Practices of Scalable Realtime Data Systems*. MEAP edition. Westhampton, NJ: Manning.

McCall, B. 2020. COVID-19 and Artificial Intelligence: Protecting Health-Care Workers and Curbing The Spread. *The Lancet Digital Health* 2 (4): e166–e167. https://doi.org/10.1016/S2589-7500(20)30054-6.

McNulty, E. 2014. Understanding Big Data: The seven V's. Accessed: 4 September 2015. Accessed: 4 September 2015. http://dataconomy.com/seven-vs-big-data/.

Miles, A., and A. Sullivan. 2010. *Understanding the Relationship Between Taste and Value in culture and Sport*. London: DCMS.

Murgia, M. 2017. Watchdog Probes Cambridge Analytica's Poll Role. *Financial Times*. Accessed: 28 April 2021. https://www.ft.com/content/7482ec7c-01c9-11e7-aa5b-6bb07f5c8e12.

Mutz, M. 2016. Christmas and Subjective Well-Being: a Research Note. *Applied Research in Quality of Life* 11 (4): 1341–1356. https://doi.org/10.1007/s11482-015-9441-8.

NHS. 2016. Want to Feel Happier? Take a Break from Facebook. *NHS*. https://www.nhs.uk/news/mental-health/want-to-feel-happier-take-a-break-from-facebook/.

Niiler, E. 2020) An AI Epidemiologist Sent the First Alerts of the Coronavirus. *Wired*. Accessed: 28 April 2021. https://www.wired.com/story/ai-epidemiologist-wuhan-public-health-warnings/.

Noble, S.U. 2018. *Algorithms of Oppression: Data Discrimination in the Age of Google*. New York: New York University Press.

Oman, S. 2013a. Review of 'Counting What Counts: What Big Data Can Do for the Cultural Sector'. Cultural Value Initiative. http://culturalvalueinitiative.org/2013/06/08/review-of-nestas-counting-what-counts-what-big-data-can-do-for-the-cultural-sector-by-susan-oman/.

———. 2013b. Tackling the Deficit: Well-Being and Cultural Participation. Presentation at *Culture, Health and Wellbeing International Conference*. University of Bristol.

———. 2015. Measuring National Well-Being: What Matters to You? What Matters to Whom? In *Cultures of Wellbeing: Method, Place, Policy*, ed. S. White and C. Blackmore. London: Palgrave Macmillan.

———. 2017. *All Being Well: Cultures of Participation and the Cult of Measurement*. PhD Thesis. The University of Manchester.

———. 2019a. *Improving Data Practices to Monitor Inequality and Introduce Social Mobility Measures: A Working Paper*. The University of Sheffield. Available at: https://www.sheffield.ac.uk/polopoly_fs/1.867756!/file/MetricsWorkingPaper.pdf. Accessed: 29 March 2021.

———. 2019b. Measuring Social Mobility in The Creative and Cultural Industries: The importance of working in partnership to improve data practices and address inequality. Sheffield: The University of Sheffield. Accessed: 29 March 2021. https://www.sheffield.ac.uk/polopoly_fs/1.867754!/file/MetricsPolicyBriefing.pdf.

———. 2020. Leisure pursuits: Uncovering the 'Selective Tradition' in Culture and Well-being Evidence for Policy. *Leisure Studies*, 39(1), 11–25. https://doi.org/10.1080/02614367.2019.1607536.

————. n.d. How Data Work in Contexts. *Living with Data*. Accessed: 29 April 2021. https://livingwithdata.org/previous-research/how-data-work-in-contexts/.

O'Neil, C. 2016. *Weapons of Math Destruction: How Big Data Increases Inequality and Threatens Democracy*. London: Allen Lane.

ONS. 2001. *60 Years of Social Survey: 1941–2001*. Norwich: HMSO.

————. 2016. *Early Census-Taking in England and Wales*. Office for National Statistics. Accessed 28 April 2021. https://www.ons.gov.uk/census/2011census/howourcensusworks/aboutcensuses/censushistory/earlycensustakinginenglandandwales.

Otterbacher, J., Bates, J., and Clough, P. 2017. Competent Men and Warm Women: Gender Stereotypes and Backlash in Image Search Results. In *Proceedings of the 2017 CHI Conference on Human Factors in Computing Systems* (pp. 6620–6631). Association for Computing Machinery. https://doi.org/10.1145/3025453.3025727.

Pearce, R., S. Erikainen, and B. Vincent. 2020. TERF Wars: An Introduction. *The Sociological Review* 68 (4): 677–698. https://doi.org/10.1177/0038026120934713.

Pellert, M., et al. 2020. Dashboard of Sentiment in Austrian Social Media During COVID-19. *Frontiers in Big Data* 3. https://doi.org/10.3389/fdata.2020.00032.

Pidd, H. 2020. 'Punishment by statistics': The father who foresaw A-level algorithm flaws. *The Guardian*. Accessed: 11 August 2021. http://www.theguardian.com/education/2020/aug/14/punishment-by-statistics-the-father-who-foresaw-a-level-algorithm-flaws.

Pink, S., and V. Fors. 2017. Being in a Mediated World: Self-Tracking and the Mind–Body–Environment. *Cultural Geographies* 24 (3): 375–388. https://doi.org/10.1177/1474474016684127.

Plunz, R.A., et al. 2019. Twitter Sentiment in New York City Parks as Measure of Well-Being. *Landscape and Urban Planning* 189: 235–246. https://doi.org/10.1016/j.landurbplan.2019.04.024.

Poovey, M. 1998. *A History of the Modern Fact: Problems of Knowledge in the Sciences of Wealth and Society*. Chicago: The University of Chicago Press.

Porter, T.M. 1986. *The Rise of Statistical Thinking 1820–1900*. Princeton: Princeton University Press.

————. 1996. *Trust in Numbers The Pursuit of Objectivity in Science and Public Life*. Princeton: Princeton University Press.

Quercia, D. et al. 2012. Tracking 'Gross Community Happiness' from Tweets. In *Proceedings of the ACM 2012 Conference on Computer Supported Cooperative Work. CSCM 2012*, ed. D. Gergle, et al., 965–968. New York: ACM.

Ram, A., and M. Murgia. 2019. Data Brokers: Regulators Try to Rein in the 'Privacy Deathstars'. *Financial Times*. Accessed 29 March 2021. https://www.ft.com/content/f1590694-fe68-11e8-aebf-99e208d3e521.

Ruckenstein, M., and M. Pantzar. 2017. Beyond the Quantified Self: Thematic Exploration of a Dataistic Paradigm. *New Media & Society* 19 (3): 401–418. https://doi.org/10.1177/1461444815609081.

Ruppert, E., J. Law, and M. Savage. 2013. 'Reassembling Social Science Methods: The Challenge of Digital Devices. *Theory, Culture & Society* 30 (4): 22–46. https://doi.org/10.1177/0263276413484941.

Savage, M. 2010. *Identities and Social Change in Britain Since 1940: The Politics of Method*. Oxford: Oxford University Press.

Scott, J.C. 1998. *Seeing Like a State: How Certain Schemes to Improve the Human Condition Have Failed*. New Haven: Yale University Press (The Yale ISPS series).

Sinclair, J. 1798. *Statistical Accounts of Scotland*. https://stataccscot.edina.ac.uk/static/statacc/dist/home.

Strain, T., K. Wijndaele, and S. Brage 2019. Physical Activity Surveillance Through Smartphone Apps and Wearable Trackers: Examining the UK Potential for Nationally Representative Sampling. *JMIR mHealth and uHealth* 7(1): p. e11898. https://doi.org/10.2196/11898.

Suzuki, M. 1992. Political Business Cycles in the Public Mind. *American Political Science Review* 86 (4): 989–996. https://doi.org/10.2307/1964350.

The Economist. 2017. The World's Most Valuable Resource Is No Longer Oil, But Data. *The Economist*, 6 May. Accessed 29 March 2021. https://www.economist.com/leaders/2017/05/06/the-worlds-most-valuable-resource-is-no-longer-oil-but-data.

Townsend, L., and Wallace, C. 2016. *Social Media Research: A Guide to Ethics*. Aberdeen: The University of Aberdeen, p. 16. https://www.gla.ac.uk/media/Media_487729_smxx.pdf.

Turow, J. 2011 Introduction. In *The Daily You: How the New Advertising Industry Is Defining Your Identity and Your Worth*, 1–12. Yale University Press.

UK Data Justice Lab. n.d. *Data Justice Lab*. https://datajusticelab.org.

United Nations. 2014. A World That Counts: Mobilising the Data Revolution for Sustainable Development. Secretary-General of the United Nations. https://www.tralac.org/images/Resources/UN_Summit/A%20world%20that%20counts%20Mobilizing%20the%20data%20revolution%20for%20sustainable%20development%202014.pdf.

———. 2015. *Indicators and a Monitoring Framework for the Sustainable Development Goals*. Launching a Data Revolution for the SDGs. Secretary-General of the United Nations, p. 233. https://sdgs.un.org/sites/default/files/publications/2013150612-FINAL-SDSN-Indicator-Report1.pdf.

Voukelatou, V., et al. 2020. Measuring Objective and Subjective Well-Being: Dimensions and Data Sources. *International Journal of Data Science and Analytics*. https://doi.org/10.1007/s41060-020-00224-2.

Whitaker, B. 2020. *The Computer Algorithm That was Among the First to Detect the Coronavirus Outbreak*. Accessed 28 April 2021. https://www.cbsnews.com/news/coronavirus-outbreak-computer-algorithm-artificial-intelligence/.

Wilmott, C. 2016. Small Moments in Spatial Big Data: Calculability, Authority and Interoperability in Everyday Mobile Mapping. *Big Data & Society* 3 (2): p. 2053951716661364. https://doi.org/10.1177/2053951716661364.

YouGov. n.d. *Brits Use of Wearable Devices (E.g. A Smartwatch or Wearable Fitness Band)*. Accessed 28 April 2021. https://yougov.co.uk/topics/technology/trackers/brits-use-of-wearable-devices-eg-a-smartwatch-or-wearable-fitness-band.

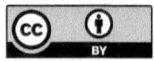

CHAPTER 6

Well-being, Values, Culture and Society

6.1 The Relationship Between Culture and Well-being

For many the arts are a real source of happiness, joy, fun, relaxation and learning. (The Director of Research at Arts Council England [Bunting 2007a, 4])

A wider definition [of wealth], associated with Ruskin, sees a nation's wealth as including personal happiness and fulfilment. It's an obviously broader view, into which culture fits more readily. (Secretary for Culture, Media and Sport [Jowell 2004, 8])

to maximise and exploit the contribution of the arts to core policies including education, health, crime, regeneration and the well-being of the population at large. (Funding agreement between Arts Council England and the Department for Culture, Media and Sport,[1] April 2003–March 2006 [DCMS 2003a, 15])

In 2007 the Director of Research at Arts Council England (ACE) reported on phase one of its first ever 'public value[2] enquiry' (Bunting 2007a). The Arts Debate gathered data from nearly 1700 contributions to workshops, in-depth interviews, discussion groups, 'deliberation' and 'open space' meetings and web discussions (Bunting 2007b, 4–5). The first of the above quotes is from one of the reports: *Stage one findings and*

© The Author(s) 2021
S. Oman, *Understanding Well-being Data*,
New Directions in Cultural Policy Research,
https://doi.org/10.1007/978-3-030-72937-0_6

next steps. It argues that the data collected in the Arts Debate prove that the arts are a source of different aspects of well-being, many of which we have already encountered in this book. If this is the case, then these data are useful for understanding how people feel about the arts, as well as how they feel about well-being.

The argument in the above quote from the Arts Debate report recalls the words of utilitarian philosopher Jeremy Bentham that we have encountered before: that the most happiness of the most people should be the aim of policy. By extension, it could be argued that if the arts are a source of happiness for many, then they are important to policy about well-being. The Research Director's statement seems to be a clear assertion of the utility of the arts to people. This 'public value enquiry' was a data gathering exercise to understand the value of the arts to people in the UK, to enable arguments *for* value in these terms. In cultural policy, 'culture' tends to refer to 'the arts' by default, and this is reinforced through institutions like ACE and activities like this. The report conjures up a relationship between culture and well-being that, even if unconsciously, is reinforced by drawing on a philosophical grounding. This relationship and the ideas behind it have become naturalised and popularised over time and are used to describe how the arts can improve life, theoretically and practically.

Three years prior to the Arts Debate, Tessa Jowell, the then Secretary for Culture, Media and Sport, published a personal essay called *Government and the Value of Culture* (2004). In this essay, also quoted above, utilitarianism is referenced directly before nineteenth-century thinker, John Ruskin (who is renowned for his thoughts *against* utility). Jowell paraphrases John Ruskin, stating that a nation's wealth should include personal happiness. Here, the culture secretary is very consciously explaining that this idea of the good society shows us how culture can demonstrate its value. Crucially, Jowell articulates the value of Ruskin's view: 'because culture fits', and 'readily', therefore cementing culture's public role. The relationship between culture and well-being, or, more specifically, the appetite to *prove* this relationship, is particularly hungry for well-being data, whilst also producing much well-being data itself. It is, therefore, a good case study for this book, which we will examine further in Chaps. 7 and 8.

This chapter looks at the relationship between culture and well-being to uncover the background to its reliance on data. It sets out the context and arguments behind the subsequent individual data case studies in Chaps. 7 and 8. Establishing 'the culture–well-being relationship' in this chapter enables three things. First, it illustrates the role of well-being data in policy evaluation by focussing on one policy sector. Second, it helps us expand on the political economy of data and data practices that we have encountered in Chap. 5. Third, it explores the specific dynamics of the economy of well-being data in a policy sector where few who work inside it consider themselves adept at data (as discussed in the Preface and Chap. 1), despite their reliance on them.

The quotes that open this chapter present evidence of how the 'culture– well-being' relationship is invoked and has become naturalised, particularly in the UK. By this I mean, there is a generally accepted view that culture (broadly defined) is good for well-being (broadly defined). We look at the lineage of this idea as something that began with philosophers and is now common sense; naturalised over time and then popularised. More specifically, these two examples from cultural policy-makers demonstrate how the relationship is *operationalised*[3] (put to use) to argue the value of culture.

We will see how this operationalisation means that these ideas can easily be co-opted to argue that culture should be included in delivering social aims. Good social policy is arguably entirely reliant on appreciating the cultural specificities of communities and broader society. However, this meaning of culture, as 'ordinary, in every society and every mind' (Williams [1958] 1989a, 4), is different from that meaning of culture which defaults to that of 'the arts' sought by the Arts Debate. We have acknowledged the slippage between definitions and ideas of well-being (happiness, quality of life, the good society, etc.) in previous chapters and will pay similar attention in terms of culture here. This slippage in meaning can be useful in arguments that defend the utility of culture as good for society. As we discover in Chaps. 7 and 8, this is important when looking at uses of well-being data.

This process is often called *instrumentalisation*[4] (Gibson 2008; Hadley and Gray 2017; Belfiore 2012) and involves 'culture' being used as a means or 'instrument' for attaining goals in other areas of society, or what are sometimes called policy areas or domains. Examples can be found in policy documents (as we have seen at the beginning of this chapter), research agendas, strategies and practitioner movements, such as the 'arts in health' movement (ACE 2007; AHRC 2021; AHSW n.d.) or the area of culture in regeneration (DCMS 2004; LGA 2020; UNESCO 2018). What we have seen through this ongoing period of instrumentalisation is the idea that the arts can be used to directly address societal problems, leading to the argument that culture is, in fact, *instrumental* to these social policy areas. Indeed, policy documents have argued that arts are so helpful in delivering positive health outcomes that they recommend that health and social care professionals should be trained in arts-based approaches (All-Party Parliamentary Group on Arts, Health and Wellbeing 2014).

This principle—that the arts are instrumental in delivering broader social projects and improving social infrastructure—has in turn been *operationalised* to advocate for funds for the arts, as part of making the case for the instrumental value of culture. This has shifted the idea of the value of culture from something belonging to everyone (Williams [1958] 1989a; Keynes 1945), to something that is valued for its social impact or for its economic contribution (Campbell 2019; DCMS 2011; National Endowment for the Arts 2018). In arguing this case, the sector is increasingly required to evaluate how much of this additional value it has generated in response to funding; for example, in the 2003 funding agreement between ACE and the government (cited above) there is a commitment to a contribution across various social policy areas as well as the 'well-being of the population at large' (DCMS 2003a, 15).

This is why the cultural sector requires evidence. It has become increasingly reliant on data for these arguments, often requiring metrics as proof. As we go on to discover, the sector is dependent on commissioning research to articulate its value, owing to gaps in data skills and resource as touched on in Chap. 1, and which this book aims to help address.

Box 6.1   The Culture–Well-being Relationship
Theorised → *naturalised* → *popularised* → *operationalised* → *instrumentalised* → *operationalised* → *metricised* → *capitalised*

The values of 'a good society', and the idea that culture is intrinsic to them, have become amalgamated into the process of valuation, which has evolved into a form of proof along the way. As Box 6.1 represents, the processes of theorising and naturalising the relationship, to operationalise this idea, have led to a need to prove this relationship exists. In turn the symbolic value of this proof to the cultural sector means that well-being data now have a financial value, and those who can work with well-being data are able to capitalise on this (Oman and Taylor 2018). This slippage of the meanings of value, values and valuation is part of the cultural value debate[5] that we introduce in this chapter.

The 'slippery' nature of culture is revealed by how the term is defined and then used. Culture can be described as something more ordinary

(Williams [1958] 1989a), all around us and in everything we do, but the same term can be used to justify the funding of artforms which are anything but ordinary, with often small numbers of people interested in participating on rare, special occasions. Culture is such a 'complicated word' (Williams [1976] 1988, 87) that it makes it difficult to write about the culture–well-being relationship. However, we can see this ambiguity operationalised, as some arguments for the value of culture will refer to broader ideas of culture, when they are arguing for the arts, as we shall see in later chapters.

As described in Chap. 1, change is seen in data, but felt in culture. In the culture–well-being relationship, data are used to ascribe *value* and culture is where *values* manifest. Recognition of the increasing value of data tends to focus on the scale of Big Data and the human rights issues of personal data. Whilst important, the effects of the fetishisation of data we have encountered throughout this book are also felt in smaller data projects highlighting the need for skills and literacy in social and cultural policy. This chapter establishes two things: first, the relationship between culture and well-being and its association with data and, second, the explanation as to why there is a market for well-being data and analysis in cultural policy as a form of social policy.

Well-being and Culture: Reviewing the Long Theoretical Lineage

to increase the happiness of men by giving them beauty and interest of incident to amuse their leisure, and prevent them wearying even of rest, and by giving them hope and bodily pleasure in their work; or, shortly, to make man's work happy and his rest fruitful. (William Morris, Aims of Art lecture, 1887, in Belfiore and Bennett 2008, 144)

The aims of art, according to William Morris, should be to improve 'man's' quality of life in numerous ways. The role of culture (broadly defined) in a 'good society' has a long history that can be traced back to ancient Greece. Culture tends to be presented in a positive light, and Aristotle's name tends to be attached to this representation. As you may remember from Chap. 2, many theoretical lineages of ideas of well-being and its measurement for policy derive from Aristotle. Yet, these ideas are not without problems when viewed from contemporary society[6] and the representation of the culture–well-being relationship as a positive one also requires context.

The theoretical lineage that culture is vital to a good society actually began in Aristotle's 'counterargument' to Plato. Plato asserted the arts were, in fact, corrupting (Belfiore and Bennett 2008, 39). This reframing of the 'honourable and dishonourable intellectual history of the arts' (Belfiore and Bennett 2008, 10) demands attention if we are to consider the culture–well-being relationship, which leans on this moment in its historical tradition.

Theories of the arts' 'deeply transformative effects for the individual and society' (Belfiore and Bennett 2008, 10) are now an assumed truth that has become naturalised and popularised. However, when this assumption is drawn on, it is the positive effects which are referred to. The noted 'dishonourable' and negative outcomes are conveniently discarded and often forgotten, especially in discussions about what culture is for and in cultural policy.

The cultural sector 'believes that it makes a real difference to people's lives' (NMDC, undated in Selwood 2010, 4) and in recent decades much effort has gone into investigating the sector's impact on individuals and how this might play out in communities, societies and nations. So intrinsic is the idea that arts are a social good, that evidence suggests cultural managers believe the sector is good for other people, even if they do not like certain artforms themselves (Stevenson 2019). Here, we will look at specific aspects of subjective well-being (happiness or feeling that life is worthwhile). We know from previous chapters that these have different theoretical lineages and subtle differences in meaning, and so how they appear in cultural policy documents warrants a revisit, before contemplating what is being captured when using data to understand or measure an aspect of well-being.

For example, Dame Liz Forgan suggested that the arts can 'cheer us up' and create forms of 'escape, comfort, understanding and reference in tough times' (ACE 2009, 3). Forgan, who became the first female chair of ACE the same year, echoes the German philosopher (dubbed the artists' philosopher) Arthur Schopenhauer's ([1818] 2000) ideas of the aesthetic experience as protective from the anguish of the human condition. Schopenhauer believed that as understanding and experience of the world develop, we experience pain and responsibility. He felt it was important for the individual to escape certain pressures of communal responsibility, and therefore this was a purpose for the arts.

To contextualise the chair of ACE's comments, she speaks from what we then thought were tough times: the immediate aftermath of financial crisis (the 2007/2008 crash). Reflecting on Schopenhauer's idea that we sometimes need to shield ourselves from tough times might cause us to reflect on who Forgan means by 'us', particularly in tension with the communal responsibilities we might want shielding from. This function of the arts—as tonic in times of difficulty—is also related to rejecting struggle. As Belfiore and Bennett (2008) point out, Schopenhauer's meaning of will remains contested, but they conclude (via Janaway 1994, 6) that 'the best way to understand the concept of "will" is to conceive it as a form of unrelenting yet blind "striving forward" for something' (Belfiore and Bennett 2008, 93–95). Does art, therefore, offer a way out of contemporary life's relentless impetus to strive forward? If so, how might these ideas of the importance of art for well-being intersect with the version of well-being as a balance of pleasure and purpose that is introduced in Chap. 2? Perhaps art allows us to escape our own will and the will of society, to be immersed in something else. Yet, this also presents a tension between the social responsibility that is implicit in culture's role in a good society and aesthetic pleasure as an escape from feeling these pressures personally.

Schopenhauer's thinking builds on that of another German philosopher, Emmanuel Kant. For Kant, aesthetic pleasure lies within the process or state of understanding. More specifically, once the aesthetic experience has captured the imagination, it enables greater insight and meaning, and this is pleasurable. Perhaps for Forgan, this is the understanding we are also able to refer back to from tough times?

Yet again there are contradictions, as the pleasure from aesthetic experiences is found in the striving for personal enlightenment. According to Kant, such awareness can only be found while in a balanced state: some sort of equilibrium of the senses. If this has been achieved, then it is possible to experience the 'enjoyment of wellbeing', but only following feeling stirred by 'the play of affects' (Kant [1790]1987, 134, cited in Belfiore and Bennett 2008, 86). Another way of looking at this is that Kant's thinking on hedonism is not about a moment of extreme pleasure (or indeed the chasing of a series of pleasures), but appreciating a moment of satisfaction, which comes after specific kinds of pleasure that lead to enlightenment. For Kant, then, it is important to recognise the feeling of satisfaction that follows this pleasure as a change in well-being.

This is starting to sound more like the language of the happiness economists from Chap. 4 who want to measure subjective well-being as an experience. However, based on this highly simplified version of Kant, the well-being caused by aesthetic pleasure (whether in a park, or in a theatre) is not a single effect, but a series of effects that happen over time. When relying on the theoretical lineages of well-being, it is important to consider that they do not always map neatly onto the concepts that economists are hoping to operationalise. This is also true for the culture–well-being relationship, and its inherent assumption that all forms of culture (or any of its chosen sub-categories, whether art, leisure, singing, food, travel) can contribute to all forms of well-being (whether they are physical health, fun, enlightenment, relaxation, empathy, escapism, social responsibility etc.).

As a result, discussion of what culture is, who it is for and how it can be instrumentalised tend to be stuck in a cyclical debate, much like the arguments performed to an audience 2000 years ago by our learned friends Plato and Aristotle in the School of Athens. As with the Arts Debate, consideration of what culture *is* or what it is for often merges with articulations of the value of culture (and often as the arts). By extension, these discussions segue into advocacy, for investment in culture as a good choice for social policy (as with the public consultation on public value referred to above) or into debates over how investment is distributed as a public service. We will return to this latter point, but first we need to establish how cultural policy became a form of social policy.

6.2   Cultural Policy as Social Policy

Cultural Policy: Operationalising the Question 'What Is Culture?'

Taking now the point of view of identification, the reader must remind himself as the author constantly has to do, of how much is here embraced by the term culture. It includes all the characteristic activities and interests of a people; Derby Day, Henley Regatta, Cowes, the twelfth of August, a cup final, the dog races, the pin table, the dart board, Wensleydale cheese, boiled cabbage cut into sections, beetroot in vinegar, nineteenth-century Gothic churches and the music of Elgar. The reader can make his[7] own list. And then we have to face the strange idea that what is part of our culture is also part of our lived religion. (T.S. Eliot, Notes Towards a Definition of Culture [1948] 1973)

In cultural policy, 'culture' tends to refer to 'the arts' by default. There are many books which consider questions of culture and many 'men of letters' have concerned themselves with its definition, with Raymond Williams and poet T.S. Eliot some of the most quoted. Understanding culture is more complicated than thinking of its definition and devising lists of what it is, however. Williams and his fellow cultural studies scholars' work on culture explains far more than its definition. Williams attempts to capture how meanings and values interact across society (1977); what he famously called 'our modern structure of meanings' ([1958] 1989a, xiii), incorporating the institutions which manage our quality of life. He is interested in how ideas of 'continuity' are determined by certain groups which define 'the tradition'.[8] He continues that it is 'the tradition' of certain groups that gets to decide what culture is ([1961] 1971, 66), and what culture will continue to be. By extension, this means that only certain people get to define culture and its role in society, as an ongoing process that repeats itself.

The definition and management of culture might make you think of some of the issues we have encountered with well-being data, particularly the penultimate section of Chap. 3. Some people get to define what they think well-being is, and what should be measured, using particular data. This essentially defines well-being, well-being data and their role in society, but also how society is managed. For Williams, the way well-being, data and culture are organised is vital to how society works, and we need to understand them all together.

Williams offers us more than a definition of culture. He presents a theory of culture, to deepen understanding of how culture *works* ([1961] 1971). He argues that to develop an understanding of culture and society, we need to incorporate and deepen:

> analysis of elements in the way of life that to followers of the definition are not "culture" at all: the organisation of production, the structure of the family, the structure of institutions which express or govern social relationships [and] the characteristic forms through which members of the society communicate. ([1961]1971, 57–58)

What he means by this is that if we want to understand culture and how it works in society, we need to look at all of the stuff around it: how it is organised, communicated and managed—in the context of how other social structures work.

A simpler way of describing this, and why it is important here, is that: to understand culture and society, we need also to understand social policy and governance in general, as well as the institutions that organise and manage them. This includes appreciating how social policy works on society, or its effects, alongside the ways that this happens. Also, good social policy and governance require a better understanding of culture and society.[9] Therefore, society and social policy—and culture and cultural policy—are interlinked and need to be understood together, and within the context of the ways they are organised. Furthermore, this book argues that data are cultural, and so we cannot fully understand well-being data without appreciating both society and culture and, as Williams explains, the institutions which manage them.

Cultural Policy: Institutions for Well-being

> It was the task of C.E.M.A. [Council for the Encouragement of Music and the Arts] to carry music, drama and pictures to places which would otherwise be cut off from all contact with the masterpieces of happier days and times: to air-raid shelters, to war-time hostels, to factories, to mining villages. (John Maynard Keynes 1945)

The naturalised relationship between culture and well-being is a consequence of the theoretical lineage of ideas of the good society we touched on above. The culture–well-being relationship has subsequently been operationalised through cultural policy as social policy in numerous ways. The above quote is from John Maynard Keynes, a key figure in economics, whose developments still inform much government policy today. Keynes invokes the culture–well-being relationship here, by describing what would happen without its preservation. He paints a mental picture where cutting off miners from masterpieces jeopardises their happiness, as that is how they access memories of happier days.

For the Victorians, the arts and culture were considered 'elevating and refining to the working man' (Bennett 2000, 1414). Public cultural institutions were established 'to resolve problematic class behaviours', with Henry Cole advocating in 1884 that 'museums should go into competition with the Gin Palaces' (cited in Bennett 2000, 1414), as 'the rapt contemplation of a Raphael' would keep wayward husbands from the tap-room (contemporary magazine [1858], cited in Bennett 2000, 1414). Even the public park emerged for those who migrated to cities during the Industrial Revolution (Gilmore and Doyle 2019). In other words, the park as we now know it was another Victorian strategy for the improvement—and regulation—of urban populations.

When culture is categorised as a solution for society, the idea is then developed and operationalised, and presented as a way to restore some form of social balance; whilst recognising that museums are 'in competition' with other ways of spending time, whether a park or a pub. Identifying problematic aspects of society and their associated pastimes has been long entwined with ideas that certain activities, and therefore the people that do them, are deficient, and lacking in the right sort of culture, or are 'uncultured'. People may lack a link to masterpieces of the past, but that does not mean that they lack culture, are 'cut off from it' or are indeed less happy as a result.

People in fact choose to not seek links to the culture described as a masterpiece and find happiness in pastimes that may suit them better. This approach to managing society by addressing the ways in which certain people 'lack' a certain kind of culture is called a 'deficit model'. It stigmatises the practices of some people, and not others, the belief being that if certain people only engaged in a particular form of cultural participation, in the same way as these other, more exemplary people do, then we could be closer to 'a good society'. This model of cultural policy still dominates contemporary UK cultural funding (Miles 2013), despite various attempts to redress it (that we encounter in this chapter).

The current framework of UK cultural policy is indebted to the Victorians and their adoption of ideas of civilising as a way to a good society. Its management is more a history of institutions, and in 1940, the Council for the Encouragement of Music and the Arts (CEMA, to become the Arts Council of Great Britain) was established. It was World War II, and British cultural life—whether professional or amateur—was thought to be retracting, as described by Keynes cited earlier. The Board of Education intervened, saying it is essential 'to show publicly and unmistakably that the Government cares about the cultural life of this country' (cited in Hewison 1995, 30). The funding agreement committed CEMA to the 'preservation in wartime of the highest standards in the arts of music, drama and painting' and 'the widespread provision of opportunities for hearing good music and the enjoyment of the arts generally' (Hewison 1995, 33).

We can see that slippage between meanings of culture here cemented in a policy document from 80-odd years ago. Where the idea of a broader 'cultural life' becomes synonymous with 'encouraging music and the arts', and that these are things 'the Government cares about'. As Hewison points out 'these essentially aristocratic, though benign, intentions are at odds with the democratic sentiments' (Hewison 1995, 33) of commentators like Raymond Williams who began questioning what and who culture was for.

These concerns of whether people are accessing culture, and who has access, have become key questions for cultural policy. As we shall see, the Department for Culture, Media and Sport (DCMS) commissioned its own survey of 'characteristic activities and interests' (to quote T.S. Eliot again), to discover who is doing what. Yet, the model of government funding remains fixated on this link between the masses and master-pieces.[10] Consequently, the institutions that formulate and deliver most of what we think of as cultural policy have become fanatical not only about ideas of cultural participation for its perceived personal and social benefits, but also how to fix 'non-participation',[11] by engaging those who are not taking part. A cynic might say that this would allow the institutions of cultural policy to gain credibility for social impact and social change by way of simply getting those who are assumed to need more culture to enter their institutions, and we shall see how that plays out in data.

The deficit model of participation, and how many people are participating as an indicator of impact, is increasingly recognised as politically and empirically problematic. Cultural institutions are beginning to address the question: how are *we* deficient, if we are not engaging communities, rather than why are certain people not engaging with us? It is also important to note that cultural participation is a distant proxy measure of any form of social change. Entering a museum will not dissolve the social structures or traumatic experiences that leave some with ill-being or social disadvantage. So, counting heads of who enters institutions generates data with many limits, yet this method was the staple of data use for some time (as we will see in more detail in Sect. 6.3). To assume anyone who does not wish to participate in a cultural offer is deficient in some way is morally dubious at best and to prescribe particular activities as any sort of cure for social ills may even be argued to be irresponsible (Oman and Edwards 2020; Oman 2019a, b), misleading and misdirecting resources.

Well-being data have been used to plug the gap between attendance numbers and the capacity of cultural institutions to deliver social policy aims. Yet, in spite of years of investment, reams of theory, research and recent evolutions in data analysis, little has changed for the better (see Brook et al. 2020). We will return to how well-being data can be used to link the masses to masterpieces and help retain how the culture–well-being relationship remains institutionalised. However, we first of all need to return to questions of how certain aspects of culture are considered good for well-being in certain contexts.

Cultural Policy: Whose Culture Is Good Culture for Well-being?

Sport and culture are widely perceived to generate social impacts. There is a long history of academic and evaluation research into the social impacts of sport and culture ... This evidence includes individual impacts (e.g. health/ fitness, mental health and wellbeing), life satisfaction, cognitive development, social skills; and broader community impacts such as social capital, increased volunteering, improved community cohesion, perceptions of quality of local area, increased educational performance, reduced crime/re-offending, reduced health care needs and economic development/regeneration.

Sport is a broad and vague term that includes a wide range of activities.

Culture is defined as a broad term which encapsulates the arts, heritage and museums, libraries and archives. (The Culture and Sport Evidence Programme (CASE) Taylor et al. 2015)

We encountered how the naturalised relationship between culture and well-being is evident in the 2003 funding agreement between ACE and DCMS quoted at the beginning of this chapter, in which it committed to 'maximise and exploit the contribution of the arts to ... the well-being of the population at large' (DCMS 2003a, 15). DCMS distributed funding to a number of arm's length bodies in 2003, responsible variously for sport, the arts, heritage and museums and libraries and archives. The 2003 funding agreement articulated the idea that via ACE, the arts have a specific and mandated role in society. That role is to address societal issues, and in doing so, improve quality of life. Essentially, the arts should help people make the most of these activities to improve their well-being.

What happened to the concern over 'cultural life' more generally, you might ask? If culture is described in cultural policy research evaluations (such as this CASE[12] example), as the activities attached to arts and cultural institutions, then what of the culture happening outside them? Why is this not also so for less institutionalised cultural engagement, recently labelled 'everyday participation' (Miles and Sullivan 2010)? CASE is 'a joint programme of strategic research led by DCMS in collaboration with Arts Council England, English Heritage and Sport England' (UK Government 2021). Originally a three-year-long project costing £1.8 million, reports have continued to be published under the CASE programme since.

Arguably two main things are going on in the way the CASE programme is framing culture. One might be that the institutionalising of certain forms of culture means that, by default, a social role must be found for such activities, if they are to receive government subsidy that could otherwise be distributed to other areas of social policy. Secondly, that evidence programmes were established in support of the activities managed by these institutions. So, more evidence is needed to justify the social role of culture, media and sport, in order to provide good reason for its subsidy. Crucially, evidence in support of these institutionalised areas is also more invested in (and more institutionalised) than broader cultural life.

The hierarchy of high art and leisure, or a more popular or vernacular culture, has been contested by cultural studies scholars such as Raymond Williams ([1958] 1989a) and Stuart Hall (various, see 1977 and McRobbie 2016). In the Leisure Studies literature, Stebbins' binary of 'casual leisure' and 'serious leisure' (Stebbins 1997, 1999) indicates that the latter is more 'important to the wellbeing [sic] of the individual and society', rather than largely non-productive leisure activities, such as 'hanging around' (cited in Blackshaw and Long 2005, 248). What are perceived to be bad choices and undesirable leisure pursuits remain a target for change, with personal and social 'happiness by design' (e.g. Dolan 2014) dominating the discourse of behavioural economics that includes many of the happiness economists we encountered in Chap. 4.

In policy terms, 'casual leisure' is often demonised. For example, the description of the 1999 reversal of Bhutan's national television ban[13] includes a story of soaring crime, drug-taking and playground violence (Layard 2006, 78). Richard Layard explains that 'a third of parents now preferred watching TV to talking to their children', warning that the introduction of television as leisure coincided with the 'deteriorat[ion of] family relationships, the strength and safety of communities and the prevalence of unselfish values' (Layard 2006, 77, 78).[14] Bhutan was the first nation to begin measuring what it calls 'gross national happiness' (GNH). In 1972, the Fourth King declared GNH to be more important than Gross National Product (GNP, similar to GDP), and from this time onward, the country oriented its national policy and development plans towards GNH. There is, of course, a longer history: the 1729 legal code, which dates from the unification of Bhutan, declared that 'if the Government cannot create happiness (*dekid*) for its people, there is no purpose for the Government to exist' (Ura 2010 via Helliwell et al. 2012, 111). Its measures incorporate the interdependence of aspects of wellbeing and the belief 'that the beneficial development of human society takes place when material and spiritual development occurs side by side to complement and reinforce each other' (Helliwell et al. 2012, 111).

The story of Bhutan maintains a persistent place in narratives of the second wave of well-being which are otherwise Euro-American centric. However, the tale we are told is often partial. Bhutan's social and cultural life was idealised in descriptions of the importance of well-being measurement as a political and social project. The innovations of the Bhutanese happiness index were greatly praised. Yet, the domains and indicators themselves are rarely discussed. As Karma Ura, President of the Centre for Bhutan Studies and GNH research, explains:

> The term subjective well-being, by which happiness is known in western literature, is telling. (Ura 2011, 1)

Ura is highlighting how happiness is an individualised concern in the West, rather than something oriented around an idea of society, and also pointing out that a fair society should be encouraged by: 'enlightenment education with respect to ethics, intellect and wisdom by its population in order to reach happiness (*dewa*)' (ibid., 2). He continues that social welfare accrues from 'unquantifiable spiritual and emotional well-being' (ibid., 2). Indeed, the Bhutanese well-being index has a whole domain called 'Cultural Diversity and Resilience', including 'native language', 'cultural participation', 'artisan skills' and 'conduct' (Helliwell et al. 2012, 115). In short, Bhutan's innovations in well-being measures incorporate many of the cultural aspects of social life that are missing from the other objective lists described in Chap. 3 from the likes of the OECD and the ONS.

Bhutan's attention to social and cultural life can be explained by the fact that—as a nation—it was less entrenched in the measurement and policy histories that informed many of the Euro-American approaches. They were therefore better equipped to capture 'culture' and 'well-being' without the institutional histories that Raymond Williams describes and as outlined in the evaluation research that opened this section. The question may not only be, 'why is Bhutan measuring different aspects of socio-cultural life than OECD countries?' We might also ask the question, 'why are OECD countries so keen to follow Bhutan and measure well-being, but not follow *how* they are measuring well-being?' If we look at the well-being agenda more generally, we find a tendency to borrow (or appropriate) aspects of a different culture and adapt them. These modifications suit institutional histories of those doing the borrowing, indeed in the case of the wellness industry, to capitalise on them. This is the case of mindfulness (borrowed from Buddhism) and yoga, of course; Western versions of both of these cultural practices have been criticised for hollowing out their meaning, even disrespecting the beliefs of the cultures that have been borrowed from.[15]

To return to the narrative of television and Bhutan's happiness and leisure policy is, of course, informed by value judgements that preconceive what is 'good' leisure for individuals and society—and what is not. These value judgements are—of course—inherited. They are evidenced by Layard using statistics but interestingly, as noted in Chap. 4, White and Dolan (2009) found that time spent with children is relatively more rewarding than pleasurable, whereas time spent watching television is relatively more pleasurable than rewarding.

What is also interesting is that the reversal of the television ban (1999) happened but one year after GNH was announced as Bhutan's objective (Layard 2006, 77) and a few years before the indicators were developed. This marks a move from simply aiming for GNH, as the Fourth King aspired to in 1972, to actually measuring it. Bhutan was becoming less culturally closed to Western developments including the television—and social indicators. Ironically, Layard notes that the impact of television on Bhutan society 'provides a remarkable natural experiment in how technological change can affect attitudes and behaviour' (Layard 2006, 7), without acknowledging that measuring society to drive objectives will also lead to cultural and societal change. Well-being indicators being a good technological development and television not, we must assume, in this value system.

Choices over what is good for well-being and what has value in these terms are cultural decisions in their own right. This can be demonstrated in Bhutan's choice of indicators when compared to other decisions that we comprehensively covered in Chap. 3. It is also worth noting that the influential Sarkozy Commission that was established in 2007 and reported in 2009 (Stiglitz et al.) references the importance of cultural specificities and recommends that each nation find its own measures of well-being (Stiglitz et al. 2009, 18). Crucially, it is not only in the inclusion of a cultural domain that Bhutan differs, but also in the relationships drawn between social and cultural values within the structures of meaning that Williams advocates (cited earlier). Bhutan also included within its education indicator 'the cultivation and transmission of values' (Ura et al. 2012, 11) suggesting that these intertwined social, cultural and religious values are at the heart of the rationale for developing the GNH index in the first place. By contrast, social and cultural values held a precarious place in the project to establish the UK's well-being index, which we return to at the end of this chapter. For now, we must turn to how social value and cultural value each has a different meaning in UK social and cultural policy.

Cultural Value and the Role of Well-being Data

As with the terms culture, well-being and social value, you will probably not be surprised to know there is no one definition of cultural value. Like so many of the other terms set out in this book, there are long debates and no clear consensus (Oakley and O'Brien 2015). Given the extent of these discussions, there is a brief overview of cultural value, acknowledging how its definition and quantification became a much-discussed problem to resolve, safe in the knowledge that the detail of these debates can be found elsewhere.[16]

The impact of culture on the economy first became a prominent feature of cultural value in the last quarter of the twentieth century. The focus on efficiency of the 'Thatcherite revolution' (Power 1994) and new public management discussed in Chap. 2 saw a focus on 'social value' as a consideration in public decision-making. In parallel, what was called the 'economic turn' instigated new methodologies for measuring culture's worth as economic returns on investment (most notably Myerscough 1988). The new possibilities for measurement enabled by new methodologies, in turn, resulted in an increasing focus on measuring value, full stop, including areas of life less readily measurable than money.

Ideas of cultural value enable continuity from economic value to instrumental approaches to *valuing* what culture and leisure activities could do for both individuals and society. Under New Labour (1997–2010), this tended to be articulated more prominently as social value (harking back to Victorian values of social and moral improvement). However, in truth, there was a growing abundance of econometrics that were taken up as proxies for cultural value.

The Department for Culture, Media and Sport (DCMS, formerly Department for National Heritage) was renamed in 1997 by the then recently elected Tony Blair and was keen to promote the idea that 'sport and culture are widely perceived to generate social impacts' (Taylor et al. 2015, 11), alongside economic impacts (see e.g. Hesmondhalgh et al. 2015). All New Labour departments inherited a civil service culture steeped in almost two decades of new public management approaches, mixing public and private provision and a commitment to using social science technologies to evaluate what worked and what did not in public administration (as discussed in Chap. 2).

Initially, the ways DCMS was required to assess its performance against social and economic goals were not demanding in terms of data or data expertise. As discussed above, it compared visitors to a range of events with the general population and used these numbers to make arguments about contributions to social aims. If the profile of people at these events grew closer to that of the general population—and less highly educated and white—then arguments were made for a contribution to social cohesion, as a 'strategic priority' (DCMS 2003b).

While not technically challenging, such assessments were hampered by the limits to the data available. It was impossible to identify how the fraction of the population going to a museum had changed in the last 12 months without a figure for the previous 12 months. The data collected on the cultural sector were partial, largely driven by specific targets generated by DCMS and related bodies.[17] Thus, they reflected the interests and management approaches nationally, as well the expertise available. Cultural value arguments were increasingly included in the rhetoric of other actors and organisations, such as local authorities. These arguments retained the two key focusses: social impact and economic multipliers. If a local authority could show their local theatres led to economic growth, or to social impact, they could make a case for greater funding. Similarly, bids for new local arts venues ordinarily entailed commitments to an evaluation of economic and social impact.

Here we see the general 'enthusiasm for numbers' (Hacking 1991, 186; Hacking 2002) discussed in Chaps. 2 and 5, manifest in a need for data expertise in the cultural sector, which was lacking, because it had not been previously required. Consequently, there was an increasing reliance on consultancies to satisfy the desire for data and evidence for policy evaluation. This was symptomatic of a shift from collecting and describing data to a more involved analysis of the data gathered, as part of the production of evidence for valuing culture. Whereas researchers once 'collected and recorded mainly quantitative data on things like the number of creative or cultural businesses in a particular area, the number of people they employed, the amount of revenue they generated and other typically economic "indicators" of cultural and creative activity' (Prince 2015, 584), this work broadened, so that by 2010, consultancies were estimating social and economic impact. This included bespoke data collection—for example, assessing the social impact of events by surveying attendees about changed perceptions (Prince 2015). It also increased the demand for understanding statistical power and significance (Prince 2014, 755). In short, the more research that was brought in, the more sophisticated it became, and the further outside the day-to-day remit of many responsible for evaluations.

Meanwhile, the need to ensure culture was part of discussions of valuation and appraisal encouraged further attempts to define cultural value. One of the most prominent is John Holden's (2004, 2006), for whom, there are different parts of society with different relations to, and needs for, culture. These different parts of society also reflect different perspectives on value: the public, the professionals and the politicians. Cultural value also takes three forms for Holden (2006), broadly representative of these groups. For example, 'intrinsic value' is the subjective experience of culture: 'intellectually, emotionally and spiritually' (Holden 2006, 14). 'Instrumental value' is how culture can be 'used to achieve social or economic purpose' (Holden 2006, 16). There is also 'institutional value' found in how people relate to cultural organisations. For example, the BBC was very concerned about its 'public value' and conducted a consultation so it could articulate its institutional value (in Holden's terms) to the public and its instrumental value in economic terms.[18] ACE's 2007 Arts Debate aimed to fulfil a similar objective (Bunting 2007a, b). However, public consultation data may not always reinforce the values of institutions and can in fact challenge them. When reanalysing the ONS' data from the national well-being debate in 2010, I also found that Holden's three groups formulate the value of culture to well-being differently. The lack of reference to arts and cultural institutions in general or specific terms by people in these data (Oman 2020) poses important questions for the cultural value debate.

The problem of cultural value is also extrinsically linked to, yet separated from, economic value, in the policy context. Cultural economist David Throsby breaks cultural value down into different elements—aesthetic, spiritual, social, historic, symbolic and authenticity value—arguing that each contributes to the overall value of a cultural object, institution or experience (Throsby 2006, 42). He maintains that cultural value is separate from economic value and, relatedly, that 'there are some aspects of cultural value that cannot realistically be rendered in monetary terms' (Throsby 2006, 42). However, he also argues that a thorough economic valuation of both the market and non-market benefits of a cultural object can offer a good indication of its cultural value, because generally 'the more highly people value things for cultural reasons the more they will be willing to pay for' them (Throsby 2006, 42; see also 2010). Some aspects of cultural value lend themselves more readily to being expressed in the language of outputs and outcomes, whilst others do not. Given the valuation tools we have are predominantly from the field of economics, perhaps the one which is most readily *measurable* is economic value. This is because it is already numerical, in a way that people's subjective experiences are not.

As we can see, the idea of culture, the policies which contain and promote it, those who work in it, its infrastructure and research, seem to both attract and resist economic analysis.[19] The proliferation of data collection and consultancy for policy appraisal included economic impact and valuation methodologies. Some of the economic valuation techniques that are used to capture the effects of culture are not yet technically sound (Rustin 2012), as will be expanded on in greater detail in the subsequent chapters (Chaps. 7 and 8). Yet, some argue the need to satisfy the demand for evidence of this kind of value has to be addressed in some way. One particular in-depth project focussed on how to overcome the gulf between what the cultural sector thought it was making culture for, and the demands of Her Majesty's Treasury (HMT) (O'Brien 2010). This report argued the need for pragmatism in presenting cultural value to secure public funding (O'Brien 2010, 8–9). It argued that 'the lack of consensus in the literature over the meaning of cultural value and how to best measure and capture cultural value suggests the potential of using established economic valuation tools' (O'Brien 2010, 15). By encouraging the sector to measure the value of culture in ways more acceptable to the hierarchies of evidence demanded by HMT, the report aimed to reconcile two cultures of evidencing cultural value. Arguably, however, this may have reinforced how very distinct they are, as well as leading to increased technocracy in the attempts of arts managers to do cultural economics or deal with more data.

Many in the sector see the value of their work as exceeding its economic value, and feel it cannot be reduced to economic considerations alone. Others argue that instrumentalising culture for social policy ends is not ethical for various reasons. It has also been pointed out that the hierarchies of cultural value (that one thing is more valuable than another to solve social problems) essentially 'define[] culture as a mechanism for the replication of inequality' (Oakley and O'Brien 2015, 5). These contestations have led to various audits of cultural value, such as the Warwick Commission for Cultural Value, which influentially cites Taylor's finding that the most privileged 8%[20] access culture (Taylor 2016, in Neelands et al. 2015). Arts Council England has commissioned numerous reviews on the subject, many of which ask for further evidence rather than using the evidence we already have. For example, the publication *The Value of Arts and Culture to People and Society* (ACE 2014) lists key themes of the value of culture as economy, health and well-being, society and education. Positioned as a rapid review of evidence, the report identifies a number of gaps, particularly regarding longitudinal data and the health and well-being evidence on cultural participation. Another example, the Arts and Humanities Research Council (AHRC) Cultural Value Project, a £2.5 million initiative over 3.5 years, supported over 70 original pieces of research initiated by the call, largely from arts and humanities research disciplines. The programme intended to improve comprehension of the value of arts and culture and the methods used to capture this value (Crossick and Kaszynska 2016). This programme has finished, but has resulted in a new Centre for Cultural Value which aims to build 'a shared understanding of the differences that arts, culture, heritage and screen make to people's lives and to society'.[21]

A recent large-scale academic project looked at how we might re-articulate 'cultural values' through understanding what people do in their everyday lives as culture, rather than thinking of cultural policy as something inherited to manage an elite idea of culture (Miles and Gibson 2016). *Understanding Everyday Participation: Articulating Cultural Values* (UEP) notably used many different types of data, collecting primary data using various methods, and analysing secondary data using different approaches. The premise was simple: understand what people were *actually* doing, and what they valued, rather than what cultural policymakers, the government, economists or the Happiness Tsar thought people *should be* doing (and then investing in programmes to get them to do what *they thought* people *should be* doing and measuring whether they did it, or not). Insights include dwindling investments in the social infrastructure presented by the local park (Gilmore 2017), or how charity shops in certain communities have been overlooked despite their specific 'relations between culture, economy and place which has effects in the social sphere' (Edwards and Gibson 2017).

As noted above, a particularly influential insight from UEP was through reanalysis of DCMS' Taking Part Survey data. Taylor found that:

approximately 8.7% of the English population is highly engaged with state-supported forms of culture, and that this fraction is particularly well-off, well-educated, and white. Over half of the population has fairly low levels of engagement with state-supported culture but is nonetheless busy with everyday culture and leisure activities such as pubs, darts, and gardening. (2016, 169)

Taking Part: The National Survey of Culture Leisure and Sport had been established in 2005 (DCMS 2006) as part of a programme of evidence generation led by DCMS. This new survey (known as Taking Part, and often shortened to TPS) aimed to collect data that would be useful to the concerns of all the sectors under DCMS' remit. Notably, the CASE programme cited above was also a part of this project. TPS asks detailed questions about what people do and where. Chapter 8 goes into greater detail about the wording of the questions, demonstrating the level of detail collected about simple pastimes, such as walking. The survey also collects demographic data and since the 2013–2014 dataset has also contained 'the ONS4' (see Table 4.3). TPS data therefore have inequality measures, well-being measures and highly detailed data about how people spend their time in terms of the variety of activities they undertake, how frequently and for how long. While DCMS have been criticised for not making enough of the survey data themselves (Bunting et al. 2019), others have analysed the data, looking at types of participation and inequality (Taylor 2016) and well-being (Fujiwara 2013; Fujiwara et al. 2015).

My PhD research was connected to the UEP project, and as discussed in Chap. 3 and briefly here, one of my approaches used free text fields from the ONS' Measuring National Well-being Debate. My research presented a reordering of data to see how people value different domains of their life, in comparison to the published findings (Table 3.1). I found that when people talk about their well-being, they tend to describe the sorts of activities that Taylor lists, rather than those subsidised by cultural policy or indeed the institutions which house them. Overall, the vast body of research presented across the UEP project indicates the limits to research on and for cultural value arguments in asserting the value of particular forms of culture.

Most examples of articulating cultural value are attached to a specific idea of cultural policy (conflated here with arts policy), as you can see above. What is key here is that in deciding what is cultural in cultural value, cultural policy practitioners (policy-makers and academics) are also ascribing value to certain activities or practices. Much like the definition of social value and well-being, as described in Chap. 2, this is a value system in and of itself: a ranking system which results in certain places, people and practices being invested in, while others are not. What is interesting is that what is thought to have caused the downfall of the social indicators movement in the 1970s was the 'bewildering array' of measures, as we discussed in Chap. 2. It was also the lack of a robust theoretical or ideological analysis, as well as the failure to establish what needed to be achieved for whom and how (Scott 2012, 36). Despite the breakdown in prior measures, and years of contestation around the limitations of metricised cultural value, however, it remains a resilient idea that is heavily invested in.

Well-being Measures: Arguing a Right to Culture?

Everyone has the right freely to participate in the cultural life of the community, to enjoy the arts and to share in scientific advancement and its benefits. (Article 27 of the 1948 United Nations Universal Declaration of Human Rights)

Before the UK's well-being measures were finalised, a national debate was administered by the ONS to decide 'what matters to you?'. The first iteration of the national well-being measures (Beaumont 2012) did not account for culture. At the time, prominent commentators from the cultural sector expressed their dismay at this outcome, with one observer concluding in a national newspaper that this was proof that 'culture was invisible' to governments (Holden 2012). In actual fact, the omission was for various reasons; in part, because there was no validated measure for culture across the UK.[22] But also, the ONS acknowledge the complexity of measuring multiple activities and wanted to avoid judgement on what should count and what not:

ONS considers that the currently proposed measures of satisfaction with the use and amount of leisure time should adequately reflect the effect of an individual's leisure time on their well-being without making a judgement that particular or specific activities are good for well-being. (Beaumont 2012, 15)

Avoiding judgement is worth reflecting on for a moment, when you think back to the discussions on who decides whose culture, and the

Victorians putting museums 'into competition' with gin palaces, for example. Despite this disinclination to 'judge', in 2014, the ONS included one of DCMS' measures of culture from TPS in the national measures of well-being.

The metric is based on whether people have 'engaged with/participated in arts or cultural activity at least three times in the last year' and notably only covers England, rather than the whole UK. While it can be contested whether this maps directly on to Article 27 of the Declaration of Human Rights, cited above, the debate (Evans 2011; Oman 2020) and its subsequent public consultation (reported in Beaumont and Self 2012) demonstrate the social importance of a measure which included socio-cultural concerns to the nation.

This makes it even more interesting to compare Bhutan's multiple measures for culture to the single indicator in the UK's well-being measures. We have encountered limitations on measuring domains of life that are relevant to well-being, and how the decisions of 'the metric makers' are largely down to deciding the metric is robust enough. The case study in Chap. 3 of the OECD composing its international index found a theoretical and moral commitment to including a measure of sustainability and yet, the measures of sustainability available were not robust enough.

There is an important tension in committing to understanding culture, community and sustainability, but arguing that these are too complex to capture. There may well be an argument that this is because these domains had not yet received the attention they deserved by Euro-American statisticians, despite the supposed influence of Bhutan. We might also wonder if it is the politicians who do not care for such domains (as Holden 2012 describes) or those who measure and research well-being?

Countering Holden's claims that culture has an invisibility problem (Holden 2012), cultural participation does feature in high-profile reports about well-being. As the influential Commission on the Measurement of Economic Performance and Social Progress highlights in its report, there is a long tradition of research emphasising the importance of leisure time for quality of life. 'This research points to the importance of developing indicators of both leisure quantity (number of hours) and quality (number of episodes, where they took place, presence of other people), as well as of measures of participation in cultural events and of "poor leisure"' (Stiglitz et al. 2009, 49).

In Europe, levels of 'access to cultural amenities was a significant predictor' of well-being in the countries measured by the European Quality of Life Survey (Chapple 2013, 98[23]). However, the same report states that the accessibility of amenities does not independently predict life satisfaction. Instead, it has a positive impact on all other outcome variables, 'particularly reducing social exclusion and stress/busyness' (Chapple 2013, 52). Therefore, there is international recognition for the role of culture in attempts to both measure and understand well-being, but capturing this is complex, especially if it is not always fully interrogated.

The slippage of the meanings of culture we encountered earlier can also be found in Holden's exasperation that culture was not going to feature in the ONS' well-being measures. He uses a broad definition of culture in the same article in which he describes its (meaning the arts) invisibility to policy-makers (2012). These slippages might, in fact, be exacerbating the lack of attention to cultural indicators in larger statistical projects.

Culture and well-being are both 'complicated' words and attempts to capture either are contested—whether this is in their definition or in data. Similarly, value and values attract and resist the numeration and research that enable the persuasive arguments people want to make. This makes these insights valuable to different groups, creating a market for this research. The fact that Bhutan measures culture and values in multiple ways in its well-being index, when OECD countries do not, is important to take away from this chapter. Yet, when these are so difficult to define, slippage in meanings is exploited and national statistics offices want to avoid these sorts of judgements, it is difficult to see a way forward.

6.3   Conclusion

As we have seen, the naturalised role of cultural life as being valuable to a good society (or national and personal well-being) has been popularised in different parts of society and instrumentalised as policy. Yet articulations of cultural participation slip between everyday and elite activities, arguably confusing claims to social impact and understanding of what I call the culture–well-being relationship.

We have reflected on the theoretical lineage behind this naturalised relationship between culture and well-being. We have problematised assumptions, and shown the diversity of these claims for happiness, social justice or indeed hiding from social responsibility. The slippery nature of culture and well-being as concepts enables the relationship to morph to the needs of whoever chooses to invoke it, whether they are cultural commentators or policy-makers. This popularisation and instrumentalisation of the culture–well-being relationship is rife in cultural policy, and at a time in which the second wave of well-being and new valuation demands from Treasury affected demands for evidence, the relationship is increasingly reliant on well-being data and expertise.

The burden of proof is enmeshed with a historical tendency to decide what is good for (other) people's well-being, and what has social and cultural value. Such relations and values are not as fixed as these approaches assume. Of course, really, one would hope that all social policy areas impact on personal, social or community well-being in one way or another; otherwise they would not require social policy-making. Ironically, the idea that well-being measures can neutrally capture technological change without making their own technological changes is highly disputable when you consider the policy histories of Chap. 2. Data are cultural and they change culture and society in ways that are not acknowledged.

The Bhutanese well-being index has a rich cultural domain, with cultural values featuring in other domains, such as education. Yet, despite acknowledging Bhutan as an inspiration to measure well-being, few indices are inspired by the GNH indicators. In the UK, the current, single well-being indicator has a limited capacity to capture even arts participation at present—let alone a broader idea of social and cultural life. The following two chapters account for some issues in the 'evidence base' of evidence-based social and cultural policy. We interrogate data, how these are used to make arguments and how we might all be better equipped to interact with well-being data to understand culture and society for ourselves.

NOTES

1. The Department of Culture, Media and Sport (DCMS) became the Department of Digital, Culture, Media and Sport in July 2017.
2. We will talk more about public value and cultural value later in this chapter, but if you want a refresher on social value, moral values and valuation, there is a section on it in Chap. 2.
3. Notably, operationalise means something slightly different in research, particularly quantitative research. Box 7.1 in Chap. 7 explains this further.
4. The academic literature looking at the process and effects of instrumentalisation are mixed. Gibson (2008) defends it, whilst many others who write on it talk of its damaging effects (i.e. Belfiore 2012; Hadley and Gray 2017).
5. The cultural value debate has been long-running, see: Crossick and Kaszynska (2016) for an overview.
6. The reliance on slavery to sustain this version of a good society, being just one. See footnotes 3 and 5 in Chap. 2 for further discussion and reading.

7. Of course, you may find yourself noting the lack of consideration of a female reader by this 'man of letters'.

Other cultural studies scholars agree with this crucial point: Dick Hebdige explains that some groups have more opportunities to make more of the rules that organise 'meaning' as how we understand the world and each other through culture (1979). This he describes as hegemony, a term borrowed from Antoni Gramsci to account for how the dominance of certain groups of societies—their ideals, morals, values—and financial value—can be sustained over time. Stuart Hall (1977, cited in Hebdige 1979) explains that hegemony can only be maintained if the 'dominant classes "succeed in framing all competing definitions within their range", so that subordinate groups are, if not controlled, then at least contained within an ideological space which does not seem at all "ideological" which appears instead to be permanent and 'natural' to lie outside history, to be beyond particular interests' (Hebdige 1979, 16).

8. For a recent take on Williams on this point, see Levine (2020).

9. Notably, for example, Arts Council England's ten-year strategy was called Achieving Great Art for Everyone (2010).

10. For discussion on issues with non-participation as an idea, see Stevenson (2016), and using Taking Part data, see Taylor (2016).

11. The CASE programme ran from 2008 and its outputs are hosted here https://www.gov.uk/guidance/case-programme#case-programme-the-resources, although only up until 2013, whereas the report cited in this chapter is from 2015. A special issue of the journal *Cultural Trends* reflected on the programme, and that publication is useful background to this story. See O'Brien (2012).

12. Until 1999 TV had been banned in Bhutan, as had public commercial advertising. Layard (2006) describes this in greater detail, acknowledging that we shouldn't generalise from one event.

13. There is a rich area of media studies which interrogates these assumptions about media consumption and 'deviance' (i.e. Eithne Quinn's work on hip hop, 2020). While Bhutan's case is an interesting 'test' environment, as it had not previously had television, other studies using longitudinal data have been unable to substantiate a link (i.e. Shi et al. 2019).

14. See Purser's (2019) critiques of 'McMindfulness'.

15. For example, in: O'Brien (2010); Oakley and O'Brien (2015); Crossick and Kaszynska (2016); Neelands et al. (2015).

16. See Selwood (2002) for a comprehensive review of cultural sector data.

17. O'Brien (2013, 122–130) covers particular case studies of public value in greater detail.

18. See Doyle (2010) for a longer discussion on how culture attracts and resists economics.

19. Note it was actually 8.7%, but was unconventionally rounded down in error to 8% when the finding was reproduced. See Taylor (2016) for more detail on the actual findings.
20. The Arts and Humanities Research Council (AHRC), Paul Hamlyn Foundation (PHF) and Arts Council England (ACE) jointly funded this call to establish a Centre for Cultural Value (CCV) to the value of up to £2 million (University of Leeds n.d.). The new centre is hosted at the University of Leeds.
21. This was partly because the work to include indicators for culture (e.g. within local authority Best Value performance indicators that had been significantly invested in during the New Labour period) was erased with the removal of such performance management strategies by the incoming Coalition government in 2010. See Gilmore (2014) for further discussion.
22. The report does not explicitly outline how 'access to cultural amenities was a significant predictor' of well-being, however. Furthermore, the question about amenities in the survey, which allows the authors to arrive at this policy recommendation, is: 'Access to amenities (including postal services, bank, public transport, culture, green space)' (Chapple 2013, 106). Green space is the most important predictor, but the report is not clear on the degree to which access to cultural amenities predicts well-being.

REFERENCES

ACE. 2007. *Strategy for the Arts Health and Wellbeing.* London: Arts Council England, p. 52. Accessed 29 April 2021. https://www.artshealthresources.org.uk/wp-content/uploads/2017/01/2007-ACE-Strategy-for-the-arts-health-and-wellbeing.pdf.

———. 2009. *Annual Review 2009.* London: Arts Council England, p. 160. Accessed 28 April 2021. https://www.artscouncil.org.uk/sites/default/files/download-file/Review%20-%20Arts%20Council%20England%20Annual%20Review%202009.pdf.

———. 2014. *The Value of Arts and Culture to People and Society.* Arts Council England. Accessed 28 April 2021. https://www.artscouncil.org.uk/publication/value-arts-and-culture-people-and-society.

AHRC. 2021. *Arts and Health, Health and Wellbeing Research Portfolio.* Accessed 29 April 2021. https://ahrc.ukri.org/innovation/health-and-wellbeing-research-portfolio/arts-and-health/.

AHSW. n.d.. *Arts & Health South West, Arts & Health South West—Home.* Accessed 29 April 2021. https://www.ahsw.org.uk/

All-Party Parliamentary Group on Arts, Health and Wellbeing. 2014. *Creative Health: The Arts for Health and Wellbeing.* Accessed 28 April 2021. https://www.culturehealthandwellbeing.org.uk/appg-inquiry/.

Beaumont, J. 2012. *Measuring National Well-Being: A Discussion Paper on Domains and Measures.* Office for National Statistics. http://webarchive.nationalarchives.gov.uk/20160106195224/http://www.ons.gov.uk/ons/dcp171766_240726.pdf.

Beaumont, J., and Self, A. 2012. *Initial Findings from the Consultation on Proposed Domains and Measures of National Well-being.* London: ONS.

Belfiore, E. 2012. "Defensive instrumentalism" and the legacy of New Labour's cultural policies. *Cultural Trends* 21 (2): 103–111. https://doi.org/10.1080/09548963.2012.674750.

Belfiore, E., and O. Bennett. 2008. *The Social Impact of the Arts: An Intellectual History.* Basingstoke and New York: Palgrave Macmillan.

Bennett, T. 2000. Acting on the Social: Art, Culture, and Government. *American Behavioral Scientist* 43 (9): 1412–1428. https://doi.org/10.1177/00027640021955964.

Blackshaw, T., and J. Long. 2005. What's the Big Idea? A Critical Exploration of the Concept of Social Capital and its Incorporation into Leisure Policy Discourse. *Leisure Studies* 24 (3): 239–258. https://doi.org/10.1080/0261436052000327285.

Brook, O., D. O'Brien, and M. Taylor. 2020. *Culture Is Bad for You: Inequality in the Cultural and Creative Industries.* Manchester: Manchester University Press.

Bunting, C. 2007a. *Public Value and the Arts in England: Discussion and Conclusions of the Arts Debate.* Arts Council England. https://www.a-n.co.uk/research/public-value-arts-england-discussion-conclusions-arts-debate/.

———. 2007b. *The Arts Debate: Stage One Findings and Next Steps.* London: Arts Council England. http://www.artscouncil.org.uk/artsdebate/ArtsDebate_ACE_stage1_report.pdf.

Bunting, C., A. Gilmore, and A. Miles. 2019. Calling Participation to Account: Taking Part in the Politics of Method. In *Histories of Cultural Participation, Values and Governance,* ed. E. Belfiore and L. Gibson, 183–210. London: Palgrave Macmillan UK (New Directions in Cultural Policy Research). https://doi.org/10.1057/978-1-137-55027-9_8.

Campbell, P. 2019. *Persistent Creativity: Making the Case for Art, Culture and the Creative Industries.* Palgrave Macmillan (Sociology of the Arts). https://doi.org/10.1007/978-3-030-03119-0.

Chapple, S. 2013. *Subjective Well-Being and Social Policy.* European Commission.

Crossick, G., and P. Kaszynska. 2016. *Understanding the Value of Arts & Culture: The AHRC Cultural Value Project.* Swindon: AHRC.

DCMS. 2003a. *Funding Agreement between Arts Council England and the Department for Culture, Media and Sports, April 2003–March 2006.* Department for Culture, Media and Sport.

———. 2003b. *Strategic Plan 2003–2006.* London: Department for Culture, Media and Sport.

———. 2004. *Culture at the Heart of Regeneration*. Department for Culture, Media and Sport.

———. 2006. *Taking Part: The National Survey of Culture, Leisure and Sport, 2005–2006; Adult and Child Data* [Data Collection]. 2nd ed. SN: 5717. UK Data Service. https://doi.org/10.5255/UKDA-SN-5717-1.

———. 2011. *Creative Industries Economic Estimates*. Department for Digital, Culture, Media & Sport. https://www.gov.uk/government/collections/creative-industries-economic-estimates.

Dolan, P. 2014. *Happiness by Design: Finding Pleasure and Purpose in Everyday Life*. London: Penguin Books.

Doyle, G. 2010. Why Culture Attracts and Resists Economic Analysis. *Journal of Cultural Economics* 34 (4): 245–259. https://doi.org/10.1007/s10824-010-9128-9.

Edwards, D., and L. Gibson. 2017. Counting the Pennies: The Cultural Economy of Charity Shopping. *Cultural Trends* 26 (1): 70–79. https://doi.org/10.1080/09548963.2017.1275131.

Evans, J. 2011. *Findings from the National Well-being Debate*. Office for National Statistics. https://docplayer.net/66842-Joanne-evans-office-for-national-statistics.html Accessed 10 August 2021.

Fujiwara, D. 2013. *Museums and Happiness: The Value of Participating in Museums and the Arts*. United Kingdom: The Happy Museum; Museum of East Anglian Life; Arts Council England. Accessed 29 March 2021. https://happymuseumproject.org/wp-content/uploads/2013/04/Museums_and_happiness_DFujiwara_April2013.pdf

Fujiwara, D., P. Dolan, and R. Lawton. 2015. Creative Occupations and Subjective Wellbeing. 15(9). https://media.nesta.org.uk/documents/creative_employment_and_subjective_wellbeing_1509_1.pdf.

Gibson, L. 2008. In defence of instrumentality. *Cultural Trends* 17 (4): 247–257. https://doi.org/10.1080/09548960802615380

Gilmore, A. 2014. *Raising Our Quality of Life: The Importance of Investment in Arts and Culture*. CLASS (Centre for Labour and Social Studies. Accessed 28 April 2021. http://classonline.org.uk/docs/2014_Policy_Paper_-_investment_in_the_arts_-_Abi_Gilmore.pdf.

———. 2017. The Park and the Commons: Vernacular Spaces for Everyday Participation and Cultural Value. *Cultural Trends* 26 (1): 34–46. https://doi.org/10.1080/09548963.2017.1274358.

Gilmore, A., and P. Doyle. 2019. Histories of Public Parks in Manchester and Salford and Their Role in Cultural Policies for Everyday Participation. In *Histories of Cultural Participation, Values and Governance*, ed. E. Belfiore and L. Gibson, 129–152. London: Palgrave Macmillan UK (New Directions in Cultural Policy Research). https://doi.org/10.1057/978-1-137-55027-9_6.

Hacking, I. 1991. How Should We Do the History of Statistics? In *The Foucault Effect: Studies in Governmentality*, ed. G. Burchell, C. Gordon, and P. Miller. Chicago: The University of Chicago Press.

———. 2002. Making Up People. In *Historical Ontology*. Cambridge, MA: Harvard University Press.

Hadley, S., and C. Gray. 2017. Hyperinstrumentalism and Cultural Policy: Means to an End or an End to Meaning? *Cultural Trends* 26 (2): 95–106. https://doi.org/10.1080/09548963.2017.1323836.

Hall, S. 1977. Culture, the Media, and the 'Ideological Effect'. In *Essential Essays*. Durham: Duke University Press.

Hebdige, D. 1979. *Subculture: The Meaning of Style*. London: Methuen.

Helliwell, J.F., R. Layard, and J. Sachs. 2012. *World Happiness Report [2012]*. Vancouver: University of British Columbia Library. Accessed 28 April 2021. http://hdl.handle.net/2429/44498.

Hesmondhalgh, D., Oakley, K., Lee, D., and Nisbett, M. 2015. *Culture, Economy and Politics: The Case of New Labour*. Palgrave MacMillan.

Hewison, R. 1995. *Culture and Consensus: England, Art and Politics since 1940*. London: Methuen.

Holden, J. 2004. *Capturing Cultural Value: How Culture Has Become a Tool of Government Policy*. London: Demos.

———. 2006. *Cultural Value and the Crisis of Legitimacy: Why Culture Needs a Democratic Mandate*. London: Demos.

———. 2012. New Year, New Approach to Wellbeing?, *The Guardian*. https://www.theguardian.com/culture-professionals-network/culture-professionals-blog/2012/jan/03/arts-heritage-wellbeing-cultural-policy.

Janaway, C. 1994. *Schopenhauer*. Oxford: Oxford University Press.

Jowell, T. 2004. *Government and the Value of Culture*. London: HMSO/DCMS.

Kant, I. [1790]1987. *Critique of Judgment*. Translated by W.S. Pluhar. Indianapolis: Hackett Publishing Company.

Keynes, J.M. 1945. The Arts Council: Its Policy and Hopes. In *The Collected Writings of John Maynard Keynes*, ed. D. Maggridge, 367–372. London: Macmillan.

Layard, R. 2006. *Happiness: Lessons from a New Science*. Penguin.

Levine, C. 2020. Raymond Williams, Marxism and Literature (1977). *Public Culture* 32 (2 (91)): 423–430.

LGA. 2020. *Cultural Strategy in a Box*. Local Government Association.

McRobbie, A. 2016. Stuart Hall: Art and the Politics of Black Cultural Production. *South Atlantic Quarterly* 115 (4): 665–683. https://doi.org/10.1215/00382876-3656081.

Miles, A. 2013. Culture, Participation and Identity in Contemporary Manchester. In *Culture in Manchester: Institutions and Urban Change since 1850*, ed. J. Wolff and M. Savage, 176–193. Manchester and New York: Manchester University Press.

Miles, A., and L. Gibson. 2016. Everyday Participation and Cultural Value. *Cultural Trends* 25 (3): 151–157. https://doi.org/10.1080/09548963.2016.1204043.

Miles, A., and A. Sullivan. 2010. *Understanding the Relationship between Taste and Value in Culture and Sport*. London: DCMS.

Myerscough, J. 1988. *The Economic Importance of the Arts in Britain*. London: Policy Studies Institute.

National Endowment for the Arts. 2018. *The Arts Contribute More Than $760 Billion to the U.S. Economy*. https://www.arts.gov/news/2018/arts-contribute-more-760-billion-us-economy.

Neelands, J., et al. 2015. *Enriching Britain: Culture, Creativity and Growth: The 2015 Report by the Warwick Commission on the Future of Cultural Value*. Warwick: The University of Warwick. https://warwick.ac.uk/research/warwickcommission/futureculture/finalreport/warwick_commission_report_2015.pdf.

O'Brien, D. 2010. *Measuring the Value of Culture: A Report to the Department for Culture Media and Sport*. DCMS.

———. 2012. CASE: The Culture and Sport Evidence Programme (Special Issue). *Cultural Trends* 21 (4): 0954–8963. https://doi.org/10.1080/09548963.2012.726788.

———. 2013. *Cultural Policy: Management, Value and Modernity in the Creative Industries*. New York: Routledge.

Oakley, K., and D. O'Brien. 2015. *Cultural Value and Inequality: A Critical Literature Review*. Arts and Humanities Research Council; The University of Leeds. https://eprints.whiterose.ac.uk/88558/.

Oman, S. 2019a. How Do You Manage with Loneliness? Observations from the Field: Problematising Participation as the Solution to Loneliness, presentation at *Thinking and Measuring Loneliness across the Life Course*. 12 June 2019, Manchester Metropolitan University. Available at: https://www.lonelinessconnectsus.org/blog/thinking-and-measuring-loneliness-across-the-life-course.

———. 2019b. Problematising Participation as the Policy Solution to 'Combat Loneliness': Policy Paper.

———. 2020. Leisure Pursuits: Uncovering the 'Selective Tradition' in Culture and Well-being Evidence for Policy. *Leisure Studies* 39 (1): 11–25. https://doi.org/10.1080/02614367.2019.1607536

Oman, S., and D. Edwards. 2020. Temporalities and Typologies of Loneliness: A Methodology to Understand New Parents, Self-Predicted Loneliness & the Role of NCT. In *Loneliness & Social Isolation in Mental Health Research Network Symposium*. London. https://www.ucl.ac.uk/psychiatry/events/2020/jan/loneliness-social-isolation-mental-health-research-network-symposium.

Oman, S., and M. Taylor. 2018. Subjective Well-Being in Cultural Advocacy: A Politics of Research between the Market and the Academy. *Journal of Cultural Economy* 11 (3): 225–243. https://doi.org/10.1080/17530350.2018.1435422.

ONS. 2011. *Measuring National Well-Being Technical Advisory Group. Office for National Statistics.* Accessed 5 April 2014. http://www.ons.gov.uk/ons/guide-method/user-guidance/well-being/measuring-national-well-being-technical-advisory-group/Notes-from-the-meeting-on-4-february-2011.pdf.

Power, M. 1994. The Audit Society. In *Accounting as Social and Institutional Practice*, ed. A. Hopwood and P. Miller, 299–316. Cambridge: Cambridge University Press.

Prince, R. 2014. Calculative Cultural Expertise? Consultants and Politics in the UK Cultural Sector. *Sociology* 48 (4): 747–762. https://doi.org/10.1177/0038038513502132.

———. 2015. Economies of Expertise: Consultants and the Assemblage of Culture. *Journal of Cultural Economy* 8 (5): 582–596. https://doi.org/10.1080/17530350.2014.974654.

Purser, R. 2019. *McMindfulness: How Mindfulness Became the New Capitalist Spirituality.* Repeater Books.

Rustin, S. 2012. The Conversation: Can Happiness be Measured?, *The Guardian.* Accessed 28 April 2021. https://www.theguardian.com/commentis-free/2012/jul/20/wellbeing-index-happiness-julian-baggin.

Schopenhauer, A. 1818. *The World as Will and Representation.* Translated by E.F.J. Payne. New York: Dover.

Scott, K. 2012. *Measuring Wellbeing: Towards Sustainability?* London: Routledge. https://www.taylorfrancis.com/https://www.taylorfrancis.com/books/mono/10.4324/9780203113622/measuring-wellbeing-towards-sustainability-karen-scott.

Selwood, S. 2002. The Politics of Data Collection: Gathering, Analysing and Using Data about the Subsidised Cultural Sector in England. *Cultural Trends* 12 (47): 13–84. https://doi.org/10.1080/09548960209390330.

———. 2010. *Making a Difference: The Cultural Impact of Museums.* London: NMDC.

Shi, L., S.P. Roche, and R.M. McKenna. 2019. Media Consumption and Crime Trend Perceptions: A Longitudinal Analysis. *Deviant Behavior* 40 (12): 1480–1492. https://doi.org/10.1080/01639625.2018.1519129.

Stebbins, R.A. 1997. Casual Leisure: A Conceptual Statement. *Leisure Studies* 16 (1): 17–25. https://doi.org/10.1080/026143697375485.

Stebbins, R. 1999. Serious Leisure. In *Leisure Studies Prospects for the Twenty-First Century*, ed. E.L. Jackson and T.L. Burton, 69–80. Philadelphia: Venture Publishing.

Stevenson, D.J. 2016. *Understanding the Problem of Cultural Non-Participation: Discursive Structures, Articulatory Practice and Cultural Domination.* Thesis. Queen Margaret University, Edinburgh. Accessed 29 April 2021. https://ere-search.qmu.ac.uk/handle/20.500.12289/7339.

Stevenson, D. 2019. The Cultural Non-Participant: Critical Logics and Discursive Subject Identities. *Arts and the Market* 9 (1): 50–64. https://doi.org/10.1108/AAM-01-2019-0002.

Stiglitz, J.E., A. Sen, and J.-P. Fitoussi. 2009. *Report by the Commission on the Measurement of Economic Performance and Social Progress*. OECD. https://ec.europa.eu/environment/beyond_gdp/download/CMEPSP-final-eport.pdf.

Taylor, M. 2016. Nonparticipation or Different Styles of Participation? Alternative Interpretations from Taking Part. *Cultural Trends* 25 (3): 169–181. https://doi.org/10.1080/09548963.2016.1204051.

Taylor, P., et al. 2015. *A Review of the Social Impacts of Culture and Sport*, 136. Department for Culture, Media and Sport.

Throsby, D. 2006. The Value of Cultural Heritage: What Can Economics Tell Us? In *Capturing the Public Value of Heritage: The Proceedings of the London Conference. Capturing the Public Value of Heritage*, 40–43. Swindon: English Heritage. Accessed 28 April 2021. https://researchers.mq.edu.au/en/publications/the-value-of-cultural-heritage-what-can-economics-tell-us.

———. 2010. *The Economics of Cultural Policy*. Cambridge: Cambridge University Press.

UK Government. 2021. *CASE Programme Guidance and Resources, National and Official Statistics*. Accessed 28 April 2021. https://www.gov.uk/guidance/case-programme.

UNESCO. 2018. *RURITAGE: Rural Regeneration through Systemic Heritage-Led Strategies, UNESCO*. Accessed 28 April 2021. https://en.unesco.org/ruritage.

United Nations. 1948. *Universal Declaration of Human Rights, United Nations*. United Nations. Accessed 28 April 2021. https://www.un.org/en/about-us/universal-declaration-of-human-rights.

University of Leeds. n.d. *Centre for Cultural Value*. School of Performance and Cultural Industries. https://ahc.leeds.ac.uk/centre-cultural-value-1.

Ura, K. 2011. *The Bhutanese Development Story*. Centre for Bhutan & GNH Studies. Accessed 28 April 2021. https://www.bhutanstudies.org.bt/publicationFiles/Monograph/mono-1en-bt-dev-stry.pdf.

Ura, K., S. Alkire, and T. Zangmo. 2012. *GNH and GNH Index*. Centre for Bhutan Studies. Accessed 28 April 2021. https://ophi.org.uk/wp-content/uploads/GNH_and_GNH_index_2012.pdf.

Williams, R. [1958]1989a. Culture Is Ordinary. In *Resources of Hope: Culture, Democracy, Socialism*, ed. R. Gable. London and New York: Verso.

———. [1961]1971. *The Long Revolution*. London: Pelican.

———. 1977. *Marxism and Literature*. Oxford: Oxford University Press.

———. [1976]1988. *Keywords: A Vocabulary of Culture and Society*. 2nd ed. London: Fourth Estate Ltd.

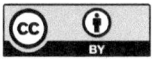

CHAPTER 7

Evidencing Culture for Policy

7.1 Well-being as Evidence for Social Policy

Now, of course we've already got some very strong instincts—even prejudices, sometimes—about what will improve people's lives, and we act on those instincts … These are instincts we feel to the core, but it's right that as far as possible we put them to the practical test, so we really know what matters to people. Every day, ministers, officials, people working throughout the public sector make decisions that affect people's lives, and this is about helping to make sure those government decisions on policy and spending are made in a balanced way, taking account of what really matters. (David Cameron, Prime Minister's Speech on Wellbeing, 25 November Cameron 2010)

Using well-being data is thought to improve how we understand human progress and development, as we discovered in the first half of this book (particularly Chap. 2). Chapter 6 looked at two further reasons to use well-being data: to evaluate policy decisions that have been made and to predict the impacts of possible policy change. In the case of cultural policy, the common rationale for using well-being data is to argue for more investment or to 'defend' (Belfiore 2012) the existing funding and status of the policy sector.

Shortly after the turn of this century, we saw an international commitment to well-being data that has been called 'the second wave of well-being' (Bache and Reardon 2013). The UK's Office for National Statistics

© The Author(s) 2021
S. Oman, *Understanding Well-being Data*,
New Directions in Cultural Policy Research,
https://doi.org/10.1007/978-3-030-72937-0_7

(ONS 2011a, 2011b) conducted a national debate so it could understand what people thought should be measured. The above quote is taken from a prime minister's speech that launched the Measuring National Well-being (MNW) programme and this debate. He talks of having instincts about what matters, but these need to be put to the test. Chapter 6 concluded with how, when the UK began measuring well-being, there was no measure for culture. This was despite the instinct that culture is good for well-being. It was also in spite of advocacy to that effect and efforts to collect more robust data, analyse them better and present compelling evidence.

Various areas of social policy have claimed their contribution to personal or societal well-being to differing degrees over the last 25 years (Oman and Taylor 2018). Notably, these appeals are rarely evaluated on their own terms (Oakley et al. 2013). The previous chapter (Chap. 6) looked at the relationship between culture and well-being because of its reliance on data and because the cultural sector[1] has sought a clear identity through arguing its value to well-being (Oman and Taylor 2018). It also discussed how this policy sector in particular often adopts what has been called a 'special case' rhetoric (O'Brien 2013), meaning it argues that it has unique or exceptional qualities. These are enmeshed in claims to the historical traditions of ideas of culture and its relationship to societal well-being (Belfiore and Bennett 2008) that have become naturalised and popularised. In other words, the relationship between culture and well-being seems almost natural, and common sense, whilst also appealing and almost taken for granted.

Alongside these processes of naturalisation and popularisation described in the previous chapter, investment in forms of research to generate well-being evidence for advocacy has also increased (Oman and Taylor 2018; Oman 2020). This form of research is often commissioned to support an argument in policy or political arenas, and we have looked at this as 'instrumentalisation' in the area of culture as social policy. This type of commissioned research is common in the UK and is meant to build an argument that a particular activity or service is good for well-being (Oman and Taylor 2018).[2] However, commissioning research to make evidence to support the value of a service, and therefore maintain its subsidy, affects the relationship between data, researcher and evidence.

How does commissioning research to support the arguments people want to, and need to make, change the nature and role of evidence in different social policy areas? How does this affect overall knowledge of 'what works for well-being'[3] in terms of social policy? Importantly, how does 'capitalising' on well-being data affect its capacity to do social good or to be good data? Do the economic value of data and their analysis change the relationship between well-being data and a good society? It is important to ask questions about research that seeks to prove something which is of financial and political value to particular groups.

In this chapter, we will look at some examples of data and evidence used to make specific arguments about the relationship between culture and well-being (the culture–well-being relationship), alongside evidence that might trouble some of the assumptions outlined previously. The examples in this and Chap. 8 are primarily focussed on cultural policy as a form of social policy. These case studies present issues for well-being data, evidence, knowledge and understanding that can be generalised more broadly to other domains of social policy, but focussing on cultural policy as one area makes the contradictions starker.

When you encounter research findings in your day-to-day life, you are most likely to see them in the media. Journalists don't often have time to sit and read a whole piece of research, and so you are likely to see the reproduction of a headline finding only. Sometimes this is directly from the researcher's own writing up, and sometimes it is reproduced second hand in others' summaries. There is an example of this in Sect. 7.4. It is less common to see the inclusion of caveats, methods, limitations and discussions when you see headline findings reproduced in the media, which limits how we understand well-being and data, as we shall go on to discover.

Can you think of a newspaper article you've read that says something like 'Loneliness is killing us' (e.g. Perry 2014) in its headline, which then moves on to clarify that this is *actually* not quite the case, the headline exaggerated the research that this article is based on and *actually* the research itself has many caveats? No, me neither. Media reporting of research is not renowned for this detail. Dramatic headlines are one thing in a newspaper article, where we have a shared understanding—to a degree—of how newspapers report information. Arguably, we have a different expectation when it comes to reading official reports. These can also lack detail on contextual information, caveats and limitations, as we discovered at the end of Chap. 4, with the testing of the ONS4 questions. This not only has a bearing on our understanding, but how we trust how data are reported. Often, it is just convenient to read headlines of research as they are presented to us, even believing they represent a body of evidence. The examples presented in the remainder of this chapter highlight that conclusive answers are difficult to find to questions about the well-being of any particular group of people, and the role of culture—or work—or leisure—in this. Crucially, looking at these examples, or 'problems' in detail, and putting them in context, generates additional well-being data to further improve understanding.

Data and Evidence in Cultural Policy

'Facts about the Arts' sets out to bring together some of the available statistics on the arts. Anyone who has the temerity to try to do this invites the scorn of those who believe that the concept of the arts itself is elusive and indefinable and any attempt to measure it cannot begin to represent its essential quality. Others, however, believe that the considerable body of material which does already exist can be gathered together and presented in such a way as to lead to a better understanding of the extent to which the arts contribute to the quality of life of the country. Amongst those potential users are Parliament, the media, the general public, and the many who have the power to influence and make decisions about the arts. (Nissel 1983, 1)

Muriel Nissel was a British statistician and civil servant, who collaboratively created 'a national survey analysing trends in social welfare' which was to become Social Trends. Social Trends (1st edition 1970) was a significant step in the history of UK statistics, as it symbolised a move away from tracking economic-only concerns to a more general concern with welfare.[4] Nissel was, therefore, key to the social indicators' movement, which coincides with what we have been describing as the 'first wave of well-being' (Bache and Reardon 2013). Nissel's quote from her book, 'Facts About the Arts: A Summary of Available Statistics' (1983), points towards this imagined clash we have encountered between the arts and data[5]: that they somehow do not go together, and yet must be put together.

Evidence is a contentious idea for those working in or interacting with cultural policy (both narrowly and broadly defined). The idea that the arts and culture have a role to play in improving quality of life is inherent to the identity of cultural policy. We saw this, of course, when the Arts Council of Great Britain was created, as discussed in the previous chapter. This idea of the culture–well-being relationship has then become operationalised in policy, by which we mean, it has been 'put to use': in order to advocate for the social purpose and even the social value of the arts; *even* the value added of 'culture' for the well-being of the wider population in various ways. So, cultural policy research will often operationalise this assumed relationship between culture and well-being in terms of value (as social impact) using quantitative evaluations, and we will look at some attempts to do that in this chapter.

Box 7.1   Operationalisation as a Process in Research
Operationalisation in research has a slightly different meaning than in everyday speech. It is the process through which you decide what you are going to measure to understand a concept. Or, more formally, it involves identifying measurable dimensions of a concept.

In this book, the main concept is well-being, of course; but along the way, we have also encountered other concepts, like poverty, social value and in this chapter, of course, culture.

How do you identify measurable dimensions of a concept? This could be designing questions that you can ask survey respondents or identifying data that are already out there (administrative data like hospital admissions are a good example). Measurement is about getting from the questions to the answers.

In some cases, it's **simple:** operationalisation could be, for example, deciding that in order to understand 'hospital capacity' you will use average A&E waiting times as the measure.

But sometimes it's **intermediate:** you might be interested in A&E waiting times overall; or average A&E waiting times for people under 18; or the percentage of people who wait more than four hours; or the longest anyone ever waited in a four-week period.

And sometimes it's **complicated:** for example, you may be calculating a scale based on responses to loads of survey questions—where the operationalisation is 'we're interested in all of these questions to get at this concept'. Think of something that looks like the PANAS Questionnaire (Fig. 4.3). Instead of lots of different feelings and emotions (as in the PANAS), imagine lots of questions that are more specific, yet similar, about your mood. This could be an operationalisation of 'anxiety' or of 'depression'.

If we want to understand the **culture–well-being relationship**—as policy, or in social impact—there are a number of ways we might **operationalise culture** and a number of ways we might **operationalise well-being**.

In statistics, operationalise, more specifically, would mean we need to find a concept from well-being data that is something measurable (a variable).

The following two chapters will investigate how the idea of a 'culture–well-being relationship' has been operationalised in policy, also looking at how it has been *operationalised* in research that is used to advocate policy decisions. This chapter problematises a number of aspects of the assumed relationship, by reconsidering how these concepts are operationalised in data. It also poses questions about why some data are utilised to reinforce long-held beliefs and values, when other data are readily available, yet are not used. Could it be that they do not allow for such a positive narrative?

Given that the value of culture is promoted for its positive relationship to well-being, and that this is partly to assure policy investment, we begin by looking at the relationship between data that capture changes in government investment in culture, and data that capture change in an aspect of subjective well-being. This exercise has two aims: to review the relationship from a different angle and to demonstrate how data can be found and used on websites that are accessible by everyone. We then look at ideas of being an artist and cultural work and compare two reports that use a similar methodology to analyse data from different countries. Again, this not only reveals something about the relationship between 'culture' and 'well-being', but also demonstrates how we can interact with research and evidence. Finally, we examine one piece of academic research that looks at 'cultural access' (participating in cultural activities) and well-being, to observe how this rendering of the culture–well-being relationship is evidenced in an academic journal article. While far from exhaustive, this chapter takes the key concerns of cultural policy: what gets funded, and to do what; who makes culture; who consumes culture; to look at them all in their own terms.

7.2   Policy Spending on Culture as Good for Society

> Wellbeing evidence can help policymakers to assess the impact of arts subsidy on wellbeing inequalities, and thus to ensure that the benefits of this spending are spread to those with lower wellbeing, including disadvantaged and underrepresented groups. (Berry 2014, 36)

The quote above is taken from a 2014 report that was written to the All-Party Parliamentary Group[6] on Wellbeing Economics. The report addressed what it called 'four policy areas' that the authors labelled: Building a high wellbeing economy: Labour market policy; Building high wellbeing places: Planning and transport policy; Building personal resources: Mindfulness in health and education; Valuing what matters: Arts and culture policy. It may strike you that these 'policy areas' seem quite different from what we have seen before—particularly in the discussion on well-being indicators and policy domains (see Chap. 3). Putting planning and transport together, for example, and foregrounding work in the economy (rather than just the financial stuff). Of course, here, we will be looking at the fact that 'arts and culture policy' is called 'valuing what matters'—recalling what we talked about in Chap. 6 and those before it, we might want to ask *who* is valuing what matters—and what matters to *who*?

On this point of what matters to who, the report advocates assessing and ensuring whether 'benefits are spread to those with lowest well-being' (cited above). Framing this statement in this way is interesting, as it seems to acknowledge that well-being (or, how different things impact on well-being) is not experienced universally. Notably, some argue that it is easier to improve the well-being of those with better well-being first (Oakley et al. 2013, 23),[7] while, of course, the Easterlin paradox implies that it is easier to improve the lives of those who are poorer using money than it is those with higher incomes (see Chap. 4 for this discussion). As you can see, the relationship between money, identifying need and improving well-being is less clear-cut than we may be led to believe.

The report does not explicitly state that policy spend does not evenly impact on people's well-being, citing evidence, so that it is clear this is a danger we should mitigate against. Instead it says we should assess *whether* it does. Its recommendations state that government should 'seek to ensure that the benefits of arts spending reach those with the lowest wellbeing, including communities with high deprivation'. This is an important point that is often glossed over. In cultural policy, it is now acknowledged that the most privileged tend to consume the most culture, they therefore benefit most as a group from the largest subsidies (Neelands et al. 2015; Taylor 2016; Belfiore 2016). The intersection of well-being and inequalities and arts spending is more complex, and one deserving of its own book. However, it seems that investigating policy spending on the arts for well-being is an issue of empirical and moral concern.

Well-being Data and Investment in Culture

For now, let's look at some well-being data to observe the relationship between culture and well-being. To be specific, we are not going to look at the concept of culture as a whole, or, as is normally investigated, the concept of participating in culture (in some way). Instead we are going to look at the money spent on culture. If advocacy for policy spending on culture is based on its positive impact on well-being, this implies that increased investment in culture is assumed to improve well-being. If this is the case, then this should be visible in some data, right? New Labour claimed a 90% increase in expenditure (in real terms) in its so-called cultural manifesto, 'Creative Britain' (in Labour 2010). You would maybe expect to be able to see a relationship between increased investment in cultural infrastructure and improved well-being as a result. You might also expect to see this demonstrated through statistics, whether they come from administrative data or from national-level surveys. Can we see this relationship in the data? How might we check?

We do not necessarily even need to find administrative data to answer the question 'Did increased spending result in increased well-being?' We can find sources that tell us about well-being over time and spending over time. The increase in spending is described in a number of other literatures, and specified in some as well, including Hesmondhalgh et al. (2015, 73):

> New Labour increased central government grants to local government from £82 billion in 1999 to £173 billion in 2010 (UK Public Spending website). This enabled local government to invest, particularly in 'cultural infrastructure' such as refurbished or completely new galleries and concert halls.

So, this means we could use the numbers published elsewhere, and simply consult well-being data, or literature, to see whether the investment identified by Hesmondhalgh and his co-authors affected well-being. However, the reference we have here indicates a credible data source for data on cultural investment, so we can use data from the UK Public Spending website and the data on well-being that would be most appropriate.

Box 7.2   Primary, Secondary and Tertiary Data
Recall from Chap. 3 that…

Primary data are collected by you or a project you are working on. In Chap. 3 we used the example of a questionnaire outside a music event in a local park.

Secondary data refer to data collected by someone else or another organisation that is made available at individual level. They will almost always be either anonymous or de-identified.[8] They are usually quantitative data but can be qualitative. In Chap. 3, I discussed reanalysing qualitative data from the Measuring National Well-being debate that was collected by the ONS.

Tertiary data consist of summaries of primary or secondary data, often called headline data. If you go to the ONS' well-being pages (n.d.), you will find headline statistics, so you do not have to do the maths yourself.

Should you want or need to find data yourself, I am sure the idea of it can feel daunting, and for many reasons. I try to tackle the most obvious ones to me in Box 7.3.

Box 7.3 Concerns with Finding Appropriate Data

1) **Where to look?:** The UK Public Spending website offers figures for year-on-year spending (tertiary data) that is a good place to start. It can be difficult to have faith in your ability to find the right data, but you can always begin by referring to how someone else has gone about it. In our case, we have started with Hesmondhalgh et al. (2015).

2) **Suitability:** There are various funding streams that subsidise 'culture', so what are you looking for?[9] As you will see in Table 7.2, I chose to use declared total government spend and Grant in Aid to ACE (being one of four arts councils in the UK). That is not to say that this is not complicated, but again, I followed how it was used in the literature and Hesmondhalgh et al. offer detailed descriptions of funding at this time (Hesmondhalgh et al. 2015, pp. 71–75) that can help you decide which is best to use. I used the clearest to me.

3) **Availability:** The availability of recent historical data that was readily available on websites may have gone through a process of archiving. This changes links and might make it difficult to find the data you have identified as useful from the literature. You can consult the UK government web archive (The National Archives n.d.) if it is government data, or data from a non-departmental government public body like the ONS or ACE. As we have already encountered, back when we were thinking about the role of methodology in data in Chap. 3, there are pros and cons to all data, but administrative data are easy to access and managed by public bodies, with strict guidelines. It is therefore a great place to explore possible relationships and patterns for further research.

4) **Assurance:** Knowing you have made the right choice can feel impossible. It is not always explicit that many choices are made in even a simple data process, like the one I describe here. The key thing is to know that most choices will have pros and cons and that there are limits to all claims of what can be known with the data and methods used. You just want to be sure to be aware of the limits, and state them when you describe your findings.

I have chosen to consult the ONS for well-being data, as their platform is most familiar to me, and therefore *feels* easiest to refer to. Going back to the choices we make about which data we choose (Table 3.1), there can be a trade-off between resources (skill, time, money) and robustness. In another situation, you might find other tertiary data more accessible. The data I use here are headline statistics, rather than the whole dataset of every response. Therefore, basic data practices (cleaning and aggregation) have already been done by those who administer the data, for ease of use by the media, government and indeed anyone who is interested. The same is true for the public spending data I have chosen.

As we have previously discovered, Life Satisfaction (LS) is probably the most popular measure of subjective well-being (see Sect. 4.5 for reasons why). While the UK's Measuring National Well-being (MNW) programme did not officially begin until 2010, the UK had national-level surveys that had a question about life satisfaction for decades. Other national statistics offices, and international statistics bodies, have also administered surveys with life satisfaction questions in. The tertiary data I use here are from the British Household Panel Survey. It followed the same representative sample of individuals—the panel—over a period of years between 1991 and 2009. The same households who took part in BHPS were asked to participate in a larger survey, called Understanding Society.[10] The same questions are asked of participants in the later survey, so data are available for after 2009.

Table 7.1 demonstrates that using data for satisfaction with life overall, as measured by the BHPS, does not show an increase in life satisfaction over time. While this is a somewhat crude attempt to use data that is readily available, it demonstrates that it can be easy to explore a fundamental question quickly and sensibly. In this case, the question might be: 'if we know that investment in a particular policy initiative or policy domain has increased substantially over time (Hesmondhalgh et al. 2015), how can headline well-being statistics help us understand the influence of investment on well-being?' As Table 7.1 shows, the increase in funding is not seen in an increase in LS scores.

There are many limits to what we can know from the data sourced—we know very little of its context in this table, for example, but it tells a clear story. As it was from an ONS summary (for ease), rather than LS data from the UK Data Service, the years represented (2002/2003–2009/2010) are those available and only a subset of New Labour's time in government exactly (1997–2010). This does not mean they are not useful.

Table 7.1 Life satisfaction data 2002/2003–2009/2010

Q: Satisfaction with life overall	2002/2003	2003/2004	2004/2005	2005/2006	2006/2007	2007/2008	2008/2009	2009/2010
Somewhat, mostly or completely satisfied	77.3	78.3	77.0	74.6	76.2	77.0	78.1	77.1

Data Source: ONS (2010a)

Table 7.2 Policy spending on the arts and life satisfaction

	2002/2003	2003/2004	2004/2005	2005/2006	2006/2007	2007/2008	2008/2009	2009/2010
LS	77.3	78.3	77.0	74.6	76.2	77.0	78.1	77.1
Total govt spend (billion)	1.59	1.84	1.77	1.96	1.94	2.03	1.88	1.97
Govt Grant in Aid to ACE (million)	289.405	324.955	368.859	408.678	426.531	423.601	437.631	452.964

Data source variable (see endnotes)

The UK government's changes in funding and policy are unlikely to see an instant impact on a national population's life satisfaction. There are likely to be lags in effects. However, as noted with the poverty data in Chap. 1, selecting your timeframe can alter the narrative about the effects of government policy, be that life satisfaction or poverty. But we can check. Hesmondhalgh et al. kindly gave us the rest of the data for Grant in Aid to ACE, as follows:

1997–1998, £186.60 million
1998–1999, £189.95 million
1999–2000, £228.25 million
2000–2001, £237.155 million
2001–2002, £251.455 million

Therefore, the increase in Grant in Aid spending was about the same in the five years that we didn't include, as in the eight years we did, and it increased quite steadily.

What if we want to ask a more complex question, or see if there is any pattern between well-being and funding? In Table 7.1 we were only exploring one dimension of data: life satisfaction over time. Table 7.2 uses the same LS data points over time with some additional rows to report data on arts funding too. This will let us see a relationship between 'amount of funding' from one set of data and the level of life satisfaction over time from another set of data. We can then plot these data over time as a line graph that looks like Fig. 7.1. A positive relationship between increase in funding and life satisfaction over time would see the lines on the graph charting a similar course, so to speak.

There is no obvious relationship between policy spend on culture in the data plotted and life satisfaction. Even if we account for the additional five years of data, life satisfaction does not appear to relate to policy spend. Interestingly, LS data from the BHPS from the longer timeframe[11] are even less inclined to show a steady increase than our subset. While the easily available data do not have all of the 13 years in which New Labour were in office, you might expect that 8 years' data would be enough to find a relationship between policy spending on the arts and life satisfaction, if there is one to find.

So, what about the limits of what we can know about the relationship? Figure 7.1 may only report life satisfaction data, but we know some other things about cultural investment, based on the literature presented so far.

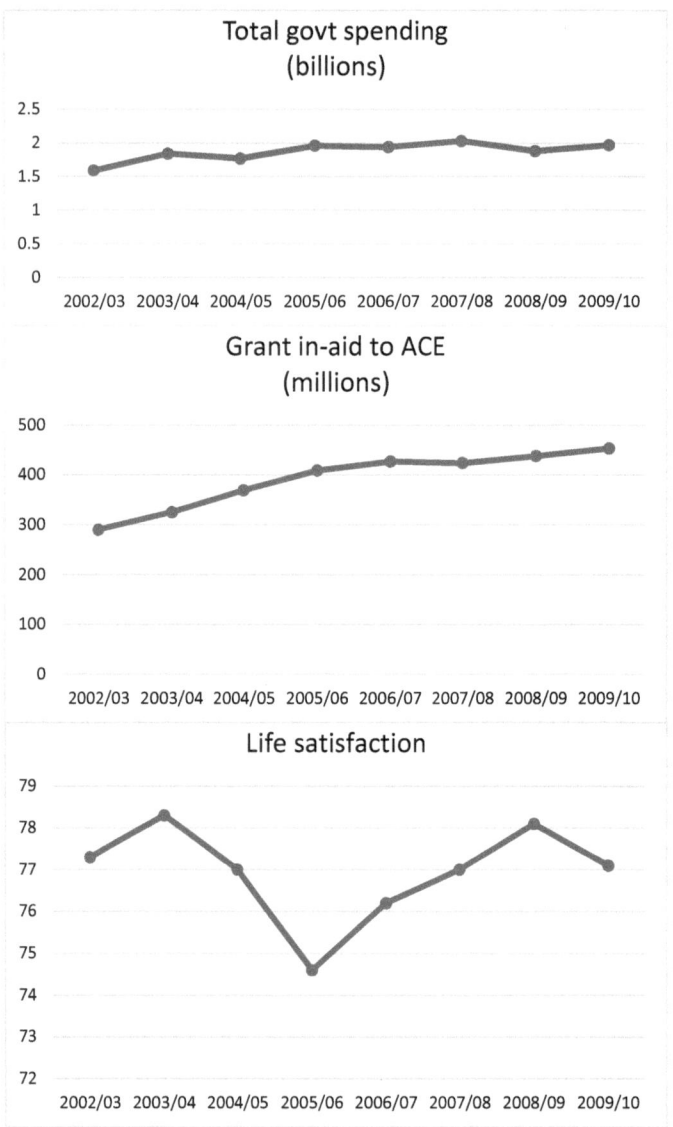

Fig. 7.1 Patterns between arts funding and life satisfaction over time. (Total spend data from UK public spending website https://www.ukpublicspending. co.uk/download_multi_year_1997_2010UKb_17c1li111mcn_F0t8nt. Grant in Aid data via Hesmondhalgh et al. 2015)

For one, we have evidence that policy spend on the arts does not reach everyone equally, because not everyone participates in the culture that this money is spent on. This *could* mean that the way that culture was funded in this timeframe would, therefore, possibly limit potential increases in life satisfaction overall across a whole population. We need to acknowledge that there is a difference between cultural participation and investment in culture.

Let's quickly return to what we have already learnt about life satisfaction data as a measure of subjective well-being. Firstly, let us consider the question: 'How dissatisfied or satisfied are you with your life overall?' This does not capture all aspects of subjective well-being. In fact, if we think back to Chap. 4 on subjective well-being and Table 4.2, with the ONS4 questions, you will remember that life satisfaction falls under one of the three dimensions of subjective well-being: evaluative. Then, it follows that there may be increases in aspects of well-being that were not captured by responses to this question. Life satisfaction data are therefore useful, and may be the most useful according to some (Layard 2006), but still limited in evaluating overall subjective well-being (if we are to follow the accepted reasoning presented so far).

So, we need to acknowledge that there are many limits to knowing the extent to which policy spending in one area can have a clear relationship with life satisfaction, and what that means for the culture–well-being relationship. There are, in fact, numerous limits to any claim that might be made for causation. The life satisfaction data could also include the effects of countless other things happening at the same time which could be counteracting the effect, if, indeed, it existed. Remember the conditions of a good measure of well-being in Chap. 3? It should

> be sensitive to important changes in wellbeing and insensitive to spurious ones. In practice, distinguishing between the two is quite a challenge and often relies on judgement based on a priori expectations. (Dolan and Metcalfe 2012, 411)

Clearly, the process I have described is not seeking a metric. All I have done here is describe the data easily available to look for a relationship between arts funding and LS. Therefore, no attempts have been made to account for confounders (which we will come to in others' research later). There are so many variables that might affect life satisfaction in a way that would be captured by life satisfaction data, that it is extremely difficult to pinpoint the impact of one aspect only in this descriptive way. People who analyse data, rather than simply describe it, will use a theory or hypothesis about pathways that shape well-being to help them create models that do this work. We will return to this in Chap. 8.

Life satisfaction is a very influential measure that we have encountered numerous times in this book. We have been measuring it for years, as it was in the first wave of well-being indicators (see Chap. 2). Realising that life satisfaction had not changed as expected with income over the years, resulted in Easterlin's paradox that was influential in the second wave of well-being as happiness economics (Easterlin 1973; Chap. 4). Life satisfaction is also measured using Big Data technologies (Chap. 5) and is thought to be the measure of subjective well-being that people most readily understand (Chap. 4). Crucially, because questions about satisfaction with life (although worded slightly differently) have appeared in numerous surveys, and for decades, we have a lot of life satisfaction data to make simple comparisons over time, as we have just seen. LS can also be used to show very powerful relationships to outcomes of well-being, such as suicide rate and the familiarity of LS, together with the prevalence of the data, make it useful for simple exercises, as we have attempted here.

We've briefly looked at ways that the relationship between different variables (different policy spend data and life satisfaction) can be plotted. This will hopefully make it a bit easier for you to engage with similar representations in future. This section also demonstrated that it is quite easy to play with data that are publicly available. You can download the data into a table, like those featured, and use a simple function in Excel to plot line graphs to look for relationships over time.

Of course, there is another key point to this section, really, and that is to problematise the assumption that the arts and culture are a priority for policy spending if you want to improve well-being (Berry 2014). If you look at historic well-being data that coincide with previous increases in policy spend, you cannot find patterns in the data that prove that this relationship exists. There are many limitations to the claims that can be made with these data. The increase in arts funding coincides with a more general increase in public spending overall, therefore it is hard to disaggregate policy spend from other things that may affect life satisfaction in this time. Another issue is that life satisfaction data only capture one aspect of well-being. I'm sure you have thought of other limits, as well. What is key is that while using data in this way may not *prove* anything, sometimes exploring data can be good enough reasons to ask questions—remember this is what Easterlin did when he found that life satisfaction did not have the relationship to income that had been long-assumed in the data he had. This is said to have changed well-being research forever—even if people still argue about it. Sometimes data help us question the status quo in productive ways. They are not only there to help certain people answer certain questions.

Policy Decisions and Investments Using Well-being Data

Lord Richard Layard (the Happiness Tsar from Chap. 4) has previously stated that 'policy is not going to be framed around [well-being] for decades, but unless you have the index you'll never get to a point where you can influence things' (Rustin 2012).[12] This is a far more measured take on well-being data and evidence being used for policy-making than suggested by the prime minister's speech that opens this chapter. Lord Gus O'Donnell, another major advocate for well-being in policy-making, is also an economist and an extremely influential civil servant.[13] He explained that same year:

> We now know much more about what drives the wellbeing of people and communities than we did 10 years ago, and our knowledge and understanding is set to increase significantly over the next few years. (O'Donnell in Legatum Institute 2012)

As recognised by the OECD and the ONS early on in their programmes to measure well-being (see Chap. 3), there was a general acknowledgement at this time that well-being measures were evolving and exploratory. So, while a simple visualisation of how life satisfaction over time might interact with arts funding or suicide rates, not all well-being measurements are equally robust, and all have limits that are not often made clear when data are expressed. This is also the case when the concept of well-being is operationalised with another concept, such as culture.

Well-being valuations are far more complex than the way tertiary or headline data were 'described' in the previous section's simple line graphs. As we discovered at the end of Chap. 6, demands from and on government departments to evaluate the impact of their decisions, evolved from the descriptive to more complicated modelling in the 2010s. These models can analyse primary or secondary data and enable a more sophisticated reading of the data. A model helps researchers understand far more complex relationships, including what might be interfering with our understanding (confounders). It can also express a relationship between two things, such as culture and well-being, in monetary terms. We will look at an example of well-being valuation modelling, and how complex this is, in greater detail in the next chapter.

Box 7.4 What Is a Model?

Earlier in this book, I stated that data don't just fall from the sky as facts. Neither do the models that analyse them. A model will probably contain assumptions about how concepts like 'well-being' and 'culture' are associated.

There are two main kinds of models: **exploratory** and **confirmatory**.

Exploratory models

These allow you to try numerous variables that *may* be associated, and see what emerges as of possible interest. In other words, you are exploring the possibilities of the data. Developments in machine learning have sped up this kind of exploratory modelling with Big Data, as we discovered in Chap. 5.

Confirmatory models

Most of the chapters in this book refer to work that aims to confirm a hypothesis. Statisticians and others who model quantitative data in this way don't just throw a bunch of variables into a model and hope for the best. Their models are designed with a theoretical foundation and that will most likely be arrived at from what we already know from previous studies about how one thing (say income) affects another, well-being, for example.

Before a good confirmatory model is designed, it is important to establish 'what counts' in the issues you are considering, and how things are expected to fit together.

In exploratory analysis, you won't need to guess how concepts fit together (although you might have an inkling), and won't need the same level of attention to the variables you pick in relation to the concepts.

An example of what a model does

A simple model might be based on the hypothesis of a positive correlation. Say, between the average wealth of a nation and its average happiness (as with Easterlin). Imperfect measures tend to be used that represent far more complex concepts like wealth and happiness. For example, variables for life satisfaction and income will not tell us all we need to know about wealth or well-being. Also, resources dictate that it is unlikely a researcher will examine the entire path between income and well-being; instead it will examine whether the two measured concepts (variables) have a statistical association.

It is likely that the relationships examined in any one study represent only small parts of a larger theory. This is not unusual, but is it always explicit when research is presented?

As Chap. 6 describes, government departments including DCMS were indeed looking at how to use well-being data in valuations[14] before Cameron's speech in November 2010 from the official launch. This is because DCMS and the areas it funds were addressing HMT's preference for valuation techniques (see O'Brien 2010). There are a couple of approaches that have been called well-being valuation. Fujiwara's (2013) seems the most influential in the UK, but other examples (Sidney et al. 2017) called well-being valuation take a different approach. Following the increase in using subjective well-being data to value the impact of services, there has been a growing number of studies investigating the impact of the arts or specific cultural organisations in this way (such as Fujiwara et al. 2014a, 2014b and Fujiwara 2013 that we look at in the next chapter). These studies use responses to subjective well-being questions in national-level surveys, together with data on, say, theatre attendance, and estimate the impact of that artform. Such valuations assess data which can tell you that people who go to the theatre are more or less likely to have answered subjective well-being questions in a particular way. The magic is in the modelling.

Important questions remain, however, when it comes to the limits of the data and the extent that valuations can advise policy; particularly when it comes to stating one thing is more valuable than another. The practice of ordering the value of one thing over another does not seem to be presenting us with findings that corroborate each other. In one study, one artform is more important than another. As we saw in Chap. 4, 'excessive TV watching' is pitted against an unspecified amount of gardening when reporting on data collected to understand how people are spending their time in lockdown and measuring their well-being (Bu et al. 2020; Mak et al. 2020; Nuffield 2021). Bias is brought to the data, which means they can be read in ways that confirm prior beliefs about what is an excessive amount in one area, but not necessary to measure about another. Consequently, this bias will feed into the presentation of findings and shape recommendations to decision-makers. In other words, ostensibly rational, neutral decisions which are supposedly made on the basis of well-being data are in danger of reproducing prior judgements and beliefs of the researchers—especially if they confirm those of the policy-maker reading the recommendations.

7.3   Well-being Data and Cultural Practice

So, we know that culture is a tricky word to define and can be measured in different ways; we know the same is true of well-being. We have looked at how we might need to think about how the concept of well-being is 'operationalised'. This is, of course, also true of culture, and the previous chapter spent some time covering different meanings and uses of culture.

What is it about culture that is being measured? This is, therefore, another question to think about, when we are trying to understand the relationship between culture and well-being. It is just as true whether we are reading the research of others, or, indeed, trying to design our own. Is it the specific activities that make culture? Different cultures? The culture wars? If it is measuring the activities that make up 'culture' (however defined), is it people who do things themselves or watch others? That is, are you producing culture (i.e. making art) or consuming it (i.e. watching Netflix)? Are you an artist or another kind of cultural practitioner who *makes* culture as their profession? Or a painter or singer in your spare time? Does singing along to the radio count the same way that being a member of a church choir does? Is it about participating with people? Does watching other people sing (because you are an audience member with people) count as participating in culture, just through watching? If so, does it make a difference if you watch it digitally—and with family or alone? What about the evidence we have seen that being outside seems to increase the relationship between different activities and well-being (MacKerron and Mourato 2013)? Should that mean that all outside arts get more money because they will have extra well-being value?

All these ways of thinking about what you might want to measure about culture for society or people actually involve quite different experiences for people. In this language of well-being valuation and data, you might find someone saying that how you operationalise culture matters for well-being effects. If you measure going to pubs or restaurants, how can you be sure that this is not a proxy for disposable income, leisure time or spending time with friends? The following might be the questions you might want to ask for cultural and social policy:

- What are you doing?
- Who are you doing it with?
- Where are you doing it?
- How long are you doing it for?
- How often are you doing it?
- How long do we expect an effect to last?
- How big should that effect be to count as impacting on well-being?

We're not going to go into arguments for what the most important aspect of cultural participation is. We have touched on these debates in Chap. 6 and acknowledged they are comprehensively covered elsewhere. Instead, as this book is about well-being data, we are going to look at how data can help answer certain questions, and what the limits to these are. We are going to compare how two different research projects answered a question about being an artist or having a creative occupation, and how that might be related to well-being.

Being an Artist and Well-being

For those of you who didn't watch Disney-Pixar's *Soul* at Christmas in 2020 (and again for those of you who didn't watch it, I'll try to not spoil it), the film places a lot of emphasis on the meaning of music for the main character, Joe Gardner. He sees music—specifically jazz—as his purpose in life. The cruel twist is that, just as Joe gets his big break, and is on the cusp of being able to make music—in a real band—not just as an elementary school teacher, this big break is jeopardised. Ironically, it is the sheer joy at his big break that leads to this twist of fate. The unfairness of Joe not getting to fulfil his potential keeps us rooting for him through a meandering journey of self-discovery. Much of the journey is watching him strive to get back to where he was, so that he is able to enjoy that big break.

The over-riding feeling for most of the movie is that, for Joe, 'making it' in music is what will make his life worthwhile. The movie goes some way to explain the moment of getting lost in music, something that positive psychologists have described as 'flow',[15] but which the movie describes as 'in the zone'. You watch Joe reflect on what he thinks amounts to his meaningless existence, like the existential philosophers before him. There is also a moment where you watch Joe, sitting on a New York sidewalk, feel the sun on his face and wonder at a helicopter seed spiralling from a tree. This—'being in the moment'—differs from flow. In flow, you are lost in your thoughts, in an activity, whereas being in the moment is about being present in your body, and is what mindfulness practice is based on. This Disney movie better describes some of the complex theoretical imaginings of well-being than thousands of years of philosophers we've come across before in this book—possibly this is of no surprise?

The drive to be able to do something creative as a job—and in the way you want—is not just the stuff of Disney films. In fact, being an artist of sorts has long been seen as desirable and holds much symbolic value.[16] Idealised representations of creative and cultural jobs include creativity and expression, autonomy and passion—or doing something you love. The realities are often far harsher: with independence comes precarity of employment; there are inequalities in opportunities to 'do what you love'. Often people end up working for money doing something associated to their creative practice—like our main character Joe being a music teacher, while awaiting his big break. Also, the rarity of opportunity to do what you love, and to be expressive and creative, often means you are expected to put up with being treated badly, or indeed to work for free, which is not an option for all.[17]

In short, the idea of being an artist is an ideal and the reality of creative occupations is quite different. While quality work is seen as important for well-being (What Works Wellbeing 2017), the *actual* quality of creative work and the anxieties that accompany the lifestyle necessary of such occupations make it an interesting case for well-being research. The idea of creative work or being an artist is filled with contradictions that deserve attention, and yet the well-being of 'creatives' and artists is less frequently looked at than you may imagine (as the publications we are about to look at tell us).

Two Reports on the Relationship Between Being an Artist or Working in a Creative Occupation and Well-being

The two reports we will turn to were published in subsequent years. Their titles and their named approaches suggest that they both contain findings from research using similar methods to answer a similar research question about the well-being of 'creatives'. This enables us to see how 'culture' can be operationalised as being and working as an artist, and how this can relate to well-being. It also continues to allow us to familiarise ourselves with looking at others' research as it appears in reports, and to think more about what might be happening under the bonnet.

Report 1, Artful Living: Examining the Relationship Between Artistic Practice and Subjective Wellbeing Across Three National Surveys was funded by the National Endowment for the Arts in the US

(Tepper et al. 2014). The research looked at different cohorts of arts practitioners and graduates in the US, using three different surveys.[18] Contrary to the received wisdom that music and the performing arts are associated with the largest increases in well-being (e.g. Fujiwara and MacKerron 2015), Tepper et al. found that fine arts and crafts consistently related to higher well-being; music did so for some groups and not others; and participating in theatre 'seemed unrelated to wellbeing'[19] in the data they had on arts practitioners and graduates (Tepper et al. 2014, 7). Overall, the authors say that there was 'strong support' that what they call 'artistic practice' is associated with higher life satisfaction and lower anxiety, as aspects of subjective well-being.

Report 2, Creative Occupations and Subjective Wellbeing is a working paper for NESTA, a UK Thinktank. This study used data from the UK's Annual Population Survey (APS).[20] This research concurs with Tepper et al. (2014) that creative occupations are associated with higher than average life satisfaction, worthwhileness and happiness, 'although most creative occupations also have higher than average levels of anxiety' (Fujiwara et al. 2015, 1). This is contrary to Tepper et al.'s findings on anxiety from their data, but is corroborated by a number of studies, including the recent book, *Can Music Make You Sick?* (Gross and Musgrave 2020).

We are going to break down the ways that these studies may seem similar, yet differ. Both Tepper et al. and Fujiwara et al. use multiple regression of cross-sectional 'national survey' data that ask subjective well-being questions from people with an artistic practice in the case of the US or a creative occupation in the case of the UK. This means that these data include variables based on questions asked by the organisations who administer the survey; the named researchers (or authors) don't ask these questions of the participants themselves. Some of the datasets used include creative practitioners and people who are not creative practitioners. This is fairly common, and the researchers simply distinguish which cases (people in the data) meet the criteria of their research question, meaning they analyse the people who have a creative occupation/artistic practice and remove those who do not form from the model.

Box 7.5   Multiple Regression and Cross-Sectional Data
What is multiple regression of cross-sectional data?
   Let's look at these separately.
   Regression analysis is common in statistical analyses. It involves estimating the relationship between a dependent variable and one or more independent variables.
   In an analysis (e.g. a regression) you distinguish between
   (1) Independent variables: that can take different values. You use an independent variable to predict the dependent variable. That is why it is sometimes called a predictor variable.
   (2) Dependent variables: that can take different values. When you are measuring your relationship, you are interested in how the dependent variable is affected by the independent variable. It is, therefore, sometimes called the outcome variable to reflect this.
   Say you are interested in **private music tuition in childhood** and **creative occupations.** You are not expecting an adult professional occupation to retrospectively generate experience of music lessons, but you might want to understand if the opportunity of private tuition affected a later career. So, **occupation would be your dependent variable**, and **music tuition in childhood would be your independent variable**.
   So, we are still interested in **private music tuition in childhood** and **creative occupations.** We have established we want to understand how the first affects the second (and not the other way around). You might decide on other things that you think predict being a creative, such as gender, which previous research may suggest affects the likelihood of entering a creative occupation. Therefore, you would bear this in mind as another possible independent variable.
   This is what makes it 'multiple' because we have now got **more than one independent variable** to predict our dependent variable.
   A regression to explain how many people work in creative occupations could be conducted with either cross-sectional or longitudinal data.
   Cross-sectional data are collected from a survey from a specific point in time, or time period. The same survey questions can be repeated, but these questions will have been asked from different people.

Box 7.5   (continued)

Longitudinal data hold information on the same people over time. This means you can ask the same questions, year on year, to see change over time. For example, you can ask people year on year if they have private music lessons. You can also have data for different questions. This is useful for our example, as we might have data on private music tuition in childhood, and data on occupation in adulthood, should the participant be around that long.

DCMS' Taking Part Survey (TPS) has a longitudinal component[21] and a cross-sectional one.

Since 2005/2006, TPS has been run on a cross-sectional basis that involves a new sample of households, which is drawn annually, and a new group of respondents who are asked the same questions. This enables researchers who use this data to say 'last year X% of the population had music lessons'. But it cannot, therefore account for change that happens to an individual, so you won't know that 'the people who stopped music lessons last year are like abc'. Given that change implies impact, this is a big deal for many of the studies we encounter in this book.

The two research projects on well-being from the US and UK that we are exploring use different samples and surveys. This means that in both studies the group in 'creative occupations' may not necessarily map onto those with an 'artistic practice' as neatly as the labels used suggest. We come back to this in the next paragraph. The UK report uses the Annual Population Survey, which contains information on people's occupation and the 'ONS4' questions that we keep encountering. Creative occupations were defined using DCMS' Creative Industries Economic Estimates (DCMS 2011) and then coded using the ONS's standard occupational classifications, called SOC codes (ONS 2010b).[22] The authors are therefore able to look at the four ONS measures: life satisfaction, worthwhileness, happiness and anxiety for the 30 creative occupations as defined by the DCMS (2011) in Table 7.3.

Table 7.3 Occupations in the creative industries

Creative industry	Creative occupations
	Description
Advertising and marketing	Marketing and sales directors
	Advertising and public relations directors
	Public relations professionals
	Advertising accounts managers and creative directors
	Marketing associate professionals
Architecture	Architects
	Town planning officers
	Chartered architectural technologists
	Architectural and town planning technicians
Crafts	Smiths and forge workers
	Weavers and knitters
	Glass and ceramics makers, decorators and finishers
	Furniture makers and other craft woodworkers
	Other skilled trades not elsewhere classified
Design: Product, graphic and fashion design	Graphic designers
	Product, clothing and related designers
Film, TV, video, radio and photography	Arts officers, producers and directors
	Photographers, audio-visual and broadcasting equipment operators
IT, software and computer services	Information technology and telecommunications directors
	IT business analysts, architects and systems designers
	Programmers and software development professionals
	Web design and development professionals
Publishing	Journalists, newspaper and periodical editors
	Authors, writers and translators
Museums, galleries and libraries	Librarians
	Archivists and curators
Music, performing and visual arts	Artists
	Actors, entertainers and presenters
	Dancers and choreographers
	Musicians

Adapted from DCMS (2011)

There are many discussions over what counts as a creative occupation using these classifications that we won't get too caught up in here.[23] However, when you imagine a town planning officer, they probably feel quite different to you from a musician. Also, realistically, the day-to-day duties of one is likely to *feel* very different than the other. A town planning officer will probably have more regular hours and a more secure contract than a cellist. You might also imagine that a cellist may have more capacity for self-expression, and feeling, well, *artistic*, than a town planner. The differences in day-to-day tasks, security, income and so on are all important external factors that will affect well-being. Therefore, these discrepancies across creative occupations (some of which may not feel that creative) may limit improved understandings of the impact these professions have on well-being, if the model treats everyone with a job defined as 'creative' (using occupational codes) as equivalent. What is key here is that it is that the categories used to break down the data (from the APS), and how they have been coded into professions (using the ONS' occupational classifications) is important context to knowing what we can understand about differences in well-being.

In contrast, the US case uses data from three surveys which target different groups. The Strategic National Arts Alumni Project (SNAAP) captures data about graduates of arts institutions. The Double Major Student Survey focusses on undergraduates who have two majors from four comprehensive institutions and five liberal arts colleges. The DDB Needham Life Style Survey (DDB) is the nation's largest and longest running annual survey of consumer attitudes. The report states that the researchers 'look specifically at responses to creative practice, life satisfaction, and "sense of control" in one's life', but it is not precisely clear whether they identified 'creatives' or looked at everyone who answered these questions. The participants across these surveys are classified as 'having an artistic practice' for different reasons. In fact, most of the secondary data analysis is of responses regarding how people do cultural activities in their spare time.

Crucially, and confusingly, the participants across the three surveys do not all actually have an 'artistic practice', in a professional sense. In fact, the authors 'use the terms artistic practice, creative engagement, and creative practice interchangeably throughout this report' (Tepper et al. 2014, 8). So, there is no analysis of the relationship between well-being and creative occupations, per se, or necessarily any differentiation between a professional artist or an amateur who 'engages' in artistic practice. Similarly, the questions used to establish aspects of subjective well-being are not the same across each survey. Table 7.4 shows the subjective well-being questions and how the 'artists' were identified across the three US surveys, alongside the UK case. Therefore, establishing what counts as 'an artistic practice' is one of the issues, and the other is establishing how subjective well-being is understood. There are therefore key differences in how these concepts were operationalised in these reports.

Table 7.4 A comparison of culture and well-being questions across the four surveys used in the two case studies

Survey name	Description of survey	Application of the survey	Culture Q	Subjective well-being question evaluative, experience/eudaimonic?
DDB Needham Life Style Survey (DDB)	The DDB Needham Life Style Survey (DDB) is the nation's largest and longest running annual survey of consumer attitudes.	In polling American adults, the surveys ask questions about—among other things, attitudes, interests, opinions, activities, product use and mass media use.	Three specific questions address creative practice, including the frequency of participation in craft projects, gardening and playing a musical instrument over the last 12 months.	SWB Q: EVALUATIVE A series of agree/disagree statements get at the issues of life-satisfaction (e.g. 'I'm much happier now than I ever was before'; 'I am very satisfied with the way things are going in my life these days'). SWB Q: EXPERIENCE To get a sense of generalised anxiety ('loss of control'), we examine several questions that address people's sense of personal efficacy (e.g. 'sometimes I feel that I don't have enough control over the direction my life is taking').
Double Major Student Survey	The survey, supported by the Teagle Foundation, assesses the link between creativity, interdisciplinarity and the liberal arts by focussing on undergraduates who have two majors.	The survey drew from a sample of approximately 1700 students from four comprehensive institutions and five liberal arts colleges, and asked them questions about demographics, academic choices, self-ratings on skills and competencies, and creativity and innovation.	Students were also questioned about their participation in artistic and creative practices, including 'played a musical instrument', 'painted, drew a picture, or made sculpture' and 'made or designed clothing, costumes, etc.' There were a total of 10 different categories of artistic and creative practices listed among the 23 activities. Students were asked to rate the frequency with which they participated in these activities.	SWB Q: EUDAIMONIC Specifically, students were asked about their positive self-image ('please check all of the adjectives that best describe yourself—'capable', 'confident', 'resourceful'); their positive social outlook; and materialistic orientation (e.g. 'it sometimes bothers me quite a bit that I can't afford to buy all the things I'd like').

				SWB Q: EVALUATIVE
Strategic National Arts Alumni Project (SNAAP)	The Strategic National Arts Alumni Project, or SNAAP, is an online survey targeted at graduates of arts institutions, which asks questions about their experiences both during and after their arts schooling.	To date, more than 100,000 alumni have been asked questions about their career path, their artistic practice (both professionally and avocationally) and their overall satisfaction with work and life. Specifically, we look at questions from the 2009 pilot survey of 4031 graduates from across 76 different arts colleges and schools.	Questions addressing personal artistic practice and the frequency with which it is undertaken. SNAAP data allow us to look at people who were once highly involved in the arts through their schooling or career, and who are no longer practising their artistic craft or are only practising it avocationally. This may reveal some information about the importance of continued artistic practice for those who valued it highly in the past and who had achieved high levels of proficiency.	Including people's response to the questions, 'in most ways my life is close to my ideal' and 'I am satisfied with my standard of living'.
Annual Population Survey (APS)	The UK's APS covers employment, unemployment, housing, ethnicity, religion, health and education.	The APS is a repeated annual cross-sectional survey of approximately 155,000 households and 360,000 individuals. Since 2011 the APS has contained the four ONS well-being questions. Waves (years) 2011–2012 and 2012–2013 are used in the analysis.	The jobs variables relate to the main job of the individual. They used the occupations as categorised by DCMS using NS-SEC (see Table 7.4).	ONS4: 'Overall, how satisfied are you with your life nowadays?' ONS4: 'Overall, how happy did you feel yesterday?' 'Overall, how anxious did you feel yesterday?' ONS4:'Overall, to what extent do you feel the things you do in your life are worthwhile?'

Adapted from Tepper et al. (2014) and Fujiwara et al. (2015)

Table 7.4 is populated with text that has largely been cut and pasted from the two reports. It contains contextual information on the nature and purpose of the surveys used (you will see that in most cases the surveys have different aims) and the wording of the questions. I have attempted to categorise the US study into Evaluative, Experience, Eudaimonic, as per the categories in Chap. 4 and Table 4.1.[24] This was easy for the ONS4 from the UK case, as these have been categorised for us already. The US case proved more difficult. The question about what Tepper et al. call 'positive self-image', while not unrelated to well-being and anxiety, fell less neatly into our categories, as designated by Dolan et al. (2011a, 2011b), the ONS or those recommended by the OECD (OECD 2013; Smith and Exton 2013).

'So what?' you may ask. Well, these two reports came out in subsequent years and with titles that imply they are researching the same relationship between culture and well-being. They may appear to have used a similar approach, listed as multiple regressions of cross-sectional data. However, there are key differences in the data they investigate. 1, they report on different countries; 2, one uses three data sources, the other uses one; 3, their operationalisation of the 'cultural occupation/artistic practice' variables are very different; 4, as are the operationalisations of subjective well-being; 5, those running the regressions (the modellers) used slightly different controls (see Table 7.5). There are numerous reasons for these differences, but mainly, remember that theories of what is good for well-being are not entirely universal, which will affect what someone wants to control for, but also the data are different, which will limit what it is possible to control for.

Box 7.6 Control Variables
Controls are control variables

Say there was a positive relationship between older people and enjoying jazz music, and a negative relationship between younger people and enjoying jazz music. A study to see if there is an association between increasing funding for jazz music and enjoyment of jazz music may find no significant difference. The differences by age would be masked because the negative (younger people) relationship and the positive (older people) relationship could cancel each other out, resulting in no overall observable relationship.

Controlling for age can better establish that 'funding jazz is likely to have a positive effect on enjoyment in older people, but not younger people'.

Table 7.5 Controls used in the two studies looking at well-being and creatives

Controls used in the report Artful Living: Examining the Relationship Between Artistic Practice and Subjective Wellbeing Across Three National Surveys	Controls used in the report Creative Occupations and Subjective Wellbeing
Age	Age
Gender	Gender
	Religion
Marital status	Marital status
	Health status
Race	Ethnicity
	Education
	Housing
Income	Income
Place of residence	Geographic region
	Date of survey
Employment status	
Children at home	

Adapted from Tepper et al. (2014) and Fujiwara et al. (2015)

When look back at Table 7.4, the survey questions generating the various forms of subjective well-being data are different. They do not use the same concepts of subjective well-being and the questions are not identically worded. The samples of creative practitioners appear to overlap conceptually at first, but they are far from identical. Therefore, we are not actually really looking at the relationship between identical things. Creative occupation or artistic practice do not strictly mean having a job that is creative in these studies, and the meanings and measures of subjective well-being are different in the data analysed.

Again, 'so what?' you may ask. Looking at the headline evidence together is the most typical way of understanding other people's data analysis and findings to construct a body of evidence. Taking a moment to compare these two reports highlights how different two studies which may appear comparable really are, as well as the difficulties in finding conclusive answers to questions about the well-being of any particular group of people, and the role of culture—or work—or leisure—in this. Looking at differences in data sources, concepts, methodology, findings and motivations provides extra data that help establish how conclusions and headline findings may have been arrived at.

The studies differ in numerous ways: the questions asked, who was asked (or included), the nature of the sample—as well as the interpretation of what being creative involves. Furthermore, the research designs were analysing different subjective experience contexts: different places, and different relationships to creative cultural engagement (e.g. professional or amateur). The two reports were also commissioned by different organisations in different countries with undoubtedly different research agendas. Therefore, while in principle, these two studies are looking at the same social issue in the same ways, they have different research questions that are applied to different contexts.

While the two studies were not designed to test each other, the two headline findings can be used together in a literature or evidence review to make a statement about what is known about being a 'creative practitioner' well-being. Notably, the UK case states: '[t]o our knowledge this is the first quantitative study that specifically analyses the connection between creative jobs and wellbeing' (Fujiwara et al. 2015, 2). The US case notes that '[a]s of yet, no one has examined the complicated relationship between creative practice and wellbeing within the US' and 'preliminary work has failed to demonstrate a robust relationship between creative practice and wellbeing in part because of limited sample sizes' (Tepper et al. 2014, pp. 8, 10). Interestingly, neither of these reports seems to have been cited much.[25] When they are cited, for example by Tiller (2014, 43), the positive impacts tend to be reported. Also Tiller (2014) reports on the benefits of 'artistic practice' as cultural participation, rather than being an artist, and others interpret Tepper et al.'s results as follows:

> Researchers have found that the more individuals participate in artistic activity, the higher they score on a variety of wellbeing. (Kemp et al. 2018, 1)
> Tepper et al. (2014) found that creating crafts, gardening, and playing a musical instrument—or personal art-making—were positively related to life satisfaction. (Kemp et al. 2018, 3)
>
> Part of the nonsignificant relationship between active arts participation and life satisfaction may be due to a perceived lack of time individuals feel they have to engage in creative practice. Hence, if they feel that time is constrained such that they do not have sufficient time to engage in artistic creation, benefits related to SWB may be minimal. (Kemp et al. 2018, 6)

This final point is of interest, as neither Tepper et al. nor Kemp et al. really pick up on the fact that it may not be that those engaged in active arts participation, as described, do not have enough spare time to do enough creative practice, but instead, that they could be—like our friend in the Disney movie—dissatisfied with the job they have. Tepper et al. say that it may be better for some graduates to walk away from their artistic practice (Tepper et al. 2014, 28), but leaving 'the industry' seems to be attributable to a lack of time for 'robust artistic life' versus 'simply dabbling in the arts'. This analysis does not incorporate what we know of the hardships of those who are full-time artists and those who are still aspiring (refer to Brook et al. 2020 for discussion on this). Given that the authors state: 'this report represents an initial exploration of the thesis that the arts are essential to a high quality of life' (Tepper et al. 2014, 28), we might question whether they were ready for an interpretation of the arts and their labour markets as bad for well-being in various ways.

Tepper et al.'s title *Artful Living: Examining the Relationship Between Artistic Practice and Subjective Wellbeing Across Three National Surveys* was misleading to some audiences, particularly in the UK, where artistic practice tends to mean working as a professional artist. Instead, it was more broadly defined to include practising an art as a hobby. Similarly, not all the creative occupations in Fujiwara et al.'s report were as closely aligned to having an artistic practice as you might assume by the term creative occupation. Ultimately, it can be more difficult to compare or synthesise studies than is obvious by the title of a report, or its headline findings. This is often not acknowledged and can limit the validity of comparisons when evidence is reviewed and synthesised.

The way that the idea of culture and well-being are operationalised in these two cases differs more than to be expected: the data and the contexts in which they were collected, or the surveys or questions which generate the variables, are not always as similar as might be assumed. When we describe findings from apparently comparable studies, it is just as important to account for the motivations and methods of these studies (their contexts) as it would be our own. This is because when we synthesise the research of others, we create new knowledge that is able to make grander claims as it appears more generalisable.

7.4   Well-being Data and 'Cultural Access'

Once we put the culture/well-being link under the right set of analytical lenses, it turns out quite clearly that 'culture counts', namely, that there is clear evidence that cultural access has a definite impact on individual psychological well being (and particularly so if cultural access occurs in a well-balanced mind–body perspective), and moreover that culture provides for some of the most effective predictors of well-being. (Grossi et al. 2012: 147)

> Among the various potential factors considered, cultural access unexpect-
> edly rankes [sic] as the second most important determinant of psychological
> well-being, immediately after the absence or presence of diseases. (Grossi
> et al. 2012, 129)

Moving national contexts again, the Italian Culture and Well-being Project used what it called 'data mining'[26] to understand the 'interaction between culture, health and psychological well-being' (Grossi et al. 2012). It is clear to see from its concluding lines that it is of interest to our exploration of how people understand what it calls the culture/well-being link. The headline outcome (also quoted above) foregrounds what it calls 'cultural access'. Interestingly, the authors claim that 'cultural access unexpectedly' appears to be the second most important thing for people's well-being, after physical health. We will return to finding the right set of lenses and a finding being unexpected at the end of this section. First, we will look at what the researchers mean by culture.

What does the report mean by 'cultural access'? The 15 'cultural activities considered in the survey' consist of 'jazz music concerts; classic music concerts; opera/ballet; theatre; museums; rock concerts; disco dance; paintings exhibition; social activity; watching sport; sport practice; book reading; poetry reading; cinema; local community development' (Grossi et al. 2012). Therefore, does 'cultural access' mean 'can you access these activities?' or does it mean 'do you do these activities?' This is a key question for cultural policy as social policy, as we have discovered a number of times in the last few chapters: for if taking part in culture becomes some kind of proxy for having access to things that improve our well-being, the word access—and the implications for fairness of who has access and who wants access are important to establish.

One of the concerns over using well-being metrics to value culture is that the models used do not include all forms of cultural life (Jones 2010; O'Brien 2010). As we know from Chap. 6, defining culture is complicated. Thus, the value of what has come to be described as 'everyday participation' (Miles and Gibson 2016), including activities, such as attending sporting events (Oakley 2011) or chatting in a local shop (Edwards and Gibson 2017) should be acknowledged in some way when valuing 'culture' as something broadly defined. Increasingly, evidence indicates that it is 'participation per se' that is good for well-being, irrespective of what one is participating in (Miles and Sullivan 2010). Likewise, when people describe what is important to them for well-being, arts and culture activities, such as formalised theatre attendance, appeared less frequently in the ONS data I analysed than a more general and everyday participation (Oman 2020). It is therefore important that well-being metrics include—or at least acknowledge if they exclude—everyday participation, together with recognised artforms, such as theatre.

The inclusion of various 'everyday' forms of participation in Grossi et al.'s model might address concerns about formal culture and everyday participation. However, can 15 activities address the concerns of O'Brien and Jones in 2010, that metrics miss some aspects of cultural life? The 15 aspects of 'cultural access' chosen by the authors are said to have resulted from a literature review. Incidentally, this review and its results are not mentioned in more than passing by the authors, so as readers we don't know why or how they came upon these 15, how many documents were reviewed before the 15 were decided, and so on.

These 15 categories of cultural access were formulated into a question that was added to a questionnaire. There is also no detail on the decisions made in this respect. The survey was conducted by an Italian pollster company called Doxa, through telephone interviews, according to the CATI[27] system, with 1500 random participants of the National Statistical Survey conducted by the Italian Statistics Bureau (ISTAT 2015). You may remember in Chap. 3 that the ISTAT is one national organisation that uses the same dimensions of well-being as the OECD. This project didn't use these dimensions of well-being.[28]

Instead, the authors describe that 'their survey collected information covering socio-demographic and health-related data' (Grossi et al. 2012, 132), together with the 15 activities as a proxy for cultural access. See Table 7.6 for these categories, as described in the article. They also describe questions from the Psychological General Well-being Index (PGWBI), which has 22 self-administered items ordinarily, but they used a trialled and tested shorter version of six items (Grossi et al. 2012, 133). As you can see in Table 7.7, these psychological questions ask very similar things to the ONS4 that we have encountered multiple times before. They are however worded slightly differently, which will have an effect on the data which may or may not be relevant to the claims made about the findings.

In order to analyse 'cultural access', the authors take the answers from the questions about how many times people have participated in a particular activity. What is intriguing is that the authors have then combined these activities into a single measure, without accounting for this in the paper's definition of 'cultural access'. Consequently, the authors seem less

Table 7.6   Variables used in Grossi et al. (2012)

Cultural access categories	Jazz music concerts
	Classical music concerts
	Opera/ballet
	Theatre
	Museums
	Rock concerts
	Disco dance
	Paintings exhibitions
	Social activity
	Watching sport
	Sport practice
	Book reading
	Poetry reading
	Cinema
	Local community development
Socio-demographic and health-related categories	Gender
	Age (years)
	Income
	Job
	Civil status
	Education level
	Geography
	Cultural access frequency
	PGWBI (average)
	Disease

Table 7.7   The Psychological General Well-being Index questions used in Grossi et al. (2012)

PGWBI: The six 'shorter version' questions	Have you been bothered by nervousness or by your 'nerves' during the past month?
	How much energy, pep or vitality did you have or feel during the past month?
	I felt downhearted and blue during the past month.
	I was emotionally stable and sure of myself during the past month.
	I felt cheerful, light-hearted during the past month.
	I felt tired, worn out, used up or exhausted during the past month.

concerned with deciphering what it is that people do (i.e. the nature of cultural access) than the frequency of cultural participation.

If we follow the recommendation that it is participation *per se* that matters for well-being (Miles and Sullivan 2010), incorporating various types of activity into a single dimension of culture could be a positive research decision. As we have already encountered a number of times, valuing one activity over another is ethically, methodologically and politically problematic. Of course, the data in and of itself do not account for all 'cultural access', or as we have described before, cultural activity. The questions can only account for the 15 activities included, missing out many social and cultural concerns, but as we saw in Box 7.4, this is not unusual in and of itself.

The analysis includes variables for aspects of cultural activity which are undoubtedly important to some people's well-being. It is in the descriptions, categories and claims where issues may arise. For example, a question on 'social activity' could end up with data including almost anything, depending on the wording of the question. We do not know the exact wording of the question, but the paper states:

> Each subject being surveyed in the study had to go through a structured questionnaire asking about the daily frequency of access to all of the activities listed. (Grossi et al. 2012, 132)

This seems to imply that the participants could define social activity for themselves, which could include leaving the house and talking to someone in a shop, which while valuable (feeling all the more valuable as I edit this book in lockdown), is not able to argue the value of investment in opera, say.

Is that a problem in and of itself? Possibly not. However, to include all social activity, and then conflate all the results to a single measure, without making this explicit in the headlines of the research may be misleading. As a consequence of these decisions, the value of 'cultural access' potentially includes the value of all social activity, as defined by different people. The authors have decided upon such a list to act as 'a proxy of individual levels of "cultural access"' (Grossi et al. 2012, 132). However, they have then combined the 15 proxies into one measure of cultural access. This could considerably inflate the impact of 'cultural access'. This is important, as, the authors state 'that there is clear evidence that cultural access has a definite impact on individual psychological well being' (Grossi et al. 2012, 147).

Combining variables into one category is an issue with the evidence base for culture and it confuses the well-being evidence base as well. The language used in findings, and reproduced in evidence reviews, assumes it argues the value of a particular idea of culture. This limits the reach of the 'discussion' aspects of academic journal articles, as much as it does our understanding. Here we see the slippage in the definitions of culture described in the previous chapter can be used to include many aspects to account for culture's impact; yet 'cultural access' comes to mean the arts when this argument is reproduced, as we shall see.

Before we move towards our conclusion, let us remind ourselves of the headline findings, again:

> The results show that, among the various potential factors considered, cultural access unexpectedly rankes as the second most important determinant of psychological well-being, immediately after the absence or presence of diseases, and outperforming factors such as job, age, income, civil status, education, place of living and other important factors. (Grossi et al. 2012, 129)

In spite of queries with the Italian Culture and Well-being Project, the headline results appear in other high-profile reviews. These include the 'Understanding the Value of the Arts and Culture' report from the AHRC's Cultural Value project (Crossick and Kaszynska 2016) and a 2020 report to the Welsh government (Browne Gott 2020). The more findings are reproduced, the more credible they seem, and the more they are reproduced. One review (Taylor et al. 2015) was commissioned by the CASE programme, which you may remember from Chap. 6. The report describes the Culture and Sport Evidence (CASE) programme as a joint programme of strategic research led by the Department for Culture, Media and Sport (DCMS) in collaboration with the Arts Council England (ACE), English Heritage (EH) and Sport England (SE). The report was of a systematic review of the literature and evidence (Taylor et al. 2015, 8) and it evaluates the above study as follows:

> Grossi (2012F) offers arguably the most authoritative review based on quantitative research, linking participation in arts with better social outcomes and impacts, including health. (Taylor et al. 2015, 71)

> [A]rts-related activities are seen as central to wellbeing by most people, according to a recent Italian study (Grossi 2012F). Among the various

potential factors considered, cultural access ranked as the second most important determinant of psychological wellbeing, immediately after the absence or presence of diseases, and outperforming factors such as job, age, income and other important factors. (Taylor et al. 2015, 75)

Even without concerns about the category of cultural access, the methods of the study did not ask people whether culture was central to anything. It asked them what they did and how they felt. There is a concern, with all social research, that if you look for a particular outcome, you are more likely to find it. Hold that thought. Because, we might want to have a think when considering others' research, whether it is putting the culture–well-being relationship under different 'lenses', until it finds the one it likes? That is until that lens, or series of lenses, finds that 'culture counts' in the way that is desired (Grossi et al. 2012: 147).

It is easy to see that the CASE review of the literature and evidence cut and pasted the findings directly from the article and, in fact, its abstract. The reason I mention this is that this is not abnormal practice. Instead, I want to highlight that it is not always clear that when a finding appears in a review commissioned by such significant body, that this does not actually qualify that the finding has been checked by that authority; there is no guarantee that the authors checked for robustness, or that it should be authoritative.

So, in presenting the impact of 'cultural access' (however defined) on well-being, research satisfies the hunger for those who want evidence of the culture–well-being relationship. This also has silly ends, fuelling the fires underneath claims such as culture can 'reduce crime' (Morris 2003) or 'tackle poverty' (National Assembly Wales 2019). The sad thing is these actions are a double-edged sword: they are popular because they seem to justify people's feelings that the arts are good for us, while at the exact same time discrediting the good evidence that is available for advocacy.

This indicates both the value of, and requirement for, a review of rigour when it comes to data and their categorisation in the empirical work underway to understand the relationship between different activities and programmes on well-being. Perhaps, even more importantly, attention must be paid to the resource in the teams synthesising and evaluating the evidence base in order to direct future research, policy and practice. It is not simply a case of levels and areas of expertise, but the resource of time to review and evaluate evidence.

This chapter has revealed that it is not hard for everyone to look a bit further—beyond the headlines—and establish potential issues. If we acknowledge that culture and well-being are slippery concepts, then how a concept such as cultural access is defined and measured requires some clarity if the evidence is going to be used politically, whether that is to justify funding or as we are increasingly seeing in this book, how resources decided by policy-makers are related to inequities of resource in society more generally.

7.5   Conclusion: Using Well-being Data to Understand Policy Questions

We began this chapter with David Cameron promising to put 'instincts we feel to the core' to 'the practical test' so that those whose decisions on policy and spending, that affect people's lives, take account of what matters. We end with concerns about impact and conflated variables. We considered data and evidence in cultural policy briefly, before looking at three components of the culture–well-being relationship that are relevant to our policy concerns. First, we looked at subjective well-being (measured as life satisfaction) over time and policy spending on culture in the UK over time. Second, we looked at different kinds of subjective well-being data and 'creatives' (broadly defined) in the UK and the US. Finally, we looked at subjective well-being and 'cultural access' (broadly defined) in Italy.

We had a play with different kinds of readily available data to look at the relationship between policy spend on culture and whether that impacts on national well-being. We considered the contexts of the data, the limits of what we can expect in terms of impact on life satisfaction as a measure and in terms of policy spend on a measure. Although these data were used descriptively, we found ourselves with questions as to why more research has not been done on the relationship between policy investment and well-being, given claims for investment based on improved well-being? This left us at a point of provocation: why are some data operationalised to understand the culture–well-being relationship, when other data are not?

We compared two studies that seemed to look at comparable groups, but reached different conclusions about the well-being of people who could be called creatives. Again, we reflected on the contexts of data, the ambitions of the researchers and the aims of the research to appreciate the limits and extents of claims that can be made. We spent some time breaking down how models and categories work, and why they are important for understanding what is being measured about culture and what is being measured about well-being. We also considered a much-cited study on the impact of what the authors call 'cultural access' on well-being. We discovered that ideas of culture and cultural access were slippery which enabled a favourable outcome. We reflected on how an outcome that might be popular, because it reinforces people's beliefs about the culture–well-being relationship, can result in the study being frequently referred to in later, and influential literature reviews.

This chapter has tried to break down some features of how these different aspects of cultural policy (investment, labour, access) are measured. It also wanted to demonstrate that these relationships can be explored simply, using easily available data. The lack of relationship between life satisfaction and GDP (the Easterlin paradox) is lauded as the starting point for a whole new area of research in happiness economics and positive psychology. Yet, the lack of relationship between life satisfaction and arts subsidy is not discussed as an important research question. We might be similarly interested in how little research has happened since the two projects on being an artist or the creative occupations, to further understanding of the complex relationship between professional creative practice and well-being.

The final question for this chapter, though, is are we using data to establish evidence or finding data to suit arguments? There are frequent calls that *more* evidence is needed to support the cause of cultural policy to argue its value as social policy. Why are there not more analyses of the data already available, even if they reveal a possibly uncomfortable relationship, as in the case of cultural funding, or other aspects of delivering social policy and well-being? Perhaps this might be where more complex relationships between well-being, inequality and culture might be explored. Despite the crudeness of tracking arts funding and life satisfaction data together, they tell a simple and effective story and definitely warrant future research. Or, at least ask questions of existing research. In the next chapter we will explore one of a number of studies that use increasingly complex quantitative techniques to express the relationship between culture and well-being differently. Thus, continuing our exploration of evidencing culture for policy.

Notes

1. The cultural sector is a broad description of cultural institutions such as libraries, heritage sites, museums and theatres. Crucially, it is not only about the buildings themselves, but all the ways people make and consume

culture and can include anything from Netflix to gaming (video games) and outdoor festivals.

2. In some ways, this may be an expected development of the aspects of well-being data usage from Chaps. 3 and 4, where part of this work is to establish a connection between, say, income and happiness (as with Easterlin 1973, see Chap. 4), or housing in the OECD index (Chap. 3).

3. 'What Works' is a programme across areas of government that is about evidence for what works in policy (Cabinet Office 2019). There is a What works for well-being centre, focussed on well-being evidence (What Works Wellbeing n.d.).

4. A review of the first edition of the associated publication stated that *Social Trends* covered 'public expenditure, leisure, personal income and expenditure, social security, welfare services, health, education, housing, justice and law' (Rose 1970, 241).

5. The above review of the first edition of publications reflecting on Social Trends lists the main areas of interest in a thought-provoking order, namely leisure is further towards the front of the list than you may expect, given what we have been led to believe are the priorities for evidence.

6. All-Party Parliamentary Groups (APPGs) are informal groups organised to investigate particular issues that might cut across government departments and involve members from different political parties.

7. You may remember in Chap. 4, we touched on the arguments against the Greatest Happiness principle and the introduction of the idea of a Utility Monster.

8. There are two helpful explanations on how data are anonymous, de-personalised or de-identified. One is here from the Future of Privacy Forum (2017). A simpler example is available from Understanding Patient Data (n.d.).

9. For discussion on these various streams, see Hesmondhalgh et al. (2015). For further discussion on how increased National Lottery spend on museums was justified in terms of increased visitors, see Selwood and Davies (2005). It is worth noting, as well, that fundraising became more professionalised in parallel, with philanthropy and private sources of investment and sponsorship also contributing.

10. As an aside while I accessed the headline data from the ONS website, the survey itself is not administered by the ONS, but in fact the Institute for Social and Economic Research (ISER) at the University of Essex. This has no bearing on my use of the data in this instance, but it is important to acknowledge the data source. Also, administration of Understanding Society is slightly more complicated than I explain in-text. Those who administer the survey have to re-sample due to what is known as 'respondent attrition' which means that members of a panel who have been recruited fall away over time and are then lost from the sample from whom

longitudinal data are being collected. This does not impact how we use the data in this chapter; however, it would be a concern were other types of claims made regarding the longitudinal qualities of the data.

11. Fitzroy and Nolan (2020) was the first article that came up in my search for life satisfaction data over these dates. Their plotting of life satisfaction over the whole period shows it is even more erratic, or, in other words, the line would be even less straight on the graph.

12. Legatum Commission Chairman Lord O'Donnell said: 'We now know much more about what drives the wellbeing of people and communities than we did 10 years ago, and our knowledge and understanding is set to increase significantly over the next few years. I look forward to working on this exciting project which could transform the way we develop policy' (Legatum 2012).

Lord O'Donnell served as the Cabinet Secretary between 2005 and 2011. Cabinet Secretary is the highest official in the British Civil Service and it is notable that he held this position under three prime ministers: Blair, Brown and Cameron.

13. Some pivotal examples from the broader DCMS evidence programme include O'Brien (2010); Matrix Knowledge Group (2010); Miles and Sullivan (2010).

14. Flow is an important concept for thinking about how subjective well-being is conceptualised as experience. Positive psychologist, Mihaly Csikszentmihalyi, in particular has spent much of his career looking into how people get lost in flow, and he studied artistic practitioners to understand 'flow' (1997). His 1975 study of the nature of enjoyment was largely based on expert cultural practitioners, such as dancers and musicians. Years later, interested in 'flow' in everyday life, Csikszentmihalyi returned to the study of creative professionals, and with colleague Nakamura, theorised 'vital engagement as a relationship to the world' that is characterised both by experiences of flow (enjoyed absorption) and by meaning (subjective significance) (Nakamura and Csikszentmihalyi 2002; Csikszentmihalyi and Hunter 2003).

15. You may remember we talked about symbolic value back in Chap. 2, where something's value is more than its material or financial value, and involves something's status.

16. See Brook et al. (2020) for compelling evidence and arguments on this matter, with nods to the more on the extensive literature on the many issues of creative labour.

17. The three national surveys were the DDB Needham Life Style Survey (DDB), the Double Major Student Survey and the Strategic National Arts Alumni Project (SNAAP). Full details of sampling can be found in the report.

18. In this book the spelling of well-being is used, unless it is a direct quote, and then the spelling of the author is used.
19. Confusingly, what is called the Annual Population Survey is actually not one survey, but a conglomerate of other surveys, as explained in Table 7.4.
20. See TNS 2011 for more information on the longitudinal element.
21. This is detailed in the report, however, for more explanation on SOC codes and the cultural sector, please also see Oman (2019).
22. A prominent recent example is Campbell et al. (2017): one of the biggest problems the author identify is the disproportionate role of IT.
23. As described in Chaps. 2 and 4, Eudaimonia is most often understood as purpose or flourishing.
24. Google scholar searches show that Tepper et al. has been cited 15 times, and Fujiwara et al., 17 times. However, of course, that does not include all the non-academic places where these reports are cited.
25. 'Data mining' might seem a bit of a reach. The sample of 1500 people would not necessarily be considered a large enough 'dataset' to warrant data mining. The novelty of the method at the time was in its complexity, because it aimed to assess the importance of lots of variables at the same time. This approach was called AutoCM and is described in the paper.
26. CATI is a computer-aided telephone system that is widely used in large-scale surveys, as well as examples such as this, where participants in large surveys are invited to participate in a smaller, specialised survey. CATI does not involve the computer doing the interviewing (as may be suggested). Instead, people, who still do the interviewing, will follow an electronic survey script. As a participant answers, the responses are recorded in the CATI system, which guides the interviewer to questions which are routed through the questionnaire based on prior responses.
27. The ISTAT implemented its well-being domains and measures in 2012, see: https://www.istat.it/it/files//2018/04/12-domains-scientific-commission.pdf for more details. Therefore, the Grossi et al. study preceded the ISTAT's new measures.

References

Bache, I., and L. Reardon. 2013. An Idea Whose Time Has Come? Explaining the Rise of Well-Being in British Politics. *Political Studies* 61 (4): 898–914. https://doi.org/10.1111/1467-9248.12001.

Belfiore, E. 2012. "Defensive instrumentalism" and the legacy of New Labour's cultural policies. *Cultural Trends* 21 (2): 103–111. https://doi.org/10.1080/09548963.2012.674750.

Belfiore, E. 2016. Cultural Policy Research in the Real World: Curating 'Impact', Facilitating 'Enlightenment'. *Cultural Trends* 25 (3): 205–216. https://doi.org/10.1080/09548963.2016.1204050.

Belfiore, E. and Bennett, O. 2008. *The Social Impact of the Arts: An Intellectual History*. Basingstoke and New York: Palgrave Macmillan.

Berry, C. 2014. *Wellbeing in Four Policy Areas: Report by the All-Party Parliamentary Group on Wellbeing Economics*. London: New Economics Foundation.

Brook, O., D. O'Brien, and M. Taylor. 2020. *Culture Is Bad for You: Inequality in the Cultural and Creative Industries*. Manchester: Manchester University Press.

Browne Gott, H. 2020. *Exploring the Relationship between Culture and Well-being*. 15/2020. Cardiff: Welsh Government. https://gov.wales/sites/default/files/statistics-and-research/2020-03/exploring-the-relationship-between-culture-and-well-being.pdf.

Bu, F., et al. 2020. Time-Use and Mental Health during the COVID-19 Pandemic: A Panel Analysis of 55,204 Adults Followed across 11 Weeks of Lockdown in the UK. *medRxiv*, p. 2020.08.18.20177345. https://doi.org/10.1101/202 0.08.18.20177345.

Cabinet Office. 2019. *What Works Network*, Public Services—GOV.UK. Accessed 2 May 2021. https://www.gov.uk/guidance/what-works-network.

Cameron, D. 2010. *Prime Minister's Speech on Wellbeing*. Cabinet Office, Prime Minister's Office. https://www.gov.uk/government/speeches/pm-speech-on-wellbeing.

Campbell, P., T. Cox, and D. O'Brien. 2017. The Social Life of Measurement: How Methods Have Shaped the Idea of Culture in Urban Regeneration. *Journal of Cultural Economy* 10 (1): 49–62. https://doi.org/10.108 0/17530350.2016.1248474.

Crossick, G., and P. Kaszynska. 2016. *Understanding the Value of Arts & Culture: The AHRC Cultural Value Project*. Swindon: AHRC.

Csikszentmihalyi, M. 1975. *Beyond Boredom and Anxiety*. San Francisco: Jossey-Bass Publishers.

Csikszentmihalyi, M. 1997. *Finding Flow: The Psychology of Engagement with Everyday Life*. Basic Books.

Csikszentmihalyi, M., and J. Hunter. 2003. Happiness in Everyday Life: The Uses of Experience Sampling. *Journal of Happiness Studies* 4 (2): 185–199. https://doi.org/10.1023/A:1024409732742.

DCMS. 2011. *Creative Industries Economic Estimates*. Department for Digital, Culture, Media & Sport. https://www.gov.uk/government/collections/creative-industries-economic-estimates.

Dolan, P., R. Layard, and R. Metcalfe. 2011a. *Measuring Subjective Well-being for Public Policy*. Office for National Statistics.

———. 2011b. *Measuring Subjective Well-Being for Public Policy: Recommendations on Measures*. London School of Economics: Centre for Economic Performance.

Dolan, P., and Metcalfe, R. 2012. Measuring Subjective Wellbeing: Recommendations on Measures for use by National Governments. *Journal of*

Social Policy, 41(2), 409–427. https://doi.org/10.1017/S004727941 1000833.

Easterlin, R. 1973. Does Money Buy Happiness? *The Public Interest* 30 (3): 3–10.

Edwards, D., and L. Gibson. 2017. Counting the Pennies: The Cultural Economy of Charity Shopping. *Cultural Trends* 26 (1): 70–79. https://doi.org/10.108 0/09548963.2017.1275131.

FitzRoy, F.R., and M.A. Nolan. 2020. Education, Income and Happiness: Panel Evidence for the UK. *Empirical Economics* 58 (5): 2573–2592. https://doi.org/10.1007/s00181-018-1586-5.

Fujiwara, D. 2013. *Museums and Happiness: The Value of Participating in Museums and the Arts*. United Kingdom: The Happy Museum; Museum of East Anglian Life; Arts Council England. Accessed: 29 March 2021. https://happymuseumproject.org/wp-content/uploads/2013/04/Museums_and_happiness_DFujiwara_April2013.pdf.

Fujiwara, D., and G. MacKerron. 2015. *Cultural Activities, Artforms and Wellbeing*. London: Arts Council England.

Fujiwara, D., Kudrna, L., and Dolan, P. 2014a. *Quantifying and Valuing the Wellbeing Impacts of Culture and Sport*. Department for Culture, Media and Sport. https://www.artshealthresources.org.uk/wp-content/uploads/2020/08/2014-Quantifying_and_valuing_the_wellbeing_impacts_of_sport_and_culture.pdf.

———. 2014b. *Quantifying the Social Impacts of Culture and Sport*. Department for Culture, Media and Sport. https://assets.publishing.service.gov.uk/government/uploads/system/uploads/attachment_data/file/304896/Quantifying_the_Social_Impacts_of_Culture_and_Sport.pdf.

Fujiwara, D., Dolan, P., and Lawton, R. 2015. *Creative Occupations and Subjective Wellbeing*. NESTA. https://media.nesta.org.uk/documents/creative_employment_and_subjective_wellbeing_1509_1.pdf.

Future of Privacy Forum. 2017. *A Visual Guide to Practical Data De-identification*. Accessed 2 May 2021. https://fpf.org/wp-content/uploads/2017/06/FPF_Visual-Guide-to-Practical-Data-DeID.pdf.

Gross, S.A., and G. Musgrave. 2020. *Can Music Make You Sick?: Measuring the Price of Musical Ambition*. London: University of Westminster Press.

Grossi, E., et al. 2012. The Interaction Between Culture, Health and Psychological Well-being: Data Mining from the Italian Culture and Well-Being Project. *Journal of Happiness Studies* 13 (1): 129–148. https://doi.org/10.1007/s10902-011-9254-x.

Hesmondhalgh, D., et al. 2015. *Culture, Economy and Politics: The Case of New Labour*. London: Palgrave Macmillan.

ISTAT. 2015. *Il benessere equo e sostenibile in Italia*. ISTAT.

Jones, S. 2010. *Culture Shock*. London: Demos.

Kemp, E., Martic, K., and Anaza, N.A. 2018. Artistic Consumption and Well-Being: A Song of Two Countries. *International Journal of Nonprofit and Voluntary Sector Marketing*, 23(4): e1612. https://doi.org/10.1002/nvsm.1612.

Layard, R. 2006. *Happiness: Lessons from a New Science*. London: Penguin.

Legatum Institute. 2012. Gus O'Donnell to Chair Legatum Institute Commission on Wellbeing Policy, Legatum Institute. *The Legatum Institute*. Accessed 20 November 2012. http://www.li.com/media/press-releases/gus-odonnell-to-chair-legatum-institute-commission-on-wellbeing-policy.

MacKerron, G., and S. Mourato. 2013. Happiness Is Greater in Natural Environments. *Global Environmental Change* 23 (5): 992–1000. https://doi.org/10.1016/j.gloenvcha.2013.03.010.

Mak, H.W., Fluharty, M., and Fancourt, D. 2020. Predictors and Impact of Arts Engagement during the COVID-19 Pandemic: Analyses of Data from 19,384 adults in the COVID-19 Social Study. *PsyArXiv*. https://doi.org/10.31234/osf.io/rckp5.

Matrix Knowledge Group. 2010. *Understanding the Value of Engagement in Culture and Sport: Summary Report*. London: Department for Culture, Media and Sport. https://assets.publishing.service.gov.uk/government/uploads/system/uploads/attachment_data/file/88449/CASE-value-summary-report-July10.pdf.

Miles, A., and L. Gibson. 2016. Everyday Participation and Cultural Value. *Cultural Trends* 25 (3): 151–157. https://doi.org/10.1080/09548963.2016.1204043.

Miles, A., and A. Sullivan. 2010. *Understanding the Relationship between Taste and Value in Culture and Sport*. London: DCMS.

Morris, E. 2003. *Speech to Cheltenham Festival of Literature*. Cheltenham.

Nakamura, J., and M. Csikszentmihalyi. 2002. The Concept of Flow. In *Handbook of Positive Psychology*, ed. C. Snyder and S. Lopez, 89–105. New York: University Press.

National Assembly Wales. 2019. *Count Me In! Tackling Poverty and Social Exclusion through Culture, Heritage and the Arts*. Cardiff: Culture, Welsh Language and Communications Committee. https://senedd.cymru/laid%20documents/cr-ld12847/cr-ld12847%20-e.pdf.

Neelands, J., et al. 2015. *Enriching Britain: Culture, Creativity and Growth: The 2015 Report by the Warwick Commission on the Future of Cultural Value*. Warwick: The University of Warwick. https://warwick.ac.uk/research/warwickcommission/futureculture/finalreport/warwick_commission_report_2015.pdf.

Nissel, M., ed. 1970. *Social Trends No. 1*. London: HMSO.

———. 1983. *Facts about the Arts: A Summary of Available Statistics*. London: Policy Studies Institute.

Nuffield. 2021. People Exercising Less and Watching More TV than in First Lockdown. *Nuffield Foundation.* Accessed 31 March 2021. https://www.nuffieldfoundation.org/news/people-exercising-less-and-watching-more-tv-than-in-first-lockdown.

O'Brien, D. 2010. *Measuring the Value of Culture: A Report to the Department for Culture Media and Sport.* DCMS.

———. 2013. *Cultural Policy: Management, Value and Modernity in the Creative Industries.* New York: Routledge.

Oakley, K. 2011. Should Happiness be the Goal of British Arts Policy?, *openDemocracy.* Accessed 29 March 2021. https://www.opendemocracy.net/en/opendemocracyuk/should-happiness-be-goal-of-british-arts-policy/.

Oakley, K., O'Brien, D., and Lee, D. 2013. Happy Now? Well-being and Cultural Policy. *Philosophy and Public Policy Quarterly,* 31(2): 18–26. https://doi.org/10.13021/G8pppq.312013.131.

OECD. 2013. How's Life? 2013 Measuring Well-being. OECD (OECD Better Life Initiative). http://www.oecd.org/sdd/3013071e.pdf.

Oman, S. 2019. *Improving Data Practices to Monitor Inequality and Introduce Social Mobility Measures: A Working Paper.* The University of Sheffield. Available at: https://www.sheffield.ac.uk/polopoly_fs/1.867756!/file/MetricsWorkingPaper.pdf. Accessed 29 March 2021.

———. 2020. Leisure Pursuits: Uncovering the 'Selective Tradition' in Culture and Well-being Evidence for Policy. *Leisure Studies* 39 (1): 11–25. https://doi.org/10.1080/02614367.2019.1607536.

Oman, S., and M. Taylor. 2018. Subjective Well-Being in Cultural Advocacy: A Politics of Research between the Market and the Academy. *Journal of Cultural Economy* 11 (3): 225–243. https://doi.org/10.1080/17530350.2018.1435422.

ONS. 2010a. *Measuring National Wellbeing: Individual Well-Being Data Tables.* Office for National Statistics. Accessed 1 October 2016. http://www.ons.gov.uk/ons/rel/wellbeing/measuring-national-well-being/discussion-paper-on-domains-and-measures/rft-individual-well-being.xls.

———. 2010b. *The National Statistics Socio-economic Classification (NS-SEC).* Office for National Statistics. Accessed 31 March 2021. https://www.ons.gov.uk/methodology/classificationsandstandards/otherclassifications/thenationalstatisticssocioeconomicclassificationnssecrebasedonsoc2010.

———. 2011a. *Initial Investigation into Subjective Well-Being from the Opinions Survey.* London: ONS.

———. 2011b. *Measuring National Well-Being Technical Advisory Group.* Office for National Statistics. Accessed 5 April 2014. http://www.ons.gov.uk/ons/guide-method/user-guidance/well-being/measuring-national-well-being-technical-advisory-group/Notes-from-the-meeting-on-4-february-2011.pdf.

————. n.d. *Well-Being*. Office for National Statistics. Accessed 30 March 2021. https://www.ons.gov.uk/peoplepopulationandcommunity/wellbeing.

Perry, P. 2014. Loneliness Is Killing Us—We Must Start Treating This Disease | Philippa Perry. *The Guardian*. Accessed 2 May 2021. http://www.theguardian.com/commentisfree/2014/feb/17/loneliness-report-bigger-killer-obesity-lonely-people.

Rose, G. 1970. Social Trends. No. 1, 1970. Muriel Nissel. *Social Service Review* 45 (2): 241–242. https://doi.org/10.1086/642719.

Rustin, S. 2012. The Conversation: Can Happiness be Measured?, *The Guardian*. Accessed 28 April 2021. https://www.theguardian.com/commentisfree/2012/jul/20/wellbeing-index-happiness-julian-baggin.

Selwood, S., and Davies, M. 2005. Museums: After the Lottery Boom, *Spiked*. Accessed 31 March 2021. https://www.spiked-online.com/2005/09/02/museums-after-the-lottery-boom/.

Sidney, J.A., et al. 2017. The Well-Being Valuation Model: A Method for Monetizing the Nonmarket Good of Individual Well-Being. *Health Services and Outcomes Research Methodology* 17 (1): 84–100. https://doi.org/10.1007/s10742-016-0161-9.

Smith, C., and Exton, C. 2013. *OECD Guidelines on Measuring Subjective Well-Being*. Paris: OECD Publishing. https://read.oecd-ilibrary.org/economics/oecd-guidelines-on-measuring-subjective-well-being_9789264191655-en#page258.

Taylor, M. 2016. Nonparticipation or Different Styles of Participation? Alternative Interpretations from Taking Part. *Cultural Trends* 25 (3): 169–181. https://doi.org/10.1080/09548963.2016.1204051.

Taylor, P., Davies, L., Wells, P., Gilbertson, J., and Tayleur, W. 2015. *A Review of the Social Impacts of Culture and Sport* (CASE: The Culture and Sport Evidence Programme). Department for Culture, Media and Sport.

Tepper, S.J., et al. 2014. *Artful Living: Examining the Relationship between Artistic Practice and Subjective Wellbeing across Three National Surveys*. Nashville: The Curb Center for Art, Enterprise, & Public Policy at Vanderbilt University.

The Labour Party Manifesto. 2010. *A Future Fair for All*. London.

The National Archives. n.d. *UK Government Web Archive*. The National Archives. Accessed 2 May 2021. http://www.nationalarchives.gov.uk/webarchive/.

Tiller, C. 2014. *The Participatory Performing Arts Literature Review*. Calouste Gulbenkian Foundation UK Branch. https://participatoryalphabet.files.wordpress.com/2014/08/participatory-performing-arts-literature-review.pdf.

Understanding Patient Data. n.d. What Does 'Anonymised' Mean?, Understanding Patient Data. Accessed 2 May 2021. http://understandingpatientdata.org.uk/what-does-anonymised-mean.

What Works Wellbeing. 2017. *Job Quality and Wellbeing, What Works Wellbeing*. Accessed 2 May 2021. https://whatworkswellbeing.org/resources/job-quality-and-wellbeing/.

———. n.d. *Homepage, What Works Wellbeing*. Accessed 2 May 2021. https://whatworkswellbeing.org/.

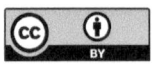

CHAPTER 8

Talking Different Languages of Value

8.1 Returning to the Culture— Well-being Relationship

The arguments of cultural value are curious, yet mundane. Chapters 6 and 7 offered glimpses of how some people argue about the value of culture one way, while others seem to speak a different language entirely. The language of data, metrics and numeric valuations of culture can feel at odds with how the majority of artists and cultural practitioners speak and think about culture. In one hand, we might hold a 2010 report of the UK's Department for Culture, Media and Sport (DCMS) (O'Brien 2010), which offers an overview of evaluation techniques, such as Quality Adjusted Life Years (or QALYs[1]). While, in the other, we might hold a copy of the Arts Council England (ACE) Strategy from the same year,[2] in which artist Jeremy Deller explains that art makes 'life worth living' (ACE 2010, 26). The report in one hand talks cost-benefit analysis, while in the other, artist Tim Etchells speaks of artistic 'value not bound up with price' (ACE 2010, 26).

Many in the cultural sector[3] are sceptical that cultural experience can be expressed in quantitative terms (Hill 2017; Oman 2013; Oman and Taylor 2018), with some being adamant that it should not be (Nissel 1983; Meyrick and Barnett 2021). Academic research on cultural metrics is equally two-sided (Belfiore 2002; Merli 2002; Selwood 2002; Gilmore et al. 2017). The gentler end of the critical scale involves damning metrics

© The Author(s) 2021
S. Oman, *Understanding Well-being Data*,
New Directions in Cultural Policy Research,
https://doi.org/10.1007/978-3-030-72937-0_8

with faint praise by stating that '[s]tatistical data well channelled can provide useful ancillary information' (Phiddian et al. 2017, 179); the harsher end involves describing 'ideas pertaining to the measurement of culture's value' as 'stupid' (Meyrick and Barnett 2017, 109).

The previous chapter outlined some differences in quantitative expressions of the culture–well-being relationship. It began with a walk through some examples of how data could be and are used to understand questions about culture and well-being. This step-by-step approach aims to open 'the black box' of well-being data (and some culture data for good measure). It is not always easy for everyone to have a practical sense of how data are used, or how they *work*, with the way that arguments and workings are generally shared. Looking closely at how analysis and valuation are presented helps understand what is going on 'under the bonnet' but can feel intimidating. Given that how people feel about these relationships is associated with their own values, the trick is to feel more confident in making value judgements for yourself.

That is why in this chapter, there is one more example of using well-being data to understand culture and their role in social policy. We are going to look in greater detail and break down these processes further again. This includes a description of how the data were collected in a national-level survey. We look at the questions, as they appear in the survey, because it can be hard to imagine the mundane contexts that data originate from when you are looking at the complex results. It is also not easy to imagine what has happened already, or indeed, what happens next.

What does research do? How does it affect the world or change things? What do well-being data become when their analyses are presented as findings, and then reproduced? We will begin to think through some of these questions by following key findings, to see how they are interpreted in the real world, to imagine data's capacity to change things. We will return to the conceptual work behind what is being measured before reflecting on what the analysis is trying to do, step by step. In this chapter I want to share that it is possible to think through what quantitative analyses are doing, without necessarily doing the maths or understanding the quantitative processes and their confusing terms.

The steps involved in data analysis like the ones in this chapter are designed on the basis of how concepts go together. It is possible to understand the research on this level, even if expressing terms in an equation feels intimidating. People may be ambivalent, even outraged at understanding aspects of well-being in numeric terms, and this is also true of trying to describe the role of an idea of culture in delivering well-being aims. Yet, numbers help us understand the extent of relationships in particular conditions; they do not necessarily decide whether that relationship exists at all. You can choose to retain that judgement for yourself.

8.2   Talking Different Languages of Value

This chapter began its life in a Manchester hotel in 2014. I was preparing a conference presentation called 'Measuring National Well-being and Cultural Participation—why don't things quite add up?' A colleague was passing as I was editing a slide with this equation on it:

He asked me what the equation was for. I was a bit taken aback, because I had assumed that while I didn't really understand what the equation was saying, that this would be immediately obvious somehow to people who work in quantitative methods, or 'Quants'. I explained that it was from a report on measuring happiness for the cultural sector, but that I didn't think that it would mean much to many I knew. As I outlined in this book's Preface, I had experienced a general lack of data confidence in the cultural sector and I imagined that most people reading a report called 'Museums and Happiness: The Value of Participating in Museums and the Arts' would struggle to make sense of the equation. In some ways, more importantly, that this equation was probably a barrier to understanding data and these valuations more generally. My colleague joked that he wasn't sure it was talking his language either,[4] and agreed it probably wouldn't make much sense to the sector.

I left the conversation with one overarching question: what does an equation like this do in this context? How does it reinforce the divide between those who see value in valuations, and those in cultural and social sectors, or people working for small charities, who maybe do not? Or perhaps, aren't sure? Could the ways that 'quants' are presented reproduce traditions called 'the Quant-Qual debate' that we touched on in Chap. 3, even outside research contexts? Is this detrimental to the ways that some people feel capable of actually reading the research reports that evidence arguments they use in their day-to-day jobs in the cultural sector? This equation triggered more questions for me and my colleague[5]: Who was this algebraic expression for and what was it *aiming* to do? How did the equation relate to the headline findings, and most importantly, whose value and values might be expressed in such a way?

I wondered if we could 'follow the data' to answer some of these questions about the equation. Which we did—in our own different ways. I mostly handled the qualitative research: I looked at the report on museums and happiness, and the cultural, policy and data histories that preceded it. This work contextualised the report in various ways, enabling us to see how it 'fit' in the general overlapping concerns of data, well-being, politics and value that we have encountered throughout this book. More specifically, these include beliefs and theories about well-being and its role in society, ambitions of the movement to establish cultural value, developments in well-being metrics, which coincided with a desire for valuation from government—and questions of data's capability remaining unanswered.

'Following the data' also included 'following the findings'. In other words, understanding context also meant researching what came after the report and how its findings were used. This gave us an idea of the impact of the report, and how it was received by different audiences. Following the findings also included reproducing aspects of the original research. My colleague led on this, the quantitative side of our project. This chapter walks you through steps in the original research about museums and happiness, as well as our subsequent project to demystify what is going on in these kinds of valuations.

Earlier in this book, I covered some of the discussions about how data tend to be presented as these neutral and objective things. This means that in some cases, it should be possible to do the same thing with the same data and arrive at the same results. This is one of the reasons why there are so many 'workings' in quantitative research—including the equation we started with: this working out is presented, so it can be scrutinised, and potentially reproduced. This is also one of the reasons why quantitative approaches are often thought to be more persuasive and robust than qualitative ones. It is not necessarily that numbers are more powerful in and of themselves; rather it is assumed that less interpretation is undertaken by the researcher. Therefore, you can work towards reproducing someone's findings by following their steps in quantitative research, in a way that you would be unlikely to do in qualitative research.[6]

This happenstance discussion about an equation in a Manchester hotel in 2014 led us to a project that wanted to understand the value of this genre of research to the cultural sector—and beyond to charities and other areas of social policy. Were there limits to understanding and presenting the culture–well-being relationship in this way? What would happen if we followed the data and processes used ourselves? The headline finding of our project is that when we reproduced these processes, we had a different finding: the monetary estimates of the relationship between participation and subjective well-being do not match across our reading and the original. Why might this be?

There are a number of reasons why two pieces of research following the same steps with the same data might offer different results. We will return to this later, but first, the aim of this chapter is to 'follow the data' on a journey of informed discovery, hoping to achieve a number of other things along the way. First, break down some of the barriers between quantitative research that helps people with their advocacy, and the practitioners who will read it and need it. Second, enable people to feel more confident with quantitative expressions and some of the language and principles of quantitative research. Third, it is a reference for people to return to, and apply to other reports they need to understand, but which 'do not speak their language'. This leads me to fourth, to help people feel greater data confidence and literacy, and perhaps enable them to make better judgements for themselves about whether more than headline findings can be useful—to them or in general.

8.3   Context: The Happy Museum and Data

The aim is to arm museums with compelling statistics to show how a healthy culture must be at the heart of a healthy society. (Tony Butler, Director Happy Museum Project and Director Museum of East Anglian Life in Fujiwara 2013, 5)

The relationship between culture and well-being has been operationalised[7] by a number of different organisations in the cultural sector. This is particularly true in the UK. Chapters 6 and 7 have covered a number of processes and projects that want to naturalise, even celebrate, this relationship. One obvious example, by virtue of its name, is The Happy Museum (n.d-b). Established in 2011, The Happy Museum focusses on more than happiness as a hedonic[8] idea; also embracing other, broader aims of the well-being agenda we covered back in Chap. 2: possibilities for sustainability, community and a sense of purpose. The Happy Museum is an advocacy organisation that has slowly grown and expanded on its activities, for example offering frameworks and training for those in the sector to understand the opportunities for the role of museums in well-being (The Happy Museum n.d-a). One of its aims was to contribute to the evidence base on the value of museums. The Happy Museum's Director, quoted above, invoked the values of culture and its relationship to a healthy society, whilst embracing the idea that this is best expressed with compelling statistics. This statement is testament to the will to progress towards bridging the gap between the languages of valuation and culture's values.

'Museums and Happiness: The Value of Participating in Museums and the Arts' was commissioned by The Happy Museum Project and funded by ACE. The equation I mentioned earlier originated from this report. It is important to say that the equation wasn't left floating alone to explain the workings, but the report contains details on why things were done and how. We will go through some of these explanations in the subsequent sections, elaborating for context and hopefully clarity. The key stated goal of the research was to 'look at the impacts of the arts on people's subjective wellbeing and health and attach values to these impacts' (Fujiwara 2013, 7). The project took a 'well-being valuation approach', which we've touched on in Chaps. 2 and 7, and which I will walk you through. As I have said before, this is not a Quants textbook, and you will not read this chapter, suddenly conversant in statistics, but it should hopefully give you a better idea of what is going on.

Taking Part Survey and the Data on Culture

'Museums and Happiness' includes findings from quantitative research that used data from the Taking Part Survey (TPS; DCMS 2010). The report explains why TPS data were chosen over other surveys, based on the different variables available, sample size and so on.[9] It points out that while this technique had been used before, it had not yet been used on this dataset.

We have talked about why TPS was established in Chap. 6: that it was part of an instrumental project by DCMS to address a need for evidence. Here, we are going to think about the data itself and the context in which it is generated. TPS covers England only, rather than the whole of the UK. It employs interviewers to go to people's homes, if they agree, of course, and interview them face-to-face with a questionnaire. The survey questionnaire asks about all different types of activities. A script asks the interviewer to request the interviewee to think in great detail, and to be specific, for example:

> Firstly, I would like you to think about all the walking you have done. Please include any country walks, walking to and from work or the shops and any other walks you may have done.

In the last four weeks, that is since [TODAY'S DATE MINUS FOUR WEEKS] have you done at least one continuous walk lasting at least 30 minutes?[10]

Were you to participate, you would be asked this, and more questions and clarifications, and finally whether your walking was 'for the purpose of health or recreation (not to get from place to place)'. The questionnaire then asks the same questions about cycling, for example; and so on. All in, you would expect to be speaking to the interviewer for about 40 minutes. In Box 8.1 you can see the museum questions from 2009–2010 survey.

Box 8.1 The Museum Questions from the Taking Part Survey 2009–2010
The museum questions[11] were phrased slightly differently from those on cycling and walking and listed below:
During the last 12 months, have you attended a museum or gallery at least once?
1. Yes 2. No -1. Don't know
In the last 12 months, have you attended a museum or gallery...?
1. In your own-time 2. For paid work 3. For academic study 4. As part of voluntary work 5. For some other reason -1. Don't know
How often in the last 12 months have you been to a museum or gallery [in your own-time] [or] [as part of voluntary work]?
1. At least once a week 2. Less often that once a week but at least once a month3. Less often than once a month but at least 3 or 4 times a year 4. Twice in the last 12 months 5. Once in the last 12 months -1. Don't know

---

To make everyone's answers analysable, all responses are combined into one dataset. Alongside questions on activities are questions about personal characteristics, for example, income, how many people live in your household, age, marriage status, whether you have children and so on. These variables allow researchers to understand how many different types of people 'take part' in different activities. These data also allow DCMS to see whether the percentages of different groups of people participating in different activities go up or down over time. These are reported on by DCMS in 'Statistical Releases', in which the results are synthesised and available for anyone to access.[12] They include information on, for example, the numbers of people who have participated in the arts in the last twelve months, and the same for sport, and so on. DCMS (n.d.) also releases a number of 'Focus On' reports each year, which they call 'short stories' (DCMS 2015a, 2). For example, in 2015[13] there were ten of these reports, including one on well-being (DCMS 2015b) and one on art forms (e.g. DCMS 2015a); in 2016, there was one on diversity (DCMS 2016).

Box 8.2 Variables: A Reminder

A variable takes different values in different situations. These values vary between cases or observations (which in this case are people but aren't always). They also vary over time or space.

So, for example, height varies across people, because some people are taller than others, but also within people over time, because people get taller as they grow up.

It is a variable because it varies. It is this change or variability that is measured, whether over time, or to compare characteristics.

In a regression, you would analyse the relationship between an independent variable, or independent variables, and a dependent variable.

Because we look at how variations in independent variables can predict values of a dependent variable,

- **independent variables are sometimes called predictor variables,**
- **dependent variables are sometimes called outcome variables.**

So, if you want to see the relationship between **age and museum attendance**, presumably, you are not expecting museum attendance to make someone age, but you might want to understand if older people are more likely to attend museums. Therefore, age would be your independent variable.

To measure the culture–well-being relationship, we need an **independent variable (for culture)** and if we wish to measure culture's relationship with well-being, then we need the chosen **well-being**

(*continued*)

Box 8.2 (continued)

variable to be the dependent variable. For ease, let us say because we want to see whether people who participate in culture have higher well-being.

*We also want to add other independent variables to make sure that **we're not inadvertently measuring other relationships as well**. For example, if married people report higher well-being on average, and are more likely to attend cultural events, we should include marital status as an additional independent variable. Without accounting for it in the analysis, marriage could be a confounding variable, meaning it could exaggerate the results. Therefore, here marriage would be controlled for, even though it is not of primary concern in the outcome.

The Well-being Data Available in the Taking Part Survey

Happiness taps in to people's emotions, technically their affective state, and hence tries to gauge people's moods at that moment. (Fujiwara 2013, 12)

As we saw in Chap. 6, part of thinking through how humans experience well-being, is acknowledging these processes are cultural and centre ideals of 'society'; they also involve imagining moments of social or cultural engagement and how they affect people on an individual level. Questions of when and how we experience particular well-being effects (or, perhaps, different kinds of well-being) are a key part of the puzzle of philosophers' thinking for centuries. As we have also seen in Chap. 4, this problem has driven recent developments in well-being measurement, arguably shaping what we have called the second wave of well-being and happiness economics. Understanding people's emotions in this way is used in various research contexts: whether using the diary reconstruction method (DRM) outlined in Chap. 4 to understand how people are doing in the day-to-day life, or to understand how a major event, such as the financial crisis of 2007/2008 or COVID-19 has impacted on people's well-being at scale.

What is hopefully clear by now is that deciphering which particular moment is actually being captured when attempting to measure an 'affective state' (such as happiness), and whether that is the moment that is relevant to your research question, has proved complex for a long time. Chapter 4's Fig. 4.1 and the related section outline how approaches to understand this differ, yet are related. 'Museums and Happiness' uses TPS data, which now include all of the UK's Office for National Statistics' four well-being questions (ONS4),[14] and has since the 2013–2014 dataset. However, the research we are looking at analysed data from 2005 to 2011, so before this change. Therefore, the question is similar, but not identical, to the ONS4 experience measures which ask about happiness and anxiety yesterday (see Table 4.2). The TPS data we are looking at in 'Museums and Happiness' understand happiness through the following question:

> "Taking all things together how happy would you say you are?" on a scale from 1–10 where 10 is described as "extremely happy" and 1 as "extremely unhappy".

The report says (as cited at the beginning of this section) that the data from this question establish someone's mood at that moment. The report continues:

> This differs to wellbeing questions that contain an evaluative judgment such as life satisfaction or eudemonic[15] wellbeing. Life satisfaction is held to contain a response about one's current emotions together with an evaluation of their life overall (how it measures up to their goals for instance) and eudemonic wellbeing questions tap in to people's perceptions of whether they are living a meaningful life. (Fujiwara 2013, 12)

If you return to Fig. 4.1 while reading this, you can see how this explanation maps onto the figure and the descriptions of approaches in Sect. 4.3 that follows it on how these measures are used. Notably, the 'taking all things together' part of the question makes it a 'general happiness' question, which is sometimes approached using Cantril's 'ladder of life' (Fig. 4.2). I say this, so you can probably imagine different ways you might answer this particular question.

There is a broader consideration with using national-level survey data to understand someone's 'happiness' in any moment. We have also encountered this before in Chap. 4, discussed in the section on experience measures. The ideal way of understanding happiness as an affective state is to ask people repeatedly during a particular day, over a period of days about how they feel in the moment. In other words, you would collect a sample of their moods and ask them what they are doing at that moment (which is why it is called the experience sampling method). This method is hard to translate into a survey because it is too time-consuming—for the interviewer and the interviewee to repeatedly ask and answer questions. This would make it too expensive to run, and difficult for many people to be available to participate in, which would then affect your sample—or, who you are talking to, and limit understanding. As an alternative, the rationale with the ONS4 experience measures is to 'replicate' or 'proxy' ESM approaches by asking respondents for their experiences and feelings relating to a whole day (yesterday).

So, let us briefly consider what is being captured by the question: these data are collected through a national-level survey and therefore at a time and in a place that is most likely completely unrelated to a museum visit. The implications of the headlines of this report is that the 'affective state' is 'gauge[d]... at that moment', but that moment is—of course—not the moment in the museum, but when the survey interviewer is in someone's home. On top of that, the question asks you how happy you feel you are overall, so it is not directing you to consider a period of time (as the ONS4 experience measures do), let alone a specific moment. So, we are beginning to encounter some limits, but this is not necessarily abnormal, because, as we know, all measures will have their pros and cons.

You may remember the difficulties in establishing whether a concert changed someone's well-being, even when you ask them immediately afterwards (Chap. 3). When the question is presented to someone by the TPS interviewer, that person may struggle to even remember the last time they were inside a museum. In truth, that is not even asked. As the box in the previous section demonstrates, the questions are about the last 12 months in general, not specifically the length of time since someone's last visit. Also, the survey did not request that they rate their happiness whilst in the museum (or before and after), but to comment on their happiness overall. Therefore, talking about measuring happiness in this way may feel confusing, because the happiness derived from visiting a museum *in-the-moment* is not what is captured directly in the data that are available for analysis. The title of the report implies that there is a relationship between museums and happiness, which at glance for some will undoubtedly confirm their belief or personal experience that museums *make them* happier, and encourage better overall well-being. This, of course, may well be true. However, we must remember that not everyone is the same, and to question what the data that are available for analysis are telling us. We must remember that it might be that—in general—people who go to museums tend to be happier than those who do not. A causal relationship may be difficult to demonstrate.

Box 8.3   Causal Inference: A Reminder

Causal inference describes the process to identify whether there is a relationship that involves the independent variable (culture) affecting the dependent variable (well-being). It means that there is an effect in the connection under study.

When looking to identify and measure causal relationships, we analyse the relationship between the cause variable and the effect variable.

To find that cultural participation is a cause of improved well-being (as the phenomenon), we need to establish that the cause precedes the effect, which means eliminating other plausible alternative causes. This is difficult because you cannot test this question in the real world.

The classic example is if we found a relationship between whether people were wearing shorts and whether they were buying ice cream, it wouldn't mean that wearing shorts caused people to buy ice cream, or that buying ice cream caused people to wear shorts. There is something else affecting this relationship that needs to be found and accounted for.

8.4   Museums and Happiness
and Other Relationships

The research reported in 'Museums and Happiness' was actually looking for more than one relationship. The equation I cited earlier in that presentation in the Manchester hotel was one of two presented in the text. The report states:

> We look at the impact on wellbeing and health of participating in and being audience to the arts and of being involved with museums and compare these impacts to other activities such as participation in sport. (Fujiwara 2013, 7)

This means, that as well as the 'general happiness' question, used in the TPS questionnaire, the researchers were also able to use other general questions on health.[16]

They also used income. We'll come back to this. But for now, we know that there are some culture variables (participating in and being an

Table 8.1 Participation variables modelled in 'Museums and Happiness'

Participation variables (the independent variables)

Museum variables	whether participants visit museums in their free time
	whether they volunteer in museums
	a measure of the number of hours spent in museums per year
	the number of museum visits per year
The non-museum variables	whether participants had done sport or other physical activity in the last four weeks
	whether participants had (in the last year) participated in each of ballet, dance, singing, playing music, painting and drawing, photography or crafts
	whether participants had (in the last year) attended exhibitions (also referred to as 'audience to arts'), opera, concerts and live music, ballet and dance

Adapted from Fujiwara (2013)

audience to), some other activities, including sport. For ease, we are going to call all of these 'participation variables'. You can find these in Table 8.1. The participation variables are the independent variables (or, you might find it easier to think of them as the predictor variables). The two dependent (or outcome) variables are health and subjective well-being.

The same process was used to calculate the relationship between visiting museums and happiness and 'has done sport or physical activity in the last four weeks' and happiness. This is a fairly simple process for someone who knows what they are doing, as they can run the same model multiple times, swapping out one participation variable for another. You might then do the same thing again with the outcome variable as health, going through the process of swapping the predictor participation variables.[17] The takeaway point is really, that we are going to proceed by talking about the processes involved in calculating the relationship between museums and happiness, for ease of understanding, but really there are multiple museum and non-museum 'participation' variables used to calculate different associations with health and happiness in this research.

To go about achieving the aims of this research: looking at the 'impact on wellbeing and health of participating in and being audience to the arts and of being involved with museums' (Fujiwara 2013, 7), a well-being valuation approach was used.[18] This approach aims to estimate 'monetary values by looking at how a good or service impacts on a person's well-being and finding the monetary equivalent of this impact' (Fujiwara 2013, 7). In order for us to engage with this process of valuation, it may be helpful to get into a mindset in which we think of participating in an activity (let's stick with museums for ease) as a 'good' or a service. By goods here we mean the same as 'trading in goods': that is, this experience has a market value; this experience can be valued in this way. That is, people can choose to spend time or money on attending museums, as opposed to on another thing, like the cinema or rock-climbing. This is a slightly different mindset, perhaps, than the idea of culture as a social good.

You have maybe spent most of this book thinking of well-being as a social good, without thinking about a social good as having a market value. In many ways, instinctively they feel opposite, as often actions to maximise something's financial value, feel at odds with a social good (we discussed this in Chap. 2 in thinking about McDonald's and the rainforest). But theoretically, all things which are good can become 'goods'. In this mindset, culture is not *just* a qualitative, incommensurable (has no common measure) experience. It is not only a way of experiencing fulfilment and happiness, but people can *choose to* consume culture, and it is something that makes them feel satisfied. This means it has utility (because it makes them happy).

Getting into this mindset helps us 'talk the talk' of valuation and imagine how culture may be quantified (in theory). When you think about it, we all have limited time to do anything, whether that is watching Netflix, going to the gym, playing video games, blowing dandelions or going to museums. Different ways of spending time might be associated with different value, but because we don't have unlimited time, we have to prioritise. The relationship between value, museums and experiential benefit is there; it is just not always readily visible to us, or something we think about.

So, if someone wants to estimate museums' impact on well-being, then they might say that they hypothesise that attending museums has a positive association to well-being, but we *know more* about the ways different types of well-being have a relationship with money. The amount of research on the relationship between income and different forms of subjective well-being far exceeds that on participation and well-being. As we discovered in Chap. 4, the relationship between income and happiness (the Easterlin paradox) is even described as the very turning point in well-being research. So, using income enables us to

1. begin to understand the relationship between museums and happiness, and
2. express this relationship in financial terms.

Of course, we have many prior estimates of the culture–well-being–money relationship to work with. This is not one undisputed value. For example, there have been thousands of studies on the relationship between income and well-being. This inevitably means that there are different approaches with different results. So, a decision has to be made by the researcher about the most suitable way to estimate the relationships they are interested in, in the specific context in which they are working. This refinement of which variables to use is standard practice, so long as the decisions made are subsequently clearly outlined and are justified and the limitations to research and the caveats to claims acknowledged and discussed.

In a valuation approach like Willingness to Pay (or another of the stated preference techniques we have previously covered in Chaps. 2 and 3), the data used are from people's responses to questions which asked them for their preferences or what they value. The questions ask people to state the value themselves for a good or service. In the simplest of terms in this example, this would be: 'how much would you be willing to pay to attend museums?' There are noted cons to asking people to attribute value themselves that are acknowledged in the report.

Page 28 of the report explains that a study in Bolton in 2005 found that people were willing to pay £33 a year for museums in Bolton. The reason this is so low, in comparison to the £3200 per year in the Museum and Happiness findings, is explained as follows. It is unlikely that people will state a high value for a currently publicly available service in case they may get asked to pay for it in the future (Fujiwara 2013, 28). This is called strategic bias. However, there is not one way that strategic bias might affect the valuation. This argument works *just as* well as saying that some people will overinflate *their* willingness to pay for a museum, knowing that the more they say it is worth, the more attractive it is to fund, and the less likely they will have to pay for it, of course. We might guess that some people would be very likely to apply a high number to their willingness to pay, by virtue of working in the cultural sector. It is not possible to be sure which way strategic bias will go in this context or indeed the motivation.

There are other issues with 'willingness to pay' and other contingent valuation methods.[19] They have limits in part because of the hypothetical nature of what you are often asking people. For example, 'existence value' is worth thinking about (and is, again, noted in the report). It is hard to imagine how much something like a museum or library is worth to you, as they exist and have value just in people knowing they are there, and some people want them to be there *in case* they—or others—want it (called option value). There is also the knowledge that they will be there for future generations. This is not the same as using these services, or being prepared to pay for them. When people are threatened with the removal of museums or libraries they do not use, they see a hypothetical value in them. Or, the theory goes that there is a value in knowing they exist at all.

The TPS data used in the 'Museums and Happiness' study did not contain people's own valuations. This means that it was not possible to have 'preference satisfaction' measures in the valuation model. Instead, it used a well-being valuation approach. The report explains that this overcomes the biases in people's own evaluations by estimating for them. The 'Museums and Happiness' report states that 'two very distinct measures of wellbeing are used' in the Bolton Study on the one hand and 'Museums and Happiness' on the other (Fujiwara 2013, 28). The report continues: 'there is no philosophical or theoretical reason why values from these methods should converge in anyway [sic]' (Fujiwara 2013, 28). This means that even though these two pieces of research are both using economic approaches to value museums and well-being, the findings should not be expected to be similar. When you think back to Chap. 7, and the importance of how culture and well-being are operationalised, versus the headline findings from reviews of evidence, you might think to yourself that this does not bode well for arguments on how much we can *know* the relationship between culture and well-being, if we cannot expect studies to have more similar results than £33 and £3200 as answer to the question 'what is the value of museums to people in terms of well-being?'

Let's return to the well-being valuation approach used here and how it can know the value of something to people without asking them. It requires a dataset to include a measure of well-being, a measure of the good we are interested in valuing [museums] and other determinants of (things we know are associated with) well-being, such as income. The logic is that say we imagine a unit of happiness as an 'HAP', and we know that £1 neatly equals exactly 2 HAPs (how convenient), economic approaches can use what we know about this relationship and apply it to understand others. The technique runs on the following rationale:

so, 1: if 'museums have a relationship with well-being that we need a value for'
and, 2: 'money has a relationship with well-being that we have a value for'
then, 3: 'how much money makes you as happy as a given unit of museums' is essentially the question.

Box 8.4   Coefficients

What they are estimating here are the coefficients behind particular types of participation. When you look up the meaning of 'coefficient', you are likely to see something like this: 'a numerical or constant quantity placed before and multiplying the variable in an algebraic expression'.

It's probably important to bear in mind that the amount of museum participation isn't how many times someone goes, how long they are there or how many people are inside a given museum. Museum participation is a variable in and of itself that will represent whatever people answered in response to the survey question, and/or how those data have been coded.

The coefficient is basically: if you increase a unit in your independent variable, how large an increase do you get in your dependent variable?

In this example, the variable 'museum participation' means 'visits to a museum a certain number of times a year', so if you increase the museum participation, how much increase in the happiness variable is there?

The variable might have values between 0 and 1 (which means the unit increase is 'goes from not doing it to doing it', and it might be continuous in hours, or could be another type of proportional increase). Say it is one of the questions from TPS in Box 8.1.

During the last 12 months, have you attended a museum or gallery at least once?

1. Yes 2. No -1. Don't know

This is either 0 or 1, for yes or no. In this instance, if people take the don't know option, they won't be included. The coefficient is how much of the variable 'attended museum or gallery' there is. So, the coefficient behind 'goes to museums or not' might be large, but that's because it only goes from 0 to 1.

However, if you have 'number of hours spent in a museum', with values lying between 0 and 1, you would expect a much smaller coefficient because the max number of hours is much more than 1.

Remember that using income is (1) a way into understanding the relationship between museums and happiness, and (2) a way to express this relationship in financial terms.

> **Box 8.5   Imagining Units of Happiness, Museums and Money**
>
> Say a HAP = 1 unit of happiness.
>
> You went to the British Museum yesterday, and your HAPs increased by 8.
>
> The day before yesterday, someone gave you £1, and your HAPs increase by 2.
>
> This suggests that going to the British Museum is equivalent to getting £4 increase in income. Or if you were to stop going to the British Museum, but were to get £4, you would stay equally happy.
>
> Once you have established this relationship, you can equate museum visitation happiness to happiness from getting more income. This is one way of valuing museums for their relationship to happiness.

In a previous study, the researcher found that 'when using lottery wins as an instrument for income... the size of the impact of income on happiness increases more than ten-fold' (Fujiwara 2013, 26). The reason why lottery wins are thought to be a good indicator for income is they are from outside of a person's day-to-day life. Theoretically, this makes it easier to determine the impact of the money on someone's happiness. You might find yourself asking 'well, how can you know how much of the happiness from the lottery win is from the increase in wealth, and how much of the happiness is from the joy of winning?' There is even a whole body of research that argues that winning the lottery doesn't impact on happiness at all.[20] However, the rationale in 'Museums and Happiness' is that it is suitable 'to get a good estimate of the causal effect of income' (Fujiwara 2013, 26).

The report also explains prior studies 'derive implausible large value estimates for non-market goods' because of this discrepancy in income (Fujiwara 2013, 26). Notably, a CASE[21] study using an income compensation approach found that going to the cinema once a year had a value of £9000 per household per year (Matrix Knowledge Group 2010a, b). The report states that

Since there is no suitable instrument for income in the *Taking Part* data we also estimate values using an income coefficient that has been multiplied by 8 (which is in the scale between 2 to 10, which is the level of bias found in the studies above, but weighted more towards 10 since the analysis of happiness data using the BHPS suggests that the true impact of income on happiness may be more than ten times larger than the OLS coefficient). (Fujiwara 2013, 26)

In simplest terms, the idea is that those previous studies are able to 'instrument for income'—which means that they can isolate the benefits of money from the benefits of being a high earner. It is important to remember that as a higher earner, you are unlikely to have data collected on how long you went to the loo; maybe you have a nicer office and get to expense your coffee, perhaps even someone else goes and gets you nice coffee from your vendor of choice? In the same way it is difficult to disaggregate the joy of winning from the impact of money, it is difficult to account for all the ways that being a higher earner *may improve* your life outside of money alone.

Returning to these previous studies, they found the discrepancy between income and lottery wins. There is therefore a number for that that can be plugged into the valuation. The report explains that this means it is therefore plausible to use people's income, as declared in the TPS, and multiply the coefficient by 8, based on the fact that the estimates between studies that 'instrument for income' and those that don't tend to differ by around this much in previous studies. This is accounted for in the report, like this:

> This is part of the reason why Wellbeing Valuation studies that do not instrument for income derive implausible large value estimates for non-market goods. (Fujiwara 2013, 26)

The report accounts for the robustness of this approach, like this:

> The wellbeing valuation techniques used here are in line with welfare economic theory on valuation (which underlies all cost-benefit analysis and SROI techniques), but we should note that these values should not be seen as amounts that people would actually be willing to pay per year for these activities. This would only be the case if people satisfy their preferences solely on the basis of what makes them happy, but other factors may impact on people's preferences and market decisions. These values should be seen as the equivalent amount of money required to create the same impact on

people's happiness and they are useful as they show us the magnitude of importance of museums and the arts to people. (Fujiwara 2013, 33)

In other words, these valuation principles are considered robust, but these values are not what people would *actually* be prepared to pay. Instead how much extra money would keep someone at their current levels of happiness if they had to stop participating. In a section called 'Key Findings', the valuations are presented as follows:

✓ People value visiting museums at about £3200 per year.
✓ The value of participating in the arts is about £1500 per year per person.
✓ The value of being audience to the arts is about £2000 per year per person.
✓ The value of participating in sports is about £1500 per year per person. (Fujiwara 2013, 8)

Using ticks for bullet points may feel an unusual way of presenting findings, especially when there are so many caveats to these estimates, particularly whether people actually *do* value museums like this, or not. More importantly, these statements imply that people value participation in these monetary terms. Again, it is not that people do not—either consciously, or unconsciously, but the presentation might be confusing to the report's audience. These are in fact what the report calls 'the compensating surplus' for these activities. In other words, according to these calculations, this is the amount of money people would in theory give up in order to undertake the activity. In other words, the finding is that on average, people who go to museums are as happy as people who don't go to museums but are paid £3200 a year more.

This can be difficult to understand when you are reading the key findings from a report as a non-expert, and especially difficult when they are presented out of context, like in a daily national newspaper. We will now look at how findings can appear in different contexts in ways that can be distracting.

8.5   Following the Findings

Even when you follow the processes involved in estimating the relationships in the 'Museums and Happiness' research, as they are broken down here, it still might be hard to see how this valuation works—from a common-sense perspective. Following the data did not find data in which people explicitly value visiting museums at about £3200 per year, and yet this is what it appears to say. This is confusing for people who are not familiar with these kinds of valuations.

These valuations were presented as Key Findings in bold in the introduction on page 8. However, the Caveats section on page 33 clearly states:

> The wellbeing valuation techniques used here are in line with welfare economic theory on valuation (which underlies all cost-benefit analysis and SROI techniques), but we should note that these values should not be seen as amounts that people would *actually* be willing to pay per year for these activities. (Emphasis in original)

The findings are partially presented in the Director's Foreword, on page 5, which states:

> By finding that the individual wellbeing value of museums is over £3000 a year, the report makes a strong case for investing in museums.

We are going to pause and follow some findings to see how and why this is important. They were reproduced partially in a number of places. The *Museums Journal* described the report as having 'found museums improve people's happiness and perception of good health, even after other factors that might be influencing them are accounted for' (Harris 2013). They also go further than the original report by claiming that visiting museums 'boosts' happiness. Notably, this exaggerates the claim of the report—not in the monetary estimates, but the idea of impact is exaggerated to become a boost, when impact was not being measured in these terms at all. This is an example of translating value and impact from one setting to another, and how it can easily be misinterpreted.

This is especially important because it is not a one-off. This is not the only report of this nature with key findings that were altered when they were reproduced. A report written to the DCMS in 2014 saw its findings become muddled before it reached the headlines. In *Quantifying and Valuing the Wellbeing Impacts of Culture and Sport* (Fujiwara et al. 2014), the authors present the key findings as:

- Arts engagement was found to be associated with higher well-being. This is valued at £1084 per person per year, or £90 per person per month.

- A significant association was also found between frequent library use and reported well-being. Using libraries frequently was valued at £1359 per person per year for library users, or £113 per person per month.
- Sport participation was also found to be associated with higher well-being. This increase is valued at £1127 per person per year, or £94 per person per month.

Much like in 'Museums and Happiness', the report for DCMS also includes estimates for many activities. Towards the end of the report, on page 29, the authors express the finding that participation in dance has the highest value of £1671 pa, followed by swimming (£1630 pa) and library visits (£1359 pa). The finding about dance appears in this form, only twice in this report, in a regression table and as a finding underneath it in bold, around two-thirds of the way through the report. In other words, it is far from a headline finding. Despite the lack of prominence of this monetary estimate in the original report, it finds itself at the beginning of a journey which results in a national newspaper headline, like this one in the *Telegraph:* 'Dancing makes people as happy as a £1600 pay rise' (Swinton 2016).

This is why following the data in different ways (and in different directions: back in time and into the future) provides valuable context. In seeing where interpretations of the findings end up, we can see the impact of claims to impact. These are attractive headlines because they feel simple to grasp, and yet, as with many headlines, they obscure the real story. In recognising the appeal of these monetary headlines, we are able to see the market value of valuations like this. We can see that the numbers—and the data practices behind them—are valuable to a sector wanting to find what the Happy Museum's director calls 'compelling statistics', as the language to articulate its value to Treasury.

However, these presentations of findings also create barriers for those who will scoff at how ridiculous an idea it is that anyone could know that 'dancing makes people as happy as a £1600 pay rise'. We must also question how helpful they are to anyone in the dancing profession who might like to understand how to translate what they do into something that is valuable to a funder. At the moment, much of what is going on behind the headlines is quite obscure for those who most need to understand and articulate this relationship for themselves. This calls into question the value of these valuations in the current context.

8.6   How Was the Value of the Relationship Between Museums and Happiness Calculated?

The previous sections have walked you through some of the contexts of the research in 'Museums and Happiness': the data, the concepts and the relationships being modelled—as well as an aside about how appealing headline findings are when they are formulated in monetary terms that appear easy to grasp. We have looked at what this example of quantitative research was aiming to do with a hypothesis on various relationships, but fundamentally: that museums improve people's happiness.

This one hypothesis emerges from a series of contexts: the naturalised relationship between culture and well-being and a hypothesis that this can be measured; a desire to isolate the qualities of museums in this relationship to argue their value; philosophical reasoning on how this is possible; prior research indicating other values that help understand the relationship in question—and prior research indicating methods and models that will be useful. We are now going to look at how the numbers were generated.

We discussed how the same model could be run over and over again, changing one variable each time. The calculations, when taken together, can model how when an individual goes to a museum, their happiness goes up because of the experience. This can account for some of the additional things that could be going on. One might be that their happiness could be going up directly because of the specific experience, and also indirectly, because their health could be getting better because their happiness has improved. So, again, it is not 'museums' that is valued, per se, but a series of variables which are different in each set of models, but some of these variables are about going to museums. I am reproducing Table 8.1, together with Table 8.2, so you can see the variables together.

As a reminder, the key findings are summarised as follows in 'Museums and Happiness' (Fujiwara 2013, 8):

- People value visiting museums at about £3200 per year.
- The value of participating in the arts is about £1500 per year per person.
- The value of being audience to the arts is about £2000 per year per person.
- The value of participating in sports is about £1500 per year per person.

Table 8.2 Variables modelled in 'Museums and Happiness' that are not about participation

Other variables

Binary variables for each of:
• marital status,
• religiosity,
• educational qualifications (having General Certificates of Secondary Education (GCSEs) and above vs not),
• sex,
• employment status,
• frequency of meeting friends (at least once a month vs less than that),
• being in London,
• satisfaction with the local area ('satisfied' and above vs less than that),
• smoking,
• ethnicity (white vs other),
• volunteering;
Scales for:
• numbers of children in the household
• and how often participants drink (from 'never' to 'every day').
• The self-rated health measure is also incorporated into the x vector.
Bands of:
• income in £5000 bands

There are four regression tables in the report that estimate the relationships between

- museum participation and happiness
- museum participation and health
- 'audience to arts'/arts attendance, arts participation and happiness
- 'audience to arts'/arts attendance, participation and health

Just to remind you, that all these variables in the regressions tables began their life around someone's kitchen table, or on their sofa, answering the questions of an interviewer, using the TPS script. Let's consider two questions again. We have already thought about the subjective well-being question. I have copied the explanations from the report as to why each variable was used in the table. It is not normal practice to display these two aspects of methodology together like this, but I find it helpful to see the what and the why (Table 8.3).

Table 8.3 Health and subjective well-being variables, questions and rationales in 'Museums and Happiness'

Variable	Question from TPS	Rationale for the question
Subjective well-being	'Taking all things together how happy would you say you are?' on a scale from 1 to 10 where 10 is described as 'extremely happy' and 1 as 'extremely unhappy'	'Happiness taps in to people's emotions, technically their affective state, and hence tries to gauge people's moods at that moment' (Fujiwara 2013, 12)
Health	'How is your health in general?' on a scale from 1 to 5 where 1 is 'very good' and 5 'very bad'	' …questions on general health will cover mental health and so we may be able to pick up some aspects of well-being or happiness that are not captured in the stand-alone happiness question' (Fujiwara 2013, 13)

Adapted from Fujiwara (2013)

It is interesting that the rationale behind using health is stated as it may pick up on mental health, which may pick up on well-being and happiness. Of course, it does not necessarily follow that responses to a health question will 'pick up' on happiness and there is much work on these complex relations. For example, Clark et al. (2018) find that measures of mental health explain more variation in well-being than measures of physical health. Again, it is not that this is not going on, but it is hard to say that it definitely is.

As the reader, you can make your own decisions on whether this question 'how is your health in general?' may be likely to collect meaningful data regarding subjective well-being for respondents. You can do this by imagining how you might answer this question, and whether you feel you would respond about your general health in a way that incorporated your subjective well-being. You might also do this for others you know well, who, for example, might identify as having poor physical health, but are generally happy, and vice versa. Again, this is not to say that because people with poor physical health are susceptible to poor subjective well-being that the health question cannot pick this up.

The other thing to remember here is that this representative sample was asked these questions between the years 2005 and 2011. When this report was written in 2013, the general public would have made less association between health and happiness. Arguably, much advocacy and attention-raising have happened in the last few years, which would possibly change how people align health and subjective well-being. Back in 2005, cultur-ally, it would have been different again. Therefore, when claims are made about how one thing picks up another, we can all think about the contexts in which the questions were asked, how we might answer them, and begin to think about the assumptions made on this basis.

Perhaps another reason that the study includes health is that it would have helped the process of comparison across the two models, in that it offers two measures of subjective well-being (according to the theory that health will pick up on subjective well-being). It will therefore be possible to check for robustness. This is because, and we should continue to bear this in mind, no measure is perfect. Having multiple measures that are shown in previous studies to be related to the relationship you want to understand will add confidence to your finding. That is, if they are all pointing in the same direction.

In summary, the research reported on in 'Museums and Happiness' compares the relationships between participation (various) and subjective well-being, and income and subjective well-being, by interpreting what the coefficients mean. In line with standard practice, assumptions about the measures of subjective well-being and everything else have been stated. So, there is a theory behind why particular variables are used, and what they can tell us (and the limits to what they cannot), and efforts have been made to communicate them. It gets confusing when the coefficient of the relationship between income and subjective well-being is then substituted with other estimates (multiplying by 8) that emerge from other reports which used different modelling techniques, different variables and con-cepts. They may also be based on other conceptualisations that may have been used in previous examples of the well-being valuation technique. The researcher also points out that this part of the process is also established, however, and has also been accepted by Treasury[22] (p. 8).

Following the key findings on page 8, some caution is advised in the report, for a number of reasons. I summarise these below (the text in brackets aims to explain the reason behind caution being required):

- arts participation and museum attendance are not randomised (without a randomised sample, claims to causation are limited)
- there are likely to be hidden factors that affect both participation and the outcome variables
  (it is not possible to isolate participation from all other possible vari-ables to be sure that the effects measured are because of participation

in museums, rather than any of a number of other things that could affect well-being)

- it is possible that the described causal relationship could be backwards (it might be that happier people tend to go to museums, rather than museums make you happier) (Fujiwara 2013, 8).

These caveats, briefly explained, are: if you really wanted to understand the relationship between museums and happiness. In a theoretically perfect world, you would engineer a sample of people that you could then randomise, making sure that half had gone to museums and half of them not, and see whether one group's happiness is higher on average at the end than the start. This is a randomised control trial (RCT) used as the gold standard in medicine to understand the effects of medication or other interventions and has become increasingly popular in policy-making (Haynes et al. 2012). Yet, such a test is not really practical or ethical in the social sciences—making it very imperfect for a well-being researcher. As I have said before, it is important to (1) use the best available data and be clear on their limitations, and (2) imagine the origins of data. For example, imagine a reality in which people were surveyed *en masse* in an RCT like this. It would be unethical for the cultural sector to force half the population into a museum and forbid the other half from going in for a year in order to model its value! Also, RCTs use placebos, so people who have not been dosed don't know. It's not as if there's a placebo version of a museum you can send people to.

When it comes to the hidden (latent) factors, the explanation in the report is useful. There are always likely to be some influences that cannot be observed in the data available.

> For example, extraverted people may be more likely to participate in the arts and also are more likely to report higher happiness and wellbeing, which means that any observed relationship between the arts and happiness may in part be driven by this personality trait rather than the act of participation itself. (Fujiwara 2013, 8)

Latent traits are personal characteristics that affect what people do, but which cannot be measured directly. So, for example, some people are more curious about the world than others. This would mean 'curiosity about the world' is your latent variable of interest, and maybe those people are both more interested in going to museums and are happier, but you can't just ask people 'how curious are you about the world?' to find out.

As a result of these typical limitations, it is hard to be sure whether it is the going to museums per se that means people are happier, or whether it's some latent trait that means that people who are more likely to go to museums are more likely to be happier. As we know, one of the key issues with the evidence base on the value of culture is that most of the research struggles to argue that 'doing culture makes you *well-er*', rather than people who are more well participate in culture.

These caveats are all threats to causal inference. Yet, as the report points out, this 'level of rigour… is anyway normally acceptable in public policy-making and policy evaluation in OECD governments' (Fujiwara 2013, 8). Therefore, the report implies that there are a number of limits to the claims that can be made, but that these limits are considered acceptable. In other words, there is a shared understanding that this is acceptable between experts who *do* valuations and experts in government who *accept them* as evidence.

Some Reasons Why Findings May Differ

As I mentioned in Sect. 8.2, we began a journey which involved understanding the contexts in which the research in 'Museums and Happiness' was undertaken. My colleague also looked at the quantitative work and used the same data, following the methodology section, to try and reproduce the results. The headline finding of the quantitative work in our project is that the monetary estimates of the relationship between participation and subjective well-being do not match across the two pieces of research. There are a number of reasons why this may be the case.

Why the difference? The second study may have recoded variables in different ways from the initial study. As we know from Chap. 3, coding ordinarily requires human decision-making on what to code how, and there is no single objectively correct way to code variables—all approaches have their own pros and cons under different circumstances. However, what follows from that is that the difference in coding, based on the way it is reported, leads to the finding being backwards. By this, I mean that there is a positive relationship between participation and happiness, but not between attendance and happiness. For example, people who play a musical instrument are happier, but people who go to concerts aren't. In short, the reports' key headlines, and their focus on the positive relationship between happiness and attending particular activities, were not the same when reproduced.

There are also questions about how 'participation' and 'audience' were operationalised in the analysis. The 'Museums and Happiness' report includes some variables and excludes others in its construction of these terms. This is another example of how models require decisions, and it is difficult to be certain that such decisions are not affected by bias, particularly regarding which variables relate to happiness and which do not. We discovered in Chap. 7 a number of ways that the operationalisation of culture and well-being is important. If the operationalisations are too narrow, and 'participation' and 'attendance' do not include all activities that we might want to be classified within these scales, then the apparent positive effects from participation could reflect something broader than just the publicly subsidised cultural sector. It may be that the positive associations of participation in publicly funded culture are similar to those of playing in a darts team or watching Eurovision with friends.

Alternatively, if the operationalisations are too broad, then the positive association between participation and happiness might be driven by one activity, or type of activity, and other activities are then undeservedly classified as being associated with happiness. For example, if dancing is associated with happiness but playing a musical instrument is not, and these two activities, along with several more, are combined into a single variable for whether or not people have participated in the arts, then dancing will be under-credited for its association with happiness, while playing an instrument over-credited. We encountered something similar in Chap. 7, where the incorporation of 'social activity' in the category called 'cultural access' with multiple other variables made it difficult to establish what the effect of cultural participation might be. We also encountered this in Box 7.6 with the hypothetical situation that young people don't like jazz music, but older people do, if you looked at everyone together you would likely find that the two groups would cancel each other out, to a degree, finding that people weren't really bothered by jazz at all.

Most importantly for the context of this book and chapter, data are not neutral, data modelling requires many human interventions, such as cleaning and coding, and experimenting with different ways to derive a relationship from the data. This leaves the processes open to human error, numerous biases and disagreements in a way that is not ordinarily accounted for. The claims made may not reflect the data collected, given the questions asked, and through careful reading we do not need to necessarily be quantitative social scientists to ask questions about where headline findings came from.

8.7   Conclusion: The Value of Valuation

Value is, in other words, both various and variable. (Throsby 2001, 28)

Where are we with our thinking on the value of valuation? If some people in the sector work in the sector because they *know* it improves happiness from their own experience, do they need proof that this is true? Even if this validation comes from research that is not immediately legible to them, is it necessary to understand the findings cited in detail? How important are the various contexts of this research and the potential limitations of its findings for those who want to use it? The *Museums Journal* described the report as having 'found museums improve people's happiness and perception of good health, even after other factors that might be influencing them are accounted for' (Harris 2013), and goes further than the original report by claiming that visiting museums 'boosts' happiness, as opposed to museum-goers being happier. While the research project aimed to contribute to the evidence base on the value of museums, its findings are extended by those who wish to see such positive results. How does this impact positively or negatively on the status of evidence in this area—and the arguments for the value of culture?

Previous chapters have explained why there is an avalanche of numbers, and the various stories of why quantitative approaches to understanding well-being tend to dominate research used in policy. Population-level understandings of well-being are necessary to understand geographic, racial and gendered disparities. Revealed discrepancies can then indicate where policy investment should focus (in theory, although these analyses were not included in the 'Museums and Happiness' research). But we must scrutinise the relationships involved in these processes—theoretically and empirically. To do this requires more people feeling like they *could* understand well-being data. This takes practice and familiarity, but most importantly, more care is needed in research and data communications to move towards more shared understandings.

This book aims to help people feel more comfortable with data by explaining what is going on. This chapter has offered snippets of a step-by-step consideration of the data contexts: their origins, how the data were used, how researchers arrived at these results, and how these findings were then used by others. We looked at all the decisions made, and how reproducing methods with the same data does not always lead to the same results. We also considered how claims were made, and findings subsequently shared. More care is required around transparency around research: even when reports are transparent, more effort could be put into *doing transparency differently*, to improve understanding and enable people to *use* research more fully. While these valuations may work for HM Treasury, there are multiple audiences for research like this, and those who present it, could try harder to speak different languages and be *more* understandable.

At the moment, this sort of research is not published in a way that makes it accessible. Instead, the culture of this kind of research more broadly tends to mean that only headline findings are accessible to cultural and social policy practitioners, who are reliant on data and expressions of data for advocacy, yet are not necessarily comfortable with their origins. Stating one thing in headline findings, but explaining how the meaning is slightly different in practice in bits and pieces further into the report is not necessarily making it as understandable as it could be, and yet it is the norm. The Happy Museum aspired to produce compelling statistics to bridge the gap of cultural values and valuations, and the research behind the report aimed to meet this challenge. However, the research met the aims of valuation, rather than the needs of those who need the research. Acknowledging this demands resource and skill in and of itself, but the culture of research for policy and social policy organisations could change to make the ways in which it uses data and discusses limitations and caveats more easily understandable.

This chapter presented one example in great detail to be a reference point for readers to come back to, to aid future understandings of how well-being data can be used. As this book has acknowledged elsewhere, there are still many issues in data and evidence that are relied on for cultural and social policy. In the age of well-being measures and measurers, it is important that we all feel able try and engage with the data and the claims on our terms—should we wish to. Given that how people feel about these relationships is imbued with their own values, the key is to feel more confident to ask questions and make value judgements for yourself.

NOTES

1. Quality adjusted life years (QALYs) are explained in Box 2.5, in Chap. 2.
2. The two valuation techniques are evaluated for their possible use in culture in O'Brien (2010) *Measuring the Value of Culture: A Report to the Department for Culture Media and Sport*. The Arts Council Strategy,

Achieving Great Art for Everyone (2010), includes a number of artists on the value of the arts, including Jeremy Deller and Tim Etchells, who are cited here.

3. If you are reading this chapter a while after reading previous ones, then the cultural sector is a broad description of cultural institutions like libraries, heritage sites, museums, theatres and so on. Crucially, it is not only about the buildings themselves, but all the ways people make and consume culture and can include Netflix and outdoor festivals.

4. I have since learnt that actually there are differences in the ways that different disciplines express characters in equations; and so, arguably they also talk different languages in this way, but we don't need to get into marginal differences between economists and statisticians here.

5. It is really hard speaking for him. If truth be told, I am not sure I knew what he was thinking, exactly, five years ago.

6. Many qualitative researchers argue that the value of context, bias and subjectivity is too important to qualitative research to enable it to be reproduced in a way that findings could be repeated.

   In quantitative research, operationalisation refers to the process through which abstract concepts, such as happiness, are translated into measurable variables. This is different from the way we use the word in day-to-day discussion. When we operationalise something, we more generally and simply put it to use. See Box 7.1 in Chap. 7 for more detail.

7. Chapters 2 and 4 are good to refer to if you need a reminder on what hedonic means.

8. If you are interested in more information on the differences across BHPS, TPS and Understanding Society at the time, and why they mattered, or indeed, want to see another example of how research like this makes decisions, do look at the original report.

9. All the questions outlined, where specifically worded, can be found in UK Data Service (2009). You can find questionnaires for each year here: https://www.gov.uk/government/publications/adult-questionnaire-taking-part-survey-2009-to-2010. It is worth being aware that TPS has a longitudinal element, which is an adapted questionnaire, as it wants to accommodate change. Therefore, the adapted questionnaire wants to also know 'why the change?' For example, 'you say you have participated more or less in this than last year. Why do you think that is?'

10. The formatting of the questions does change slightly over time, as adaptations and improvements are made. Again this is from the 2009–2010 schedule, available at: https://www.gov.uk/government/publications/adult-questionnaire-taking-part-survey-2009-to-2010.

11. The statistical release page is currently in DCMS (2013).

12. Focus on reports from 2015 can be found in DCMS (2015b).

13. Table 4.3 shows a selection of the surveys that the ONS4 have been added to.
14. This book uses the alternative spelling of 'eudaimonic'.
15. TPS also now asks more specific, subjective questions about whether people put an increase in activities down to improved or worsened health. This question is only in the longitudinal version of the survey which has been going on since 2012. It has small differences to the version of the survey used in 'Museums and Happiness'.
16. Perhaps confusingly, the calculation is slightly different for health in 'Museums and Happiness' (it does not include income), but you *could* swap the outcome variables in principle.
17. The report tells us that a similar approach was used in the CASE (Culture and Sport Evidence) programme (DCMS 2010), but with different data. The CASE programme used the BHPS study to value: sport, going to the cinema and going to concerts (as the variables available). It also used data from life satisfaction questions to measure well-being, rather than 'happiness' as with our case study here.
18. A really clear discussion of the limits of contingent valuation methods can be found in Throsby (2001, Chapter 5).
19. The first and most famous of these studies is Brickman et al. (1978). However, as with other previous examples of wealth and happiness, the evidence is not universal.
20. For more information on the Culture and Sport Evidence (CASE) programme, see Chap. 6.
21. HM Treasury is the government's economic and finance ministry, maintaining control over public spending, setting the direction of the UK's economic policy and working to achieve strong and sustainable economic growth. https://www.gov.uk/government/organisations/hm-treasury.

REFERENCES

ACE. 2010. *Achieving Great Art for Everyone: A Strategic Framework for the Arts.* London: Arts Council England. https://collective-encounters.org.uk/wp-content/uploads/2019/10/Achieving_great_art_for_everyone.pdf. Accessed 31 March 2021.

Belfiore, E. 2002. Art as a Means of Alleviating Social Exclusion: Does It Really Work? A Critique of Instrumental Cultural Policies and Social Impact Studies in the UK. *International Journal of Cultural Policy* 8 (1): 91–106. https://doi.org/10.1080/102866302900324658.

Brickman, P., D. Coates, and R. Janoff-Bulman. 1978. Lottery Winners and Accident Victims: Is Happiness Relative? *Journal of Personality and Social*

Psychology 36 (8): 917–927. https://doi.org/10.1037//0022-3514.36. 8.917.

Clark, A.E., et al. 2018. *The Origins of Happiness: The Science of Well-Being over the Life Course*. Princeton University Press. https://press.princeton.edu/books/hardcover/9780691177892/the-origins-of-happiness.

DCMS. 2010. *Taking Part: The National Survey of Culture, Leisure and Sport, 2008–2009; Adult and Child Data* [Data Collection]. UK Data Service. https://core.ac.uk/display/74280823. Accessed 28 April 2021.

———. 2013. *Taking Part: Statistical Releases*. Department for Digital, Culture, Media & Sport. https://www.gov.uk/government/collections/sat%2D%2D2. Accessed 31 March 2021.

———. 2015a. *Taking Part 2014/15, Focus on: Art Forms*. London: Department for Culture, Media and Sport. https://assets.publishing.service.gov.uk/government/uploads/system/uploads/attachment_data/file/802735/Y10_Art_forms_-_FINAL.pdf.

———. n.d. *Taking Part 2014/15: "Focus On…" Reports*. Department for Digital, Culture, Media & Sport. https://www.gov.uk/government/statistics/taking-part-201415-focus-on-reports. Accessed 31 March 2021.

———. 2015b. *Taking Part 2014/15, Focus on: Wellbeing*. London: Department for Culture, Media and Sport. https://assets.publishing.service.gov.uk/government/uploads/system/uploads/attachment_data/file/476510/Taking_Part_201415_Focus_on_Wellbeing.pdf. Accessed 31 March 2021.

———. 2016. *Taking Part focus on: Diversity*. London: Department for Culture, Media and Sport. https://assets.publishing.service.gov.uk/government/uploads/system/uploads/attachment_data/file/593993/Focus_on_diversity_final.pdf.

Fujiwara, D. 2013. *Museums and Happiness: The Value of Participating in Museums and the Arts*. United Kingdom: The Happy Museum; Museum of East Anglian Life; Arts Council England. https://happymuseumproject.org/wp-content/uploads/2013/04/Museums_and_happiness_DFujiwara_April2013.pdf. Accessed 29 March 2021.

Fujiwara, D., L. Kudrna, and P. Dolan. 2014. *Quantifying the Social Impacts of Culture and Sport*. Department for Culture, Media and Sport. https://assets.publishing.service.gov.uk/government/uploads/system/uploads/attachment_data/file/304896/Quantifying_the_Social_Impacts_of_Culture_and_Sport.pdf.

Gilmore, A., H. Glow, and K. Johanson. 2017. Accounting for Quality: Arts Evaluation, Public Value and the Case of "Culture Counts". *Cultural Trends* 26 (4): 282–294. https://doi.org/10.1080/09548963.2017.1382761.

Harris, G. 2013. Report Finds Visiting Museums Boosts Happiness. *Museums Association.* https://www.museumsassociation.org/museums-journal/news/2013/04/18042013-economist-report-finds-museums-boost-happiness/. Accessed 31 March 2021.

Haynes, L., et al. 2012. *Test, Learn, Adapt: Developing Public Policy with Randomised Controlled Trials.* SSRN Scholarly Paper ID 2131581. Rochester, NY: Social Science Research Network. https://doi.org/10.2139/ssrn.2131581.

Hill, L. 2017. "Only a Fool or a Knave" Trusts Quality Metrics, Say Academics. *ArtsProfessional.* https://www.artsprofessional.co.uk/news/only-fool-or-knave-trusts-quality-metrics-say-academics. Accessed 31 March 2021.

Matrix Knowledge Group. 2010a. *Understanding the Drivers, Impact and Value of Engagement in Culture and Sport: Technical Report for the Systematic Review and Database.* London: Department for Culture, Media and Sport. https://assets.publishing.service.gov.uk/government/uploads/system/uploads/attachment_data/file/88448/CASE-systematic-review-technical-report-July10.pdf.

———. 2010b. *Understanding the Value of Engagement in Culture and Sport: Technical Report.* London: Department for Culture, Media and Sport. https://assets.publishing.service.gov.uk/government/uploads/system/uploads/attachment_data/file/88450/CASE-Value-technical-report-July10.pdf.

Merli, P. 2002. Evaluating the Social Impact of Participation in Arts Activities. *International Journal of Cultural Policy* 8 (1): 107–118. https://doi.org/10.1080/10286630290032477.

Meyrick, J., and T. Barnett. 2017. Culture Without "World": Australian Cultural Policy in the Age of Stupid. *Cultural Trends* 26 (2): 107–124. https://doi.org/10.1080/09548963.2017.1323840.

———. 2021. From Public Good to Public Value: Arts and Culture in a Time of Crisis. *Cultural Trends* 30 (1): 75–90. https://doi.org/10.1080/09548963.2020.1844542.

Nissel, M. 1983. *Facts About the Arts: A Summary of Available Statistics.* London: Policy Studies Institute.

O'Brien, D. 2010. *Measuring the Value of Culture: A Report to the Department for Culture Media and Sport.* DCMS.

Oman, S. 2013. A True Snapshot of Life? *ArtsProfessional.* https://www.artsprofessional.co.uk/magazine/261/article/true-snapshot-life. Accessed 31 March 2021.

Oman, S., and M. Taylor. 2018. Subjective Well-Being in Cultural Advocacy: A Politics of Research Between the Market and the Academy. *Journal of*

Cultural Economy 11 (3): 225–243. https://doi.org/10.1080/17530350. 2018.1435422.

Phiddian, R., et al. 2017. Counting Culture to Death: An Australian Perspective on Culture Counts and Quality Metrics. *Cultural Trends* 26 (2): 174–180. https://doi.org/10.1080/09548963.2017.1324014.

Selwood, S. 2002. Measuring Culture. *Spiked.* https://www.spiked-online. com/2002/12/30/measuring-culture/. Accessed 30 March 2021.

The Happy Museum. n.d-a. About – Happy Museum Project. *The Happy Museum.* http://happymuseumproject.org/about/. Accessed 2 May 2021.

———. n.d.-b. The Happy Museum Project. *The Happy Museum.* https://happymuseumproject.org/. Accessed 2 May 2021.

Throsby, D. 2001. *Economics and Culture.* Cambridge: Cambridge University Press.

UK Data Service. 2009. Taking Part: England's Survey of Leisure, Culture and Sport 2008–09: Adult Questionnaire. *UK Data Service.* https://doc.ukdataservice.ac.uk/doc/6530/mrdoc/pdf/6530tpyr4_adult_questionnaire_2008-09.pdf. Accessed 31 March 2021.

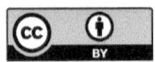

CHAPTER 9

Understanding

9.1 Understanding, Well-being and Data

We started this book with a preface: a personal note on why and how it came about. This included reflections on some of my experiences of coming to understand data and well-being—not only my direct experiences, of course, but my observations of people I know and have met, and how they interact with data issues and well-being issues. I argued this book was for friends, family and acquaintances on Facebook. For my students from courses across theatre studies to data sciences to social policy. For the data practitioners I work with in the cultural sector and for the hundreds of people I have spoken to about their well-being and/or their data in my research.

Given that most of these people are people I have met, the preface also points to how this book is based on my understanding of these issues. It often uses UK cases and relates them to more general problems, international contexts, lessons learnt and some of those that remain. Perhaps in another ten years, I will be writing about these issues from a different place again. I have been honest about how I came to know data and theories about well-being. I found it hard to find all I needed in order to be confident that I understood what I needed to understand.

Because there is a need to understand well-being and data together across many areas of society, this book is written for anyone. You are told to write a book with a specific reader in mind, but this is hard when you

© The Author(s) 2021   351
S. Oman, *Understanding Well-being Data*,
New Directions in Cultural Policy Research,
https://doi.org/10.1007/978-3-030-72937-0_9

are writing about big problems and your audiences are multiple. Given the aims of this book, it had to address everyone, but knowingly; aware that not all its parts are everybody's cup of tea. It is therefore up to the reader which bits they want to read, and what they wish to pass on. All I could do was write for what I *understood* to be (1) the needs and (2) the desires to grasp these issues better or, indeed, differently. But the needs and issues are various, so one size can't always fit all if you want to address understanding of the broader concerns. So, to return to all the people I wrote this book for, I want it to be clear that everyone can contribute to how we could understand the issues, and *differently*. What if we looked at the issues from someone else's perspective, or approached them in an alternative way?

I want to close this book by focussing on understanding for all these reasons, and more. The title *Understanding Well-being Data* might imply that we were simply going to try and understand well-being, data and 'well-being data'. Its subtitle 'improving social and cultural policy, practice and research' implies, of course, that I aspire for this book to change big things in society for the better. Really, this book has more modest aspirations to improve understanding in small ways—and who knows, perhaps these small ways can make their own differences. Whether it enables anyone who reads it to think about things they had not thought of before, or from a different perspective.

I have been talking about understanding in relation to data in a few ways for a while now (i.e. Oman 2019a, b): first, as in how we acquire knowledge; second, as how we share understanding; third, how these *work* with becoming a *more understanding* society. When I have summarised my findings on how people understand data, I have also suggested that we might think of this on a scale of knowing at one end, and feelings on the other (Oman 2019b, c). These qualities of understanding are in essence what well-being data should be about. Collecting data to inform how we might be more understanding of people's needs and experiences to do better for them and society.

How do data, well-being—and data *about* well-being, help us with these two concerns of understanding? In many ways, that is what this book is about. We are going to touch on what understanding means, explaining it through another case study: this time one of my own experiences of watching people try and understand what data are doing. But more generally, how the social sciences can adopt a more understanding position.

9.2   Meanings of Understanding

understanding | ʌndə'standɪŋ |.

noun *[mass noun]*.

1 the ability to understand something; comprehension: *foreign visitors with little understanding of English.*

• the power of abstract thought; intellect: *a child of sufficient intelligence and understanding.*

• an individual's perception or judgement of a situation: *my understanding was that he would find a new supplier.*

2 sympathetic awareness or tolerance: *he wrote with understanding and affection of the people of Dent.*

[count noun] an informal or unspoken agreement or arrangement: *he and I have an understanding | he had only been allowed to come on the understanding that he would be on his best behaviour*

adjective

1 sympathetically aware of other people's feelings; tolerant and forgiving: *a kind and understanding man | people expect their doctor to be understanding.*

2 *archaic* having insight or good judgement. (Oxford Lexico n.d. [bold and italics in original])

Sympathy This was first used to express 'understanding between people'; it came via Latin from Greek *sumpathés* (from *sun-* 'with' and *pathos* 'feeling'). (Cresswell 2010, 432 [bold and italics in original])

Now that I spend some of my time in academic research meetings, I am party to conversations on how we understand what understanding means. As you can see above, people who write dictionaries also think about these things. Ironically, people talk about academics living in ivory towers—not caring about what people think and feel; but for some of us, that is *so* much of what we think about. For example, I am a co-investigator on a research project called Living With Data (n.d.).[1] In project meetings (perhaps you can picture it?), we academics have spent quite a lot of time discussing what we mean by understanding and knowing. How they differ and overlap and how our understanding may be different from people in their day-to-day lives. This was also a conversation point in a recent project meeting with our Advisory Group[2] made up of experts from across public sector, civil society, advocacy and research.

One of the experts on the Advisory Group suggested that perhaps understanding was such a 'complicated'[3] term that maybe we might want to ask people what they understand by understanding. At this point, we all took a moment to laugh (kindly at ourselves, I like to think) and concluded that while this is important, 'ordinary' cultural understandings of the word understanding were a simpler experience. What I meant by this in the meeting, and still do now, was that most people move through life not really thinking about what the word 'understanding' *means* but are familiar with its meaning.

Understanding is a process by which we come to know something, the amount of or the depth of knowledge we have about something. At the same time, *being* understanding involves empathy, and putting yourself in someone else's position. Shared understanding, on the other hand, requires the sharing of knowledge with someone in a way that you know they will understand *it*.

Hence, understanding is both knowing and feeling—crucially it is as much about 'understanding between people' (as cited at the beginning of the section) as it is to grasp knowledge about something. As this book has explained, data and the way science and social science knowledge are constructed are also about having a shared understanding of how things are done: how to collect and analyse data in the 'right way' is a matter of discipline and tradition, which are not universal. This can lead to differences in interpretation of both well-being and how to use data across disciplines. How do those who work with data share their understandings with those who don't? Often this is done quite badly, or without thought, care and empathy.

More care is given to sharing understanding in other areas of life. When you ask a child 'do you understand?' after you have told them off for doing something and explained why: you are asking, do you understand why I had to tell you off? Have you learnt why what you were doing was dangerous or wrong? You are asking them to appreciate things on an emotional level and on a cognitive level—whether this is successful or not, is another matter. Understanding is both an emotional and cognitive exercise for all of us: we gain knowledge through understanding, and we become more understanding of others through experience.

You may remember that this idea of developing understanding is one of the age-old arguments for the benefits of aesthetic and cultural experiences in Chap. 6. Watching a film or reading a book can help us understand other people's lives, and culture's contribution to well-being is often argued because of its capacity to increase empathy. Philosophers have long seen the moment where we come to understand something as a pleasurable moment, as well as one that brings purpose and meaning to our lives. This is an idea of how understanding improves personal well-being; while of course, knowledge and understanding are seen as contributing to the development of good societies, thus improving well-being at population level. If this is indeed the case, then there is a strong case that more care and attention should be paid to understanding as good for well-being.

Using data about well-being should fulfil all of the functions of understanding: caring for and appreciating the conditions of others, building knowledge of what to do to improve it—and sharing these understandings. As an aside, it should also involve learning from mistakes. Yet, as we have discovered in this book, the limitations of 'following the data' are not always admitted to, but instead, often dodged around. First of all, I want to return to the importance of understanding in data. As with the rest of this book, we are going to use a case study to look under the bonnet of the data. While not strictly well-being data, this case study does show how simple processes of everyday data collection can feel 'hostile', and unsympathetic.

The Case for Understanding in Data

In 2018, I began a large-scale qualitative research project to understand data and diversity in the cultural sector. More specifically, Arts Council England (ACE)[4] wanted to introduce additional questions to its existing equality monitoring processes.[5] The research was undertaken in partnership with ACE to advise on how to improve data in the sector and introduce the potential new data to measure inequality better.

Inequality and inequality data are contentious issues across the UK cultural sector.[6] Commitment to social inclusion is integral to the sector's identity and values, as this book has argued. However, qualitative and quantitative data reveal, first, the failure to achieve diversity goals in terms of who gets to participate in, and work in the arts (Brook et al. 2020) and, second, the amount of missing data from administrative processes (DC Research 2017; Oman 2019c). What does 'missing data' mean? In this instance, it means a gap where there should be a value. For example, all those households who did not complete the census in March 2021 become missing data, and so people were hired to knock on your door to remind you to complete the census. Missing data reduce the accuracy of understanding that is possible from data, which can affect government decision-making, including how resources are allocated.

An example of missing data in the cultural sector equality monitoring story can be found in organisations that refused to ask people about their sexuality. One organisation I spoke with heartily believed that this question was irrelevant to their workplace, especially as they had such good LGBTQI representation in their senior workforce. They therefore did not collect these data, or report them to ACE for a sector-wide picture. Linked to this are longstanding discussions between people who don't like feeling audited by existing data collection processes that aim to understand inequality issues. It feels like this organisation took a pretty understanding position, then. However, an organisation may *think* it is being sensitive to people's privacy in not asking them the question and may not *think* it has issues of discrimination, but how could it *know?* When asked about their sexuality in a subsequent sub-study at this organisation, one person wrote that they were relieved this issue was finally being looked at, as they had experienced discrimination. Understanding what is best for knowledge and understanding is therefore far from easy.

We can see a disconnect emerging: between collecting data for good, but it feeling bad while it is happening. This tension has exacerbated issues related to data practices and diversity practices in the sector that required attention—and at the same time. How can the sector know how to change, when it doesn't know what changes to make and where? Data and research can help answer these questions in different ways, but research *on* data needed to be done first.

The thrust of the empirical research I was doing was to understand how inequality data currently worked in organisations funded by ACE and, crucially, how this might be improved (in terms of data quality and process). In essence, this was very much a project to understand the complexities of the existing context before we might know what to do to improve it. To do this, I collected and analysed many different types of data[7] to help me understand the main problems across various areas and layers of the sector, and in different ways. You may remember that in Chap. 3 we covered how different kinds of data help us understand things from different standpoints. I describe the value of understanding a complex issue like this 'in the round' (Oman 2021, forthcoming). Here, I needed to capture the complex ecosystem of data collection and analysis that informs inequality policy in the publicly funded cultural sector.

As well as various desk-based policy research, 15 organisations that were funded by ACE, called National Portfolio Organisations (NPOs), were sampled. Each NPO was chosen for a balanced distribution of geography, size of organisation, size of grant from ACE, discipline area (i.e. dance or visual arts) and social mission (i.e. reaching local working-class communities or working with disabled performers). In each NPO, I undertook participant observation, interviews with experts in data or diversity and focus groups with staff who held no management responsibilities in these areas.

One crucial aspect of this as a project was to improve understanding of how people *feel* about questions that are used to gather data about class and social mobility alongside other inequalities[8] that are protected by the Equality Act (2010). So, I am going to concentrate on my focus groups here—as these were about how people understood data in their everyday lives. People were grouped together in teams within their workplace and asked to fill in 'fake' equality monitoring forms. When I say fake, I mean that they were fabricated through bringing questions used elsewhere onto one form for people to answer, and then reflect on them. It was hoped that this would help me understand the data differently, through looking at the questions that generate them through other people's eyes.

The context and set-up were important, because, as I keep saying, context is central to people's understandings of data and how they work. It is also vital to researchers' understanding. Context is—again—another one of those 'contested concepts' (Gallie 1956). It is often discussed as a problem for the researcher: qualitative researchers need to be sensitive to the contexts they are researching. The same is true of evaluative research, irrespective of your approach, a researcher should understand as much about the contexts they are evaluating as possible. It is an important concern in data studies, with the concept of 'contextual integrity' proposed as a framework for good practice when it comes to using personal data and protecting privacy (Nissenbaum 2009). So what *is* context? In this book, it is all of the *whos, wheres, whats, whens, hows and whys*, as well as the *how much?* and the *so whats?* and *what nexts?* Context is, therefore, vital in how we understand how people feel about data more generally—and how data get *used*, more specifically. It is also vital to sharing understandings of data, which we will return to in a bit.

Keeping context at the forefront of the research design and analyses enabled interesting insights into how the data *work*. People's reflections on the questions used to gather these data offered new understanding on their utility and their accuracy. After asking everyone to complete these 'fake'[9] equal opportunities forms, we spent time discussing how people felt about the questions: how they were formatted, what they were asking—and any other reactions. People indicated that they felt a combination of the types of understanding defined by the dictionary (mentioned earlier), of data and data processes, in which they could see benefits and harms that I discuss below.[10]

I categorised four main issues, which touch on the differing aspects of understanding we have encountered above. I grouped people's responses into political, personal, practical, proxy (Oman 2019b see below; Oman forthcoming-a). When I say political issues, I refer to those who raised objections to collecting these data in this way as an issue of public concern. These sorts of responses are characterised by people asserting it is not right to collect these data like this, from a position of sympathy and shared understanding. I used the term 'personal issues' to explain people's responses which described how the process was, or could be, hurtful for, or to, themselves and others. These data were seen as too private, and the processes could disproportionately affect some more than others. There were a number of practical issues raised, including people not knowing the answer to the questions, or not being able to answer using the categories provided. This probably feels very familiar to many of you who have tried to fill in a questionnaire and not been able to make your answer fit the form. There was a lack of shared understanding between the person asking the question and the lives of the people trying to complete it. Despite the importance of all the responses across categories, I want to focus on the final category, 'proxy', below.

You may remember, a 'proxy' is an indirect measure of something. The example I gave in Chap. 2 is that someone's income does not necessarily tell you about their quality of life directly, but because the relationship has been long-studied, assumptions are made about well-being using what we know about how income relates to well-being. Or so the theory goes. Another example from Chap. 5 is that 5% of teachers were sacked in Washington, D.C., as a result of a determined mayor wanting to turn-around the city's underperforming schools. However, the teachers were judged and then let go off the back of a complex and flawed algorithm, called a value-added model which 'define[d] its own reality and use[d] it to justify their results' (O'Neil 2016, 7). The idea was that 'the numbers would speak more clearly and be more fair', but those who interacted with these models, numbers and judgements said, 'I don't think anyone understood them' (O'Neil 2016, 5). The example of the use of proxies in managing schools is more complex than the class metric in the arts question I outline above, but the premise is the same: these proxies categorise people, telling someone else something about performance, identity and background, and are not often presented in a way that is easy to understand.

In the case of equalities data, personal characteristics are used to understand class and social mobility, but it is not as simple as measuring something like age. Class tends to be categorised in bands, but the meaning and dividing lines between these bands (e.g. working class and middle class) are not universally understood by people. People are notoriously bad at self-defining their class (O'Brien 2018). This means that a direct measure of class using self-definition is unlikely to be accurate. Instead, asking people questions about their lives can indirectly establish aspects of privilege and disadvantage as a result of their socio-economic status, or their class. Some obvious questions might be to do with the house people live in, their salary—or another one that is popular is what newspaper you read. You probably have a different picture in your head for a person reading the *Sun* (a UK right-wing tabloid) than you do, say, the *Guardian* (a UK left-wing broadsheet). These questions get at different indicators of class: salary, wealth and cultural consumption, for example, and have all been shown to have different pros and cons.[11]

Although the class proxy questions that were trialled in these group discussions were new to many answering these equality monitoring forms, they have long-established methods with their own institutional histories. Many of the questions have been used for decades in sociological measures of social mobility (Goldthorpe and Hope 1972). One question asks for the occupation of the main wage earner in your household when you were 14. It is considered a more accurate measure of class than income or self-identification or any of the other proxy options (O'Brien 2018; Brook et al. 2020). This question is part of a schema that informed the National Statistics Socio-Economic Classification (NS-SEC) system used for half a century (ONS 2010). The schema identifies someone's class origins by way of the school they attended, whether their parents attended higher education, and parental occupation at 14. While policy and data experts consider these questions most able to produce the most robust metric, the latter question in particular was queried in every one of my focus groups, because of these issues of understanding as political, practical, personal or proxy.

Returning to the findings on the proxy question, what were the issues with it? People by and large understood that this was a proxy question—even if they did not understand what is meant by the term 'proxy'. Let me explain: one person said, 'I know that you are trying to get at something, but I don't know what it is, exactly'. The participant grasped that what their mum or dad did for a job years ago was not *really* the important thing for the researchers who would be looking at this data to understand class and social mobility. But they could not work out what the connection was between what they were being asked and inequality. What did it mean in the context of equality monitoring in *their* workplace at *that* moment, many years later. They found themselves in a process of trying to understand what the proxy question was doing, but it did not quite make sense to them.

Wanting to understand the rationale behind the question was not an isolated incident. There was a palpable moment in most of these group discussions where someone, or numerous people, identified that these are not neutral processes. There was more going on than met the eye and they wanted to understand. I was asked numerous questions by participants in almost every group, such as 'What are you trying to get at?', 'Why has this question been worded like this?', 'Why my parents? What have they got to do with my job now?', 'Why the employment of only one?' 'Why employment at all?' and, most frequently, 'Why 14?' and 'What about the information about my life that this question does not capture?' It is clear that this proxy question that aims to produce robust, objective data provokes many more questions when it comes into play with ordinary understandings. The key thing to learn from this was that many people did not feel comfortable answering the question for various reasons, but largely this was because they did not understand what *it* was doing, or how the data would be useful. They couldn't imagine what would happen next or how it would be valuable.

As a researcher doing research for a policy organisation, I was asked to make recommendations on what to do next. So, my key recommendation was to improve communications about *what* was happening when people gave their data (Oman 2019d). Essentially, context is not only important to understanding how data work in context for the researcher, but communicating these contexts is vital to move towards a shared understanding of how data work and why they are important.

It seemed clear that people needed to know why a question is being asked and what that question does, and why. They also craved to understand why *these* personal, intimate data are important to share. The question was not a question about questions, in so much as a question about data. Given the nature of the proxy was so far removed from everyday understandings of what the aim of using these data was, this is understandable.

People in the focus groups were (or at least claimed to be) committed to helping address issues of inequality, which is typical of people working in this sector (Brook et al. 2020). In other words, the people I spoke to by and large had the empathy part of understanding down, but equality monitoring processes were not designed for *shared* understanding.

Remember that well-being data or inequality data are data about us. Yet, it is not common practice to help people understand what *their* data can do and how their data can improve anything. Cultivating communications about the *whats, whys, whos, hows* and *so whats* and *what nexts* is important to increase public understandings and trust (Oman 2019c, d). We are seeing increasing attention to public engagement with data (Kennedy et al. 2020). Yet, to date,[12] this work is not necessarily concerned with how people come to understand data, and is still too focussed on how the tech/media company or the government wants people to engage with what they are doing.

The recommendations I made as a result of the inequality research aimed to not only improve understanding of why measuring class was important, but to be more understanding when collecting data (Oman 2019d). As a director of a major museum said to me while I was setting the research up:

> This [understanding inequality] is a project of care. It's about trying to make the sector a better place for everyone, but somehow, the way it is done is the opposite. Its unfriendly, and I think, can feel hostile. (Oman forthcoming-b)

Interestingly, this sentiment that people collecting data don't care about people was quite common in the UK's Measuring National Well-being debate (2010–2011). The quote below was one I chose to illustrate that you got the feeling when reading the comments people wrote in the free text fields, that people who completed the debate survey felt that the survey authors were talking a different language from them. They were almost from two different cultures.

> Your [sic] talking to people about their lives, not selling them a product. Empathy and understanding with how you word your surveys will make people actually give a damn and 'want' to take part as they believe (rightly or wrongly) that they will be listened too [sic] and their opinion might just count for something. (Oman 2015, p. 82)

Being more understanding when collecting data reduces these 'hostile' conditions of data collection in a project of social justice and well-being (Oman 2019c, 2015). Those who want data, especially to improve things, need to be mindful of the well-being of those whose data they need. They need to be more understanding of those whose data they ask for, and they need to take account of the personal nature of these kinds of questions and the experience of being asked questions about your identity and your background (Oman 2019a). They also need to move towards an idea of shared understanding of data and inequality.

Context should not only be a concern for researchers to improve their understanding on their terms, but needs to account for sharing understanding more broadly. We encountered this in Chap. 8, where research to understand the culture–well-being relationship is designed to prove this relationship and presented in a way that speaks to decision-makers. When in fact work should be done in social, cultural and charity sectors so that research is designed to work with and speak to the sector that wants to better understand the value of the work it does. Again, this means moving towards more shared understandings of data and their processes.

Subsequent to my research with ACE (Oman 2019c) and policy recommendations (Oman 2019d), this advice now features in the Social Mobility Commission's new guidelines on collecting data (SMC 2021). The focus on the questions rather than the data is more people-centred:

> Asking someone what their socio-economic background is can seem like a personal question to ask, and some people may not be used to being asked it.
> In order to build trust, help employees understand why the question is being asked—to help get a better picture of the socio-economic diversity in the business. People need to hear a purpose.

This movement towards being understanding when collecting data to understand society is an important one, and one that has been little acknowledged up to this point in much large-scale data collection: whether that data are about well-being or inequality. Crucially, those marginalised by inequalities are most at risk of suffering from ill-being as a result of data (Data Justice Lab n.d.; Kennedy et al. 2020). While the government statistical service (GSS) has a pledge for statistics for 'public good' (GSS n.d.), this still does not formally[13] account for being understanding of the public in data's collection, analysis and use.

9.3   DATA USES AS BARRIERS TO UNDERSTANDING

Beyond the arguments I have just made about how a lack of understanding can lead to bad data practices that are bad for well-being, I also argue that they lead to bad data. If people cannot answer the questions in a survey for practical, personal or political reasons, or because they feel uncomfortable that they do not know enough about why the data are important and what is happening with them (as is the case with the proxy questions), you jeopardise possibilities for good data, instead ending up with missing or incorrect data.

What we have also encountered in this book is how data uses lead to a lack of understanding more broadly. As in the case with Google Flu Trends we covered in Chap. 5, if you do not consider the variety of contexts in which people will type the symptoms of a pandemic illness, you will not appreciate the limits to your method. This is a barrier to understanding. Similarly, if those modelling the data on COVID-19 'in the community' are not aware of the fact that it is more difficult to collect tests from high-rise flats in poorer communities, whose data are missing? How might that hinder understanding of inequalities and the pandemic, if the data are to be analysed to answer those questions? Context is important to understanding. If you don't think about *who* is missing from your missing data, how can you know *how* important the missing pieces are? How can you know how limited your understanding is?

The gift of search engines offers us access to so much more information—daily—as we go about our business. We can playfully search to prove a family member wrong at Christmas—'no that's not the same so-and-so that was in that thing. You're thinking of this one…'—or cheat at the local pub quiz. However, the lists of information it presents us with are not always a simple single answer to a closed question. Searches of course enable you to put a proxy term in and see what the search comes up with. But there often are millions of results.

Search engines have been designed to learn what we might be looking for, based on information they have on our previous searches (and everyone else's). This means that a search engine wants to understand what we might want to know. Yet, as we discovered in Chap. 1, the search engine does not only gather data on us and show us results back in some sort of neutral process. Instead, it makes decisions on what it will recommend we look at as a result of our search terms. As Noble explained, if you typed in the phrase 'black girls' as recently as 2011, you were shown indecent images. This is not a question and answer process, but rather one of selection and assumption.

Instead, search engines try to understand what we might want to find by making associations that may be very different from our own way of understanding things, or indeed what we are imagining we might find. Returning to an important point from Chap. 1, it is possible that being shown an association subconsciously changes an aspect of our understanding of what people do, or what they look like. Data and data practices can change culture. This is potentially dehumanising and can lead to the opposite of greater understanding—or, indeed the good society. We must design data practice, along with the ways in which we engage with data, more responsibly to ensure that well-being is improved through this engagement.

9.4   FOLLOWING THE DATA: HOW WE HAVE COME TO UNDERSTAND WELL-BEING DATA IN THIS BOOK

We have covered a number of different understandings of well-being and data in this book, as well as considered their impact on, and relevance to, culture and society. We have identified how ideas of well-being differ and transcend time, place, culture and religion. We have encountered how people feel about well-being in their everyday life, and projects to try and understand this phenomenon, as well as the understandings of those responsible for people's well-being, such as those in government. We have also considered how people interact, even *live* with data in their everyday lives, but are not always sure they *understand* them.

We have followed the data into 'disciplines', as groups of academics and professionals who look at the world in a particular way, and tend to agree on certain methods to understand it. We have considered how experts understand well-being across research disciplines (including economics, social and cultural policy, social statistics and philosophy), and how they work together in sub-disciplines, and in practice. For example, many economists look for trends in what people value over time and what that means for well-being. This book has presented documents as data to analyse what well-being economists (and other disciplines) value and how that changes over time. We found indications that happiness psychology as a new discipline suited the ends of those eager for 'a new science of happiness', but that when it came to deciding on data processes, some psychologists felt their expertise was overlooked. We found that economics has traditionally held much sway with policy-making institutions, but not necessarily made their ideas and principles accessible to all. Of course, these issues are not specific to economics, but most disciplines using data to understand well-being can lose sight of shared understanding, or *being* understanding.

In Chap. 5, some of the pros and cons for writers on different Big Data approaches were synthesised. Notably, Tables 5.1, 5.2 and 5.3 indicate that these concerns tended to reflect on the utility of data for the data scientists, or whoever else might want to use them. They did not account for whose data they were and how ethical these approaches might be. Given that Big Data are often collected in ways that are not obvious to people, what could be done better to ensure shared understanding?

There are moves towards greater fairness, accountability and transparency in data uses. Yet, *following* a data controversy and watching how these principles *work* in practice demonstrate that much effort remains to establish what a shared understanding of these values look like in practice. We briefly considered the case of the algorithm that decided on students' A level grades, in lieu of an exam under COVID-19 restrictions in the UK. The outcome was contentious, but the regulator (Ofsted) insisted this was the fairest way to approach the problem. Yet as the headline premises behind the decision-making method emerged in the press, the process became a national scandal; notably, because of the impact on young people's futures and current well-being. There were then calls for transparency and accountability, but when the algorithm's methodology was published, the 319-page document was not legible to many and was only even manageable to a very select few.

Transparency could involve showing everyone everything, but how does this compromise understanding? What does that mean when the data and the actions surrounding their use are complex, highly detailed and outside of everyday understandings? Chapter 8 reviewed one research project using valuation with well-being data, step by step. It *followed the data* backwards, to understand the contexts from which they and the study originated. It also *followed the findings* forwards to understand how the research was interpreted in other contexts. The report explained that these methods were accepted by experts in government. However, the chapter found that when the methods were reproduced, using the same data, the findings differed, so what does that mean for shared understanding of experts. The chapter also showed that when the findings were reproduced in the media, they were misinterpreted to say that museums boost happiness, which was not how the research was presented in the report. What does that mean for shared understanding with non-experts in data?

Shared understandings are difficult, when within the same field. In Chap. 7, we encountered two research projects which were ostensibly looking at 'subjective well-being' in a similar population: people with an artistic practice and people with a creative occupation. We found that while the term 'artistic practice' indicates a level of professionalisation, this was not what the research was necessarily looking at. Similarly, that creative occupants didn't need to be creative at all—as we might understand the word—according to the UK government's Department for Culture, Media and Sport. We also found very different data were used to understand the concept of subjective well-being in these studies. What does that mean for how we join-up and share understanding of the well-being of different groups?

We have discovered that the meaning of well-being changes as the nature of data changes, and desire for data evolves and demands for data analytics increase. We have looked at well-being as it is understood as various measurements, and the benefits of understanding well-being at scale and over time, and have witnessed how knowledge and information can be gained, but also how some meanings can be lost by these exercises. Context that ties the data to the people it is about is removed, to enable patterns to become visible at scale, and yet context is rarely accounted for in narratives of the benefits of these data and their uses.

We have seen how well-being data are data about us—they are our data. They require our interactions, often our time, and are used to make decisions that are ostensibly on our behalf, but we may disagree with. We have seen how they change the workplace, how people were managed in COVID-19 and even the TV programmes we end up watching or the music we listen to. We have seen the growth of apps to track our well-being and tell us how to live better or walk more steps, and the market value of these apps increased considerably in this last decade. We have also witnessed how lucrative well-being data can be when their analysis has value to a policy sector, government or, in the case of a pandemic, the whole world.

We have also found indications that despite the fact we are 'living with data' (Living With Data), we don't all necessarily grasp what is happening with our data and what they do for and against us in our day-to-day lives. Unpacking various types and forms of well-being data (data about well-being) and touching on the possible impacts that data and their uses have on our own well-being, and society more generally, is crucial to grasping some of the contexts of data that get obscured. So, understanding well-being data can help us understand data better. But more than that, contextualising well-being data—discovering the *whos, whats, wheres, whens, hows* and *whys*, as well as the *so whats* and the *what nexts*—offers insight into politics and policy. It also helps us understand how research and knowledge may claim to *know* things, but that these claims may have limits.

There are limits to the promise of data: what they can achieve for society is not always good. Technical progress in data and their handling are not always a development for good. The fetishisation of data and proof of value (as with the case studies of social and cultural policy) prove that attachments to data in society are flawed, opening up a market for data practices that shifts the relationship between researcher and data. Our attachment to ideas of novelty and innovation, as with the case of 'the new sciences' and Big Data also blindside us to their limits. These are a few of the growing concerns in critical data studies, but need to be a bigger concern in all studies of well-being, across social policy, social statistics, sociology, economics, psychology and so on. There is an opportunity to take what we are learning in critical data studies and well-being studies to help the social sciences consider how it might adopt a more understanding position.

We need to return to how we understand how data are understood and how they can make us a more understanding society. Context matters: where data come from, who they are for and about, where they go and for what purpose. But context matters for more than researchers and more effort should be placed on how it can improve shared understanding, and being a more understanding society. Without acknowledging the limits in capacity, or indeed possibilities for understanding, the *What Next?* or *How can we do it better?* questions will not be answered properly for well-being.

NOTES

1. The full name of the Living With Data project (because we love a colon in academia) is: Living with Data: knowledge, experiences and perceptions of data practices.
2. It is not only the OECD and ONS projects about data that have an Advisory Group. Many research projects do. The current Living With Data Advisory Group is here: https://livingwithdata.org/advisory-group/.
3. Remember that Raymond Williams describes culture as 'one of the two or three most complicated words in the English language', this is actually an issue of understanding: 'This is so partly because of its intricate historical

development, in several European languages, but mainly because it has now come to be used for important concepts in several distinct intellectual disciplines and in several distinct and incompatible systems of thought' (Williams [1976] 1988, 87).

4. ACE is a non-departmental public body (NDPB) and the largest funder of the arts in England. ACE wanted to introduce a measure of social mobility or class inequality to its data-monitoring processes. I was asked to conduct research and to recommend a new inequality metric.

5. There has been pressure on organisations and the public sector to collect workforce demographic data as a result of the Equality Act 2010 and the Equality and Human Rights Commission Employment Statutory Code of Practice (EHRC 2015). This typically involves 'Equal Opportunities' forms that draw on the same questions as national surveys, although the formatting and wording may differ. In the cultural sector, equality of access to jobs and access to commercial content, such as cinema visits, or publicly funded culture, such as the BBC's broadcasts, is ascertained using national-level survey data, consumer insight data and these mandatory monitoring processes. The BBC has, for example, added proxy questions to its data processes to understand the class of its workforce—in line with recent Civil Service developments (BBC 2017; Cabinet Office 2016).

6. There is so much rich evidence on lack of diversity in the sector, although the arguments about this and data are summarised in Brook et al. (2020) and Oman (2019c); it is crucial to acknowledge the wider research across film, museums, television and broadcast, music, theatre and so on.

7. More detail on the data and the methodology can be found in Oman 2019c and Oman 2021, forthcoming.

8. The Equality and Human Rights Commission Employment Statutory Code of Practice (EHRC 2015) has also placed pressure on organisations and the public sector to collect workforce demographic data, again of protected characteristics. These are currently listed as age, disability, gender reassignment, marriage and civil partnership, pregnancy and maternity, race, religion or belief, sex and sexual orientation (EHRC n.d.).

9. It is important to acknowledge that, as these questionnaires were fabricated, and while the context was comparable in some respects, the context *was* different to how one would normally complete an Equality Monitoring form. The complexities of this are discussed in Oman (forthcoming-a) and are touched on in the working paper (Oman 2019c). Much care and attention were also paid to protecting participants who did not want to have personal conversations with colleagues.

10. In the working paper (Oman 2019c), which is open access, I outline these concerns, challenges and issues in greater detail.

11. Dave O'Brien (2018) in Arts pro explains this well

12. However, this will change, as it is one of the aims of the Living with Data project (and others) I've mentioned elsewhere in this chapter.
13. To be fair, there is good work happening in this area, it has just not been formalised yet.

References

BBC. 2017. *BBC Equality Information Report 2016–17*. London: BBC, p. 53. https://downloads.bbc.co.uk/diversity/pdf/equality-information-report-2017.pdf.

Brook, O., D. O'Brien, and M. Taylor. 2020. *Culture Is Bad for You: Inequality in the Cultural and Creative Industries*. Manchester: Manchester University Press.

Cabinet Office. 2016. Civil Service Pilots New Social Mobility Measures, Community and Society—GOV.UK. Accessed 29 April 2021. https://www.gov.uk/government/news/civil-service-pilots-new-social-mobility-measures

Cresswell, J. 2010. *Oxford Dictionary of Word Origins*. Oxford: Oxford University Press.

Data Justice Lab. n.d. *Data Justice Lab, Data Justice Lab*. Accessed 28 April 2021. https://datajusticelab.org/

DC Research. 2017. *Mapping Museum Data in England: Arts Council England Final Report*. United Kingdom: Arts Council England. Accessed 29 March 2021. https://www.artscouncil.org.uk/sites/default/files/download-file/Mapping%20Museum%20Data%20-%20Final%20Report.pdf.

EHRC. 2015. *Employment: Statutory Code of Practice, Equality and Human Rights Commission*. Accessed 29 April 2021. https://www.equalityhumanrights.com/en/publication-download/employment-statutory-code-practice.

———. n.d. *Protected Characteristics, Equality and Human Rights Commission*. Accessed 29 April 2021. https://www.equalityhumanrights.com/en/equality-act/protected-characteristics.

Gallie, W.B. 1956. Essentially Contested Concepts. *Proceedings of the Aristotelian Society* 56: 167–198.

Goldthorpe, J.H., and K. Hope. 1972. Occupational Grading and Occupational Prestige. *Social Science Information* 11 (5): 17–73. https://doi.org/10.1177/053901847201100502.

GSS. n.d. Public Good. *Glossary*. Accessed 29 April 2021. https://gss.civilservice.gov.uk/about-us/glossary/#public-good.

Kennedy, H., Oman, S., Taylor, M., Bates, J., and Steedman, R. 2020. *Public Understanding and Perceptions of Data Practices: A Review of Existing Research*. Sheffield: The University of Sheffield. https://livingwithdata.org/project/wp-content/uploads/2020/05/living-with-data-2020-review-of-existing-research.pdf.

Oxford Lexico. n.d. Definition of Understanding by Oxford Dictionary on Lexico. com, Lexico Dictionaries | English. Accessed 29 April 2021. https://www. lexico.com/definition/understanding.

Living with Data. n.d. *Living with Data, Living with Data.* https://living-withdata.org/.

Nissenbaum, H. 2009. *Privacy in Context: Technology, Policy, and the Integrity of Social Life.* Stanford University Press.

O'Brien, D. 2018. Tackling Class Discrimination, Arts Professional. Accessed 17 May 2021. https://www.artsprofessional.co.uk/magazine/article/ tackling-class-discrimination.

O'Neil, C. 2016. *Weapons of Math Destruction: How Big Data Increases Inequality and Threatens Democracy.* London: Allen Lane.

Oman, S. 2015. Measuring National Well-Being: What Matters to You? What Matters to Whom? In *Cultures of Wellbeing: Method, Place, Policy,* ed. S. White and C. Blackmore. London: Palgrave Macmillan.

———. 2019a. *#CreativeCase Webinar: Digging into Socio-economic Diversity.* Arts Council England (Arts Council England). Accessed 29 April 2021. https://www.youtube.com/watch?v=c1RncRZbh5E.

———. 2019b. How Do People Feel about Inequality Metrics? How Do They Work in Cultural Organisations?, presentation at Data Nord, 17 June 2019, Copenhagen.

———. 2019c. *Improving Data Practices to Monitor Inequality and Introduce Social Mobility Measures: A Working Paper.* The University of Sheffield. Available at: https://www.sheffield.ac.uk/polopoly_fs/1.867756!/file/ MetricsWorkingPaper.pdf. Accessed 29 March 2021.

———. 2019d. *Measuring Social Mobility in The Creative and Cultural Industries: The Importance of Working in Partnership to Improve Data Practices and Address Inequality.* Sheffield: The University of Sheffield. Accessed 29 March 2021. https://www.sheffield.ac.uk/polopoly_fs/1.867754!/file/ MetricsPolicyBriefing.pdf.

———. 2021, forthcoming. *Re-performance: A Critical and Reparative Methodology for Everyday Expertise and Data Practice in Policy Knowledge.* International Review of Public Policy.

———. forthcoming-a. A Question of Class and Culture: How Equality Metrics Work for the Creative Public Sector.

———. forthcoming-b. The Affective Practices of Public Sector Data Workers: The Case of the Arts.

ONS. 2010. *The National Statistics Socio-economic Classification (NS-SEC).* Office for National Statistics. Accessed 31 March 2021. https://www.ons.gov.uk/ methodology/classificationsandstandards/otherclassifications/ thenationalstatisticssocioeconomicclassificationnssecrebasedonsoc2010.

SMC. 2021. *Social Mobility Data Masterclass—#AskTheQuestion—SMC.* Social Mobility Commission. Accessed 29 April 2021. https://socialmobilityworks. org/blog/social-mobility-data-masterclass-why-you-need-to-askthequestion/.

UK Government. 2010. *Equality Act 2010.* Statute Law Database. Accessed 29 April 2021. https://www.legislation.gov.uk/ukpga/2010/15/contents.

Williams, R. [1976]1988. *Keywords: A Vocabulary of Culture and Society.* 2nd ed. London: Fourth Estate Ltd.

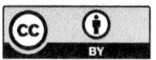

Index[1]

---

[1] Note: Page numbers followed by 'n' refer to notes.

© The Author(s) 2021   373
S. Oman, *Understanding Well-being Data*,
New Directions in Cultural Policy Research,
https://doi.org/10.1007/978-3-030-72937-0

: